Top 100 Diagnoses in Neurology

Core Features, Synopses, Illustrations and Questions for Rapid Review and Retention

Top 1 0 0 Diagnoses in Neurology

Core Features, Synopses, Illustrations and
Questions for Rapid Review and Retention

Ilya Kister, MD, FAAN

Associate Professor
Department of Neurology
Neuroimmunology Fellowship Director
NYU Grossman School of Medicine, New York

José Biller, MD, FAAN, FACP, FAHA, FANA

Professor and Chair
Department of Neurology
Loyola University, Chicago
Stritch School of Medicine

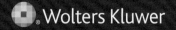
Wolters Kluwer

Philadelphia • Baltimore • New York • London
Buenos Aires • Hong Kong • Sydney • Tokyo

Acquisitions Editor: Chris Teja
Development Editor: Ariel S. Winter
Editorial Coordinators: Ingrid Greenlee and Sean Hanrahan
Editorial Assistant: Brian Convery
Marketing Manager: Phyllis Hitner
Production Project Manager: Kim Cox
Design Coordinator: Stephen Druding
Art Director, Illustration: Jennifer Clements
Manufacturing Coordinator: Beth Welsh
Prepress Vendor: TNQ Technologies

9 8 7 6 5 4 3 2 1

Printed in China

Library of Congress Cataloging-in-Publication Data

ISBN-13: 978-1-975121-11-2

Cataloging in Publication data available on request from publisher.

shop.lww.com

Dedication

I dedicate this book to my family, especially to my parents, who raised me with a sense of wonder, a love for learning, and a desire to try, as the poet put it, "in everything, to reach the inner core"; and to my uncle, who opened up new vistas for me. I would also like to acknowledge my dear children—Sh-Y., A., R., Y., and R.—for the selfish reason that it will give me pleasure to show them their initials printed in a book, and especially thank my son A., who would express concern about the slow progress of writing and gently prod me on by asking "how many chapters did you write already?" My wife asked not to be acknowledged, and this is fortuitous as I would not know how to adequately express my appreciation for her.

Ilya Kister

This book is dedicated to my patients who have given me the privilege to pursue lifelong learning medical education.
To my family with love.

José Biller

Preface

In arriving at a clinical diagnosis, think of the five most common findings (either histori-cal, physical findings, or laboratory) found in a given disorder. If at least three of these five are not present in a given patient, the diagnosis is likely to be wrong.

C. MILLER FISHER

Following the advice of C. Miller Fisher, we sought to identify the five most common findings for one hundred of the more common and important neurologic diagnoses. These five features are the nucleus around which knowledge of neurologic diseases can crystallize and grow. The choice of "5" is congruent with the idea that the human cen-tral memory store is limited to five meaningful items.

This book is not a textbook in the traditional sense, rather it is designed to supply students of neurology with a broad knowledge base that can be retained and further built upon. The book can also serve as a reference for busy clinicians—both neurol-ogists and nonneurologists—who can peruse the relevant chapter to quickly refresh their memory of a specific diagnosis and ascertain whether their patient's presentation satisfies Fisher's "three-out-of-five" rule. As such, this concise book should hopefully be useful to students and practitioners alike.

By identifying a small number of the cardinal features of the most relevant neuro-logic conditions, we hope to provide our readers with the confidence to make cogent neurologic diagnoses and to inoculate them against neurophobia, a dangerous and all-too-prevalent condition, whose cardinal manifestation is fear and confusion about all things neurologic.

We hope you enjoy our book and welcome your comments and suggestions at ilya.kister@nyulangone.org and jbiller@lumc.edu.

Cowan N. The magical mystery four: how is working memory capacity limited, and why? *Curr Dir Psychol Sci.* 2010;19(1):51-57.

Jozefowicz RF. Neurophobia: the fear of neurology among medical students. *Arch Neurol.* 1994. 51(4):328-329.

C. Miller Fisher (1913-2012), a Canadian-American neurologist, made seminal contributions to vascular neurology and described many important neurologic conditions (Miller Fisher syn-drome; normal pressure hydrocephalus transient global amnesia). The citation of Fisher's rule is from Caplan LR. Fischer's rules. *Arch Neurol.* 1982;39(7):389-390.

Table of Contents

Freely-available, high-quality Internet resources

How to use this book

This book is divided into anatomical (Diseases of the Spinal Cord), etiological (Vascular Disorders), and semiological (Nonepileptic Paroxysmal Disorders) sections. This division, while logical, is to some extent arbitrary as many entities could be placed in more than one section. Each section begins with "A Very Brief Introduction," aimed to provide the reader with an essential clinical context for further discussion of specific diagnoses.

A chapter may be devoted to a specific disease (giant cell arteritis) or syndrome (cavernous sinus syndrome), and, rarely, broader clinical categories (cerebral hemorrhage). On occasion, a chapter includes two disorders if juxtaposition could facilitate recall (polymyositis and dermatomyositis). A chapter title is followed by a subheading that broadly defines each entity and often specifies etiology and special population affected. The prevalence of each condition is coded with the help of a bar icon to the left of the chapter title. "Three bars" indicate that the condition is relatively common, present in at least one in a few hundred individuals; "two bars" implies relatively uncommon—in the order of one in a thousand; and "one bar" implies a very rare condition—one in many thousands. The "ambulance" icon next to some diagnoses alerts the reader that this condition must be evaluated and treated emergently in order to prevent irreversible neurologic disability.

Unlike the "Top 100" billboard songs that are chosen based on objective criteria—sales, radioplay, etc—the choice of "Top 100" diagnoses depended entirely upon the authors' discretion. Preference was given to adult neurologic conditions that clinicians in Western countries are most likely to encounter. Very rare disorders were only included if treatable or if they illustrate an important neurologic concept. Thus, Lambert-Eaton myasthenic syndrome (LEMS) is included because it is a classic paraneoplastic disorder and because recognition of LEMS may lead to an earlier diagnosis of occult malignancy. Wernicke encephalopathy, also very rare, is included because prompt treatment with thiamine will forestall devastating neurologic sequelae.

The core of each chapter is five **Core Features**, succinctly formulated to enable rapid review and retention. Important caveats, additions, and clarifications are contained in the subheadings under each core feature entry. **Synopses** seek to interconnect the ostensibly disparate core features, to fit them together as parts of one puzzle, and to provide additional background material. **Illustrations** showcase key concepts and findings in order to make them more memorable. **Questions for Self-Study** are designed to test readers' understanding of the subject, and also introduce important material not covered in the chapter. Readers are encouraged to come up with their own answers, either individually or in a study group, before cross-checking their answers with standard references and suggested reviews (at least one high-quality, freely accessible reference is listed at the end of each chapter, and additional high-quality resources are listed under **Free Internet Resources** at the end of the book). **Challenge Questions**, more conceptual in nature, may hopefully challenge even seasoned practitioners.

Peripheral Nervous System and the Innervation of the Upper Extremities

TOP 1 0 0

A Very Brief Introduction to the Peripheral Nervous System and Innervation of the Upper Extremities

> The sophist Pausanias, a native of Syria, who came to Rome, complained of numbness in his fifth and fourth fingers, and half of the middle finger of his left hand. … I inquired from him as to all which had happened previously, and I learned, among other details, that on his route to Rome, having fallen from his chariot, he was struck upon his upper back in the region of the spine; and that the point of impact had seemingly healed, while numbness of his fingers was progressing… I ordered that the medications which had been applied to his fingers be applied instead to the point of trauma and the man healed rapidly. The physicians do not even know that there are specific roots of nerves, which distribute to the skin of the upper limb allowing sensation, and other roots, which form branches moving muscles.

Galen*

The nervous system is traditionally divided into *central* (cerebrum, brainstem, cerebellum, and spinal cord) and *peripheral* (roots, plexuses, nerves, neuromuscular junction, and muscles) anatomical compartments. The first five sections of this book cover disorders of the peripheral nervous system (PNS), starting with a section on common disorders of the upper extremities.

Basic understanding of the innervation of the upper extremities is necessary to formulate a logical differential diagnosis. Innervation of the arm is effected via five spinal nerve roots (C5, C6, C7, C8, and T1). Each nerve root supplies a specific area termed "a dermatome."

---

*Claudius Galen of Pergamum (CE second century), an outstanding Greek anatomist and physician, authored over 100 medical books, many of which served as definitive textbooks of medicine until the Renaissance. The anecdote of the "fallen sophist" recounted in the epigraph is illustrative of Galen's astute understanding of neuroanatomy as much as of his failure to avoid the traps of post hoc fallacy and false generalization. (Cited from Awad IA. Galen's anecdote of the fallen sophist: on the certainty of science through anatomy. *J Neurosurg.* 1995;83(5):929-932.)

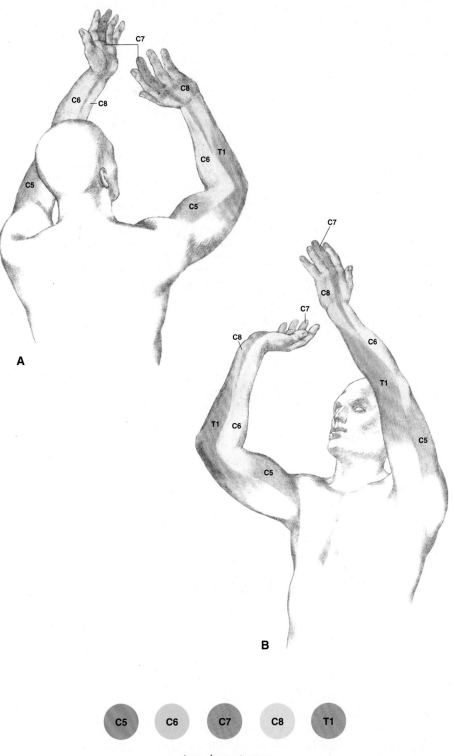

Arm dermatomes.

The dermatomes of the upper extremities are easy to remember if one keeps in mind that the "middle root" of the five cervical nerve roots—C7—supplies the middle finger (and not much else). The two "upper" cervical nerve roots supply sensation to the "upper" (lateral) surface of the upper extremity, while the two "lower" cervical nerve roots supply sensation to the "lower" (medial) surface of the upper extremity in more or less symmetric fashion with the upper dermatomes.

These five cervical nerve roots form the brachial plexus, traditionally divided into trunks, divisions, cords, and branches as shown below:

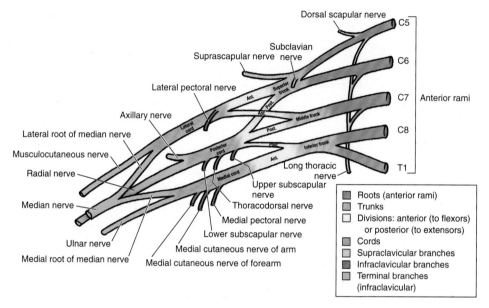

Schematic of the brachial plexus. (Reprinted with permission from Agur AMR, Dalley AF. *Grant's Atlas of Anatomy*. 15th ed. Philadelphia, PA: Wolters Kluwer; 2020:Figure 6.25.)

Because few clinicians can retrieve the mental image of the brachial plexus with all its ramifications at the bedside, we propose a simplified scheme that matches each of the five roots with their five respective terminal branches and their main motor functions. The "top 5" of the brachial plexus are as follows:

Root	Nerve	Muscle	Function
C5	Axillary	Deltoid	Shoulder extension
C6	Musculocutaneous	Biceps	Elbow flexion
C7	Radial	Triceps	Elbow extension
C8	Median/ulnar	Flexor digitorum	Finger flexion
T1	Median/ulnar	Dorsal interossei	Fingers spreading out

This scheme associates each root with one "main" nerve and muscle supplied by that root. In reality, more than one nerve root contributes fibers to each nerve, and each nerve supplies more than just one muscle. This scheme can hopefully be retained in implicit (motor) memory if motor testing of the arm systematically tests the five motor functions of the five nerve roots, as shown below:

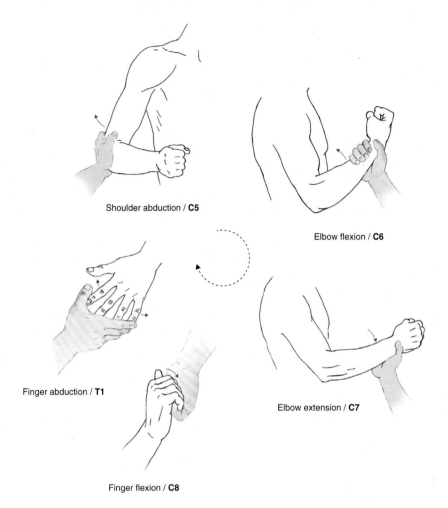

Shoulder abduction / **C5**

Elbow flexion / **C6**

Finger abduction / **T1**

Elbow extension / **C7**

Finger flexion / **C8**

Practical guide to upper extremity strength testing.

When faced with patients with motor/sensory deficits of an upper extremity, clinicians must first seek to determine the lesion location: Are the deficits due to muscle, nerve, plexus/root, spinal cord, or brain involvement? The most commonly implicated causes are mononeuropathies due to nerve compression syndromes, further discussed in Chapters 1-3, and radiculopathies discussed in Chapter 4. The brachial plexus is a relatively uncommon location of injury. Deficits arising from brachial plexus lesions are illustrated with examples of neonatal brachial plexus injuries (Chapter 5). It is quite rare for neurologic deficits limited to one upper extremity be the result of a lesion within a spinal cord or brain, as lesions in the central nervous system (CNS) typically cause a pattern of deficits extending beyond a single limb.

1 Carpal Tunnel Syndrome

Compression mononeuropathy of the median nerve at the wrist is the most common nerve entrapment syndrome

CORE FEATURES

1. Pain involving the wrist and radial (thumb) aspect of the hand.
   Pain is often nocturnal, waking the patient up from sleep; pain may radiate beyond the area of median nerve distribution to involve the whole arm.
2. Tingling and numbness in the distribution of the distal median nerve.
   This area comprises the tips of the thumb, index and middle fingers, and the radial half of the ring finger.
3. Tingling may be reproduced by flexing the wrist 90° for 60 seconds with elbows extended (Phalen sign) or percussion where the median nerve enters the carpal tunnel (Tinel sign).
4. Weakness of ABduction of the thumb.
   Testing of the abductor pollicis brevis muscle is shown below. Atrophy of the thenar eminence—median nerve–innervated muscles at the base of the thumb—may be present in advanced cases.
5. Nerve conduction studies (NCS) of the median nerve show delayed or absent sensory responses.
   The median nerve is stimulated distal to the carpal tunnel over the index finger and the response recorded proximal to the carpal tunnel at the level of the wrist.

SYNOPSIS

Lifetime prevalence of carpal tunnel syndrome (CTS) is approximately 5%. The distal median nerve carries sensation of the tips of digits 1 to 4 and supplies motor function to several small hand muscles, of which the most commonly tested is the ABductor pollicis brevis. To identify the area of sensory loss, ask patients to draw on a picture of a hand where they experience tingling and numbness. Some variability is to be expected, but when the affected area is well outside the distribution of the median nerve—if it involves the fifth finger or the ulnar aspect of the forearm—a diagnosis of CTS is doubtful. Pressure and stretching on the nerve within the carpal tunnel can reproduce the pain and tingling (Tinel and Phalen signs) and may explain nocturnal awakening if the wrists are bent inward during sleep. Velocities on NCS are slowed because the median nerve is demyelinated within the carpal tunnel. In more extreme cases, there is also axonal loss that can account for the electrophysiologic signals to be completely blocked.

FIGURES

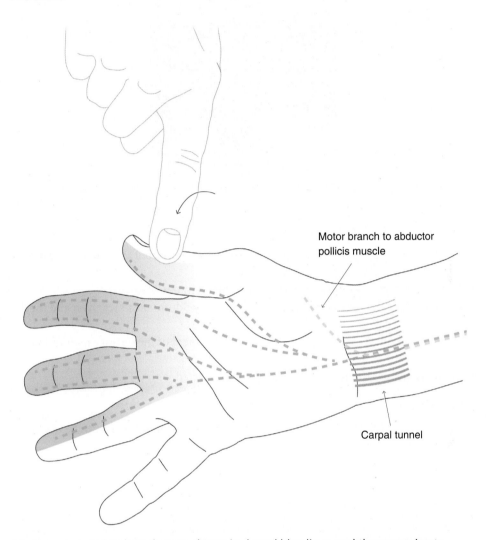

Motor branch to abductor pollicis muscle

Carpal tunnel

Median nerve and its branches are shown in dotted blue lines, and the approximate location of carpal tunnel, in striped lines. Area corresponding to sensory loss in CTS is shaded in blue. Abductor pollicis brevis is usually weak in CTS (examiner presses thumb down toward the palm to test thumb abduction).

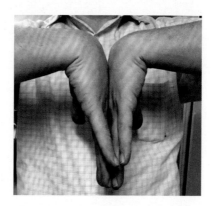

Hand position in Phalen test; if positive, it is highly suggestive of CTS.

QUESTIONS FOR SELF-STUDY

1. Demonstrate on your wrist where the carpal tunnel is located and name the different anatomical structures running through it.
2. Explain how to differentiate CTS from de Quervain tenosynovitis.
3. Explain why CTS may cause thenar atrophy but seldom numbness over the thenar eminence.
4. What is the conservative approach to the management of the sensory manifestations of CTS?
5. What are the common medical conditions associated with CTS?

CHALLENGE

Explain the anatomic basis as to why CTS may in some instances account for weakness of muscles innervated by both the ulnar and median nerves.

REFERENCES

Chammas M, Boretto J, Burmann LM, Ramos RM, Dos Santos Neto FC, Silva JB. Carpal tunnel syndrome – part I (anatomy, physiology, etiology and diagnosis). *Rev Bras Ortop*. 2014;49(5):429-436. [free online resource]
Olney RK. Carpal tunnel syndrome: complex issues with a "simple" condition. *Neurology*. 2001;56:1431-1432.
Padua L, Coraci D, Erra C, et al. Carpal tunnel syndrome: clinical features, diagnosis, and management. *Lancet Neurol*. 2016;15(12):1273-1284.

2 Ulnar Neuropathy

Compression of the ulnar nerve at the elbow is the second most common upper extremity entrapment neuropathy

CORE FEATURES

1. Pain over the medial aspect of the elbow and forearm.
   Pain worsens after a prolonged period of elbow flexion or elbow pressure.
2. "Pins and needles" sensation involving the fourth and fifth digits.
   Tingling may also be present over the ulnar side of the dorsum of the hand and palm.
3. Positive Tinel sign.
   Tapping or palpation of the medial aspect of the elbow elicits tingling and local sensitivity in the ulnar nerve distribution. The sensitivity of this clinical sign is limited because mild paresthesias may be elicited in unaffected individuals as well.
4. Weakness in pushing digits away from the midline (digit ABduction).
   Testing of the abductor digiti minimi is shown below. Thumb abduction is not affected as it is mediated by the median nerve.
5. Froment prehensile sign indicates weakness of ADduction of the thumb.
   When the patient is asked to hold a piece of paper between their thumb and index fingers, they will flex the thumb to compensate for thumb adduction (Froment prehensile sign).

SYNOPSIS

During elbow flexion, the ulnar nerve is stretched between the medial condyle of the humerus and the olecranon and may be compressed over the medial condyle in the elbow or more distally, within the cubital canal. Compression of the ulnar nerve leads to referred pain at the elbow and forearm, sensory loss and tingling in ulnar nerve–innervated areas of the hand and fingers, and weakness in ulnar nerve–innervated muscles (abductors of all digits except the thumb and adductor of the thumb). Long-standing ulnar nerve damage can lead to atrophy of the hypothenar and first dorsal interosseous muscles.

FIGURES

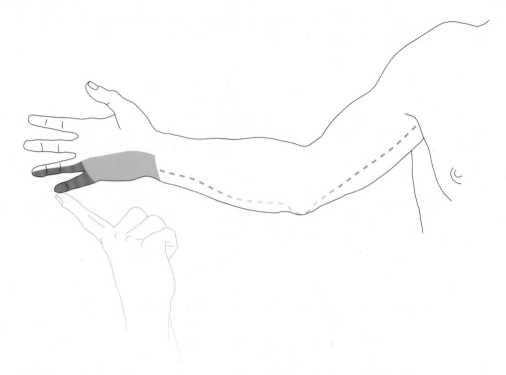

Ulnar nerve is traced from its origin in the brachial plexus (dotted line). Pattern of sensory loss when ulnar nerve is compressed at the elbow is shown in blue. Abductor digiti minimi is often impaired in ulnar palsy (examiner is pushing little finger toward ring finger to test little finger abduction).

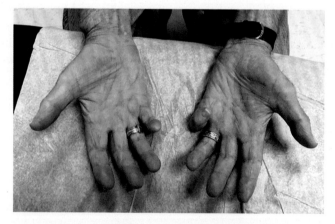

Bilateral ulnar neuropathies in a patient with type 1 diabetes mellitus, coronary artery bypass graft, and end-stage renal disease. Note the hypothenar atrophy and bilateral Dupuytren contractures of the fifth digits. Electrodiagnostic studies were consistent with bilateral ulnar neuropathies superimposed upon a polyneuropathy.

QUESTIONS FOR SELF-STUDY

1. Identify on your elbow the location of the medial condyle and the olecranon. Can you reproduce sensory symptoms in an ulnar distribution by gentle pressure over the medial condyle?
2. What is the conservative approach to the management of the sensory manifestations of ulnar neuropathy at the elbow?
3. A professional cyclist develops symptoms of ulnar neuropathy. Where is the ulnar nerve most likely to be compressed? What neurologic findings might be helpful in differentiating an ulnar neuropathy at the elbow from an ulnar neuropathy at the wrist? (Hint: consider where the branch supplying the sensory innervation of the dorsum of hand comes off the ulnar nerve.)
4. What neurologic findings might be helpful in differentiating ulnar neuropathy at the elbow from C8 radiculopathy?
5. What elbow position is more sensitive for recording a decrement in ulnar nerve velocities across the elbow: flexion or extension? Why?

CHALLENGE

Both the abductor digiti minimi (abduction of the fifth digit) and the first dorsal interosseous (abduction of the second digit) are innervated by the ulnar nerve. What condition should you consider if there is atrophy of the first dorsal interosseous (weakness in the abduction of the index finger), but not of the hypothenar region (no weakness in the abduction of the little finger)? (Hint: this unusual pattern of hand muscle atrophy is known as "split hand.")

REFERENCES

Caliandro P, La Torre G, Padua R, Giannini F, Padua L. Treatment for ulnar neuropathy at the elbow. *Cochrane Database Syst Rev.* 2012;(7):CD006839. [free online resource]
Staples JR, Calfee R. Cubital tunnel syndrome: current concepts. *J Am Acad Orthop Surg.* 2017;25(10):e215-e224.

3   Radial Nerve Palsy

Compression neuropathy of the radial nerve at the spiral groove of the humerus ("Saturday night palsy").

CORE FEATURES

1. History consistent with radial nerve compression at the spiral groove of the humerus. Common scenarios include sleeping with the arm stretched while inebriated; improper arm positioning while under anesthesia; and humeral fracture.
2. Inability to extend the wrist and fingers.
3. Preserved ability to flex wrist and fingers.
   Finger abduction and handgrip may appear affected because some of the non–radial nerve–innervated muscles responsible for these movements work best in the wrist-extended position. (You can test this observation by trying to spread your fingers with the wrist flexed and wrist extended.)
4. Sensory loss over the extensor aspect of the forearm, dorsum of the hand, and thumb.
5. Normal elbow extension.
   Elbow extension may be affected if the radial nerve is compressed proximally to the spiral groove, as in cases of "crutch paralysis," because the nerve lesion is then proximal to the take-off of the branch to the triceps muscle.

SYNOPSIS

Radial nerve palsy at the spiral groove of the humerus results in the readily recognizable wrist and finger drop. The finding of sensory deficits limited to the extensor surface of the forearm and hand confirms the suspicion of radial nerve palsy. Injury to the radial nerve or its branches proximal to the spiral groove of the humerus may cause weakness in elbow extension and decreased triceps reflex. Injury to radial nerve distal to the spiral groove may cause finger drop without wrist drop. Injury to the nerve near the wrist, often from aggressive handcuffing, leads to sensory loss over the radial aspect of the dorsum of the hand and base of the thumb ("cheiralgia paresthetica") but no motor deficits.

FIGURES

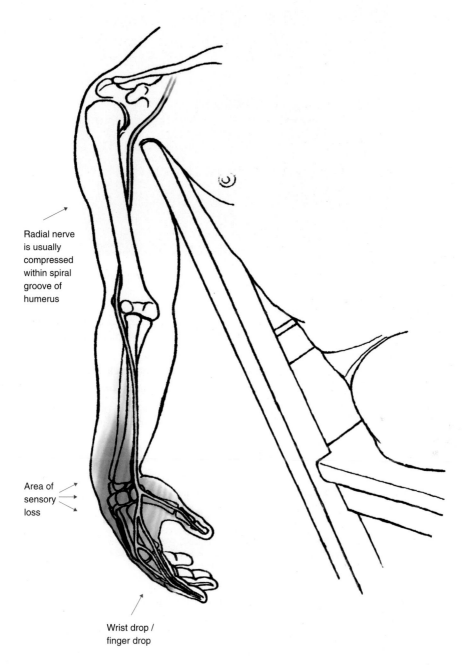

Radial nerve
is usually
compressed
within spiral
groove of
humerus

Area of
sensory
loss

Wrist drop /
finger drop

Radial nerve is traced from its origin, the brachial plexus (yellow). Pattern of sensory loss when radial nerve is injured at the spiral groove is shown in purple.

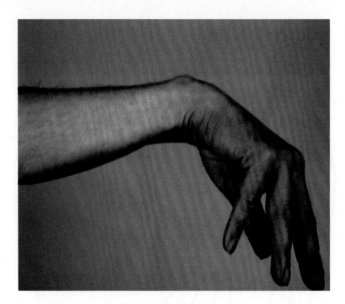

Right wrist drop in a patient with radial nerve palsy.

QUESTIONS FOR SELF-STUDY

1. Which findings help to differentiate a wrist drop due to a stroke from a wrist drop due to a radial nerve palsy?
2. A patient presents with finger drop without a significant wrist drop. The sensory examination is normal. What is the most likely site of nerve compression? What is the name of the syndrome?
3. What are the expected sensory deficits resulting from radial nerve compression at the (1) axilla; (2) humerus; and (3) wrist?
4. A 50-year-old smelter develops microcytic anemia, abdominal pain, and bilateral wrist drop. What diagnosis could best explain all these findings?
5. Match each nerve entrapment syndrome with an activity commonly associated with the respective mononeuropathy:

Neuropathy	Activity
A. Median nerve at the wrist (CTS)	Professional cycling
B. Ulnar neuropathy at the wrist	Knitting
C. Ulnar neuropathy at the elbow	"Windmill" pitching in softball
D. Radial nerve palsy	Holding a drill in position

CHALLENGE

Describe three of the most common nerve injuries resulting from misplaced intramuscular injections. (Hint: Two of them involve nerves of the arm, and one involves the nerve of the leg.)

REFERENCES

Bumbasirevic M, Palibrk T, Lesic A, Atkinson HDE. Radial nerve palsy. *EFORT Open Rev.* 2017;1(8):286-294. [free online resource]

Hobson-Webb LD, Juel VC. Common entrapment neuropathies. *Continuum (Minneap Minn).* 2017;23(2, Selected Topics in Outpatient Neurology):487-511.

4 Neonatal Brachial Plexus Injuries

Injuries to plexus resulting from failure to deliver shoulder during birth (shoulder dystocia)

CORE FEATURES

The table below summarizes three of the best-described patterns of brachial plexus injury. Erb palsy, with or without C7 root involvement, accounts for approximately 85% of neonatal plexus injuries.

		Erb Palsy ("upper")	Klumpke Palsy ("lower")	Pan-Plexopathy
1	Roots	C5, C6, C7	C8, T1	C5, C6, C7, C8, T1
2	Motor deficits	Shoulder abduction, elbow flexion, internal arm rotation (wrist extension if C7 is involved)	Intrinsic hand muscles	Complete arm and hand paralysis
3	Sensory deficits	Lateral arm and forearm	Medial arm and forearm	Whole arm
4	Arm posture	"Waiter's tip" when C7 root is involved (as seen in figure below)	"Claw hand" because ulnar-innervated muscles are predominantly affected	"Flail arm" appearance
5	Horner syndrome	Absent	May be present	May be present

SYNOPSIS

Neonatal upper brachial plexus injury results from traction on the brachial plexus when the shoulder is pulled away from the head. Lower brachial plexus injury results from traction on the plexus when the arm is pulled away from the body as shown in figure below. The pattern of motor weakness can be reconstructed if one remembers that "waiter's tip" posture is the result of upper brachial plexus injury (extended elbow, flexed wrist, and externally rotated arm). Thus, this type of upper plexus injury results in weakness of muscles that flex the elbow, extend the wrist, and internally rotate the elbow. A "claw hand" posture is the result of lower brachial plexus injury since ulnar-innervated muscles are predominantly affected. Early identification of neonates/infants with brachial plexus injuries and referral for multidisciplinary rehabilitation and (rarely) surgery can substantially improve long-term outcomes.

FIGURES

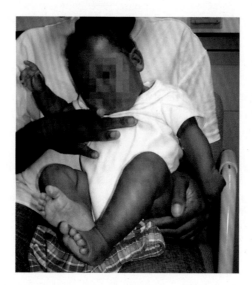

An infant with Erb palsy: left arm is adducted and internally rotated and forearm is pronated ("waiter's tip"). (Courtesy of Joseph Piatt, MD.)

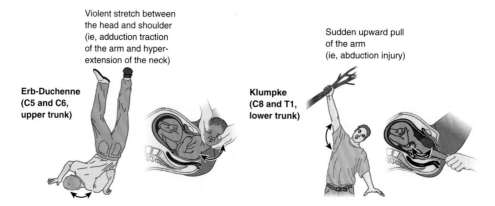

Patterns of injury in upper and lower brachial plexus palsies. (Reprinted with permission from Moore KL, Dalley AF, Agur AMR. *Clinically Oriented Anatomy.* 7th ed. Philadelphia, PA: Wolters Kluwer Health/Lippincott Williams & Wilkins; 2014:729:Figure 20.3B.)

QUESTIONS FOR SELF-STUDY

1. Falling asleep on a park bench with an arm overstretched and pressed against the back of the bench in a drunken stupor can result in a radial nerve palsy (Saturday night palsy, see the previous chapter) or upper brachial plexus injury ("Friday night palsy," Sathornsumetee et al., 2016). How can you differentiate these two entities based on the pattern of motor weakness?
2. A 40-year-old patient presents with acute onset of severe pain and patchy muscle weakness involving the right arm and shoulder. There is no history of trauma. Neurologic examination suggests brachial plexus injury. What rare syndrome should be considered in this setting?

3. A 70-year-old man with a history of lung cancer treated with radiation therapy presents with pain in the right axilla and weakness of intrinsic right-hand muscles. What are the two most likely causes of brachial plexus injury in this patient? What historical features may help differentiate one etiology from the other?

4. A healthy 50-year-old woman presents with left arm pain and weakness. The weakness is worse when raising her left arm. On examination, there is weakness and atrophy of intrinsic left-hand muscles. Electromyographic (EMG) studies/NCS support the diagnosis of brachial plexopathy. What potentially treatable cause of lower trunk brachial plexopathy should be considered? What additional ancillary testing needs to be performed to confirm the diagnosis?

5. A football defenseman had a bad "stinger" during a tackle and now complains of right shoulder and arm pain and arm weakness. He recovers fully over the course of several days. What is the likely neuroanatomic basis for these symptoms? What is the presumed mechanism of injury? (Compare your answer with Kuhlman et al., 1999.)

CHALLENGE

When assessing a patient with a potential brachial plexus injury, it is of the importance to examine for any asymmetry in pupil size and width of the palpebral fissures. Explain how a brachial plexus injury could cause a droopy eyelid and miosis. Why are these findings only seen with lower, but never with upper brachial plexopathies?

REFERENCES

Ferrante MA. Brachial plexopathies: classification, causes, and consequences. *Muscle and Nerve*. 2004;30:547-568.

Kuhlman GS, McKeag DB. The "burner": a common nerve injury in contact sports. *Am Fam Physician*. 60(7):2035. https://www.aafp.org/afp/1999/1101/p2035.html. [free online resource]

Sathornsumetee S, Morgenlander JC. Friday night palsy: an unusual case of brachial plexus neuropathy. *Clin Neurol Neurosurg*. 2006;108(2):191-192.

Smith BW, Daunter AK, Yang LJ, Wilson TJ. An update on the management of neonatal brachial plexus palsy-replacing old paradigms: a review. *JAMA Pediatr*. 2018;172(6):585-591. [free online resource]

5 Acute Cervical Radiculopathies: C6 and C7

Compression of cervical nerve roots is most commonly due to degenerative cervical spine disease

CORE FEATURES

The table below compares clinical features of the two most common cervical radiculopathies: C6 radiculopathy (affected nerve root compressed between the C5 and C6 vertebrae) and C7 radiculopathy (affected nerve root compressed between the C6 and C7 vertebrae).

		C6 Radiculopathy	C7 Radiculopathy
1	Motor	Elbow flexion	Elbow extension
2	Sensory deficit	Lateral forearm, thumb, index finger	Middle finger (not reliably present)
3	Depressed or absent muscle stretch reflex	Brachioradialis and biceps reflexes	Triceps reflex
4	Pain radiation pattern	Along the upper lateral aspect of the arm into the first two digits. Pain may be reproduced with the Spurling maneuver	Along the dorsal aspect of the arm, through the elbow and into the third digit
5	MRI cervical spine	Lateral disk herniation at C5/C6 or bony protrusion into the intervertebral foramina at C5/C6	Lateral disk herniation at C6/C7 or bony protrusion into the intervertebral foramina at C6/C7

SYNOPSIS

When a nerve root is compressed, motor, sensory, and reflex functions subserved by the involved root are affected. In theory, a simple nerve root lesion should produce a dermatomal sensory loss and a myotomal pattern of muscle weakness. (A myotome is a group of muscles innervated by single nerve root.) In practice, however, the relationship between the nerve root level and clinical findings is not always straightforward because "twigs" from one nerve root may join the neighboring nerve root such that compression of one nerve root will cause partial sensory-motor deficits in the distribution of a neighboring root. Furthermore, a posterior disk herniation may impact the spinal cord as well as the root, causing symptoms of spinal cord dysfunction.

Acute cervical disk herniation without weakness is managed with nonopioid analgesics, muscle relaxants, and physical therapy. Symptoms resolve within weeks in up to 90% of cases. Significant motor deficits, cervical spine instability, and failure of conservative therapy are indications for surgery.

FIGURES

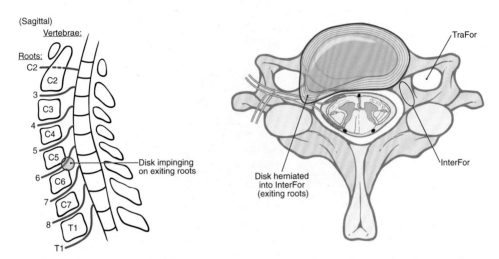

Schematic of C5-C6 right disk herniation. (Reprinted with permission from Haines DE. *Clinical syndromes of the CNS.* Part I: herniation syndromes of the brain and spinal discs. In: Haines DE, Willis MA, Lambert HW, eds. *Neuroanatomy Atlas in Clinical Context: Structures, Sections, Systems, and Syndromes.* 10th ed. Philadelphia, PA: Wolters Kluwer; 2019:297-308:Figure 9.16.)

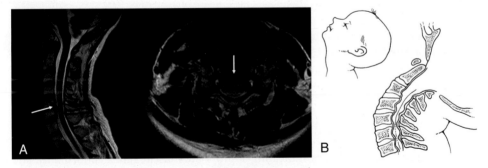

A, A 31-year-old woman with a C5/C6 midline disk herniation (arrows) on sagittal and axial T2 MRI of cervical spine. B, Schematic figure illustrates how extension of neck can worsen symptoms of radiculopathy by narrowing spinal canal. (Modified from Regenbogen VS, Rogers LF, Atlas SW, Kim KS. Cervical spinal cord injuries in patients with cervical spondylosis. *AJR Am J Roentgenol.* 1986;146(2):277-284. Copyright © 1986 American Roentgen Ray Society.)

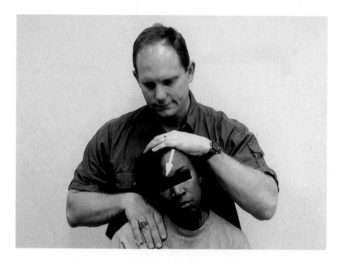

Spurling test is performed by laterally flexing, rotating, and compressing the patient's head toward the side of the symptoms. Spurling test causes the pathologic foramen to compress the nerve root and reproduces the radicular pain. This test is specific, but not sensitive for cervical radiculopathy. (Reprinted with permission from Wainner RS, Fritz JM, Irrgang JJ, Boninger ML, Delitto A, Allison S. Reliability and diagnostic accuracy of the clinical examination and patient self-report measures for cervical radiculopathy. *Spine (Phila Pa 1976)*. 2003;28(1):52-62.)

QUESTIONS FOR SELF-STUDY

1. There is an overlap in pain patterns due to C6 radiculopathy and carpal tunnel syndrome, but the patterns of sensory and motor deficits are different. Name two motor tests that can differentiate CTS from C6 radiculopathy.
2. Explain why Spurling maneuver replicates radicular symptoms. What other provocative tests can be used to test for cervical radiculopathy?
3. 65-year-old man presents with symptoms of chronic C6 radiculopathy. Examination shows diffuse hyperreflexia, bilateral Babinski signs, and a slightly stiff gait. What condition must be suspected in this clinical scenario?
4. Complete the above table by indicating appropriate muscle, reflex abnormality, and sensory testing for the uncommon C5 and C8 radiculopathies.
5. What are the noncompressive causes of cervical radiculopathy?

CHALLENGE

Do you expect sensory nerve conduction studies to be affected by a lateral disk herniation proximal to DRG? Explain your answer.

REFERENCES

Carette S, Fehlings MG. Clinical practice. Cervical radiculopathy. *N Engl J Med*. 2005;353(4):392-399.
Caridi JM, Pumberger M, Hughes AP. Cervical radiculopathy: a review. *HSS J*. 2011;7(3):265-272. [free online resource]
Rubinstein SM, Pool JJM, van Tulder MW, Riphagen II, de Vet HCW. A systematic review of the diagnostic accuracy of provocative tests of the neck for diagnosing cervical radiculopathy. *Eur Spine J*. 2007;16(3):307-319. [free online resource]

Innervation of
the Legs

TOP 100

A Very Brief Introduction to the Innervation of the Legs

The cerebrospinal water … penetrates into dural sleeves of nerve roots; hence is apt to accumulate in the sheaths of the sciatic nerve and so give pain along its course. Such pain, weakness, and limping may be cured; if necessary by vesicants and caustics to draw out the hydrops.

Domenico Cotugno*

The legs are innervated by lumbar (L1-L5) and sacral nerve roots (mainly S1 and S2). The sensory lumbar nerve roots supply most of the sensation to the anterior, medial, and lateral sides of the leg starting at the level of the inguinal region and extending down to the dorsum of the foot. The sacral nerve roots supply most of the sole of the foot and the posterior aspect of the leg. Each nerve root supplies a specific area termed "a dermatome".

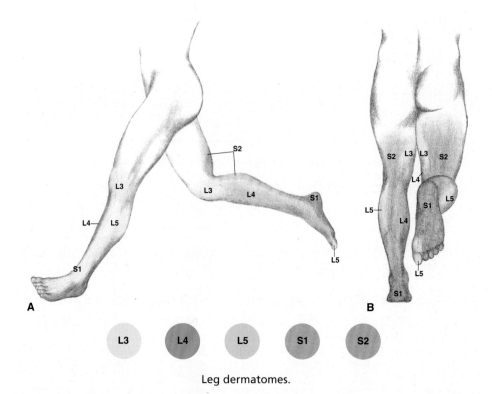

Leg dermatomes.

*Domenico Felice Antonio Cotugno (1736-1822), an Italian physician, was the first to attribute sciatic pain to spinal root pathology and to differentiate it from arthritic hip pain. Although Cotugno's suggestion that sciatic pain was due to buildup of cerebrospinal fluid is no longer accepted, his discovery of cerebrospinal fluid—tucked in the middle of a treatise on sciatica—was of singular significance. For a long period after his death, "sciatica" was referred to as "Cotugno syndrome" and cerebrospinal fluid as "Liquor Cotugni." Citation is from Pearce JM. A brief history of sciatica. Spinal Cord. 2007;45(9):592-596.

The lumbosacral nerve roots exit from the vertebral foramina and enter the psoas muscle to form the lumbosacral plexus. All the nerves that innervate the leg derive from the lumbosacral plexus. Some of the nerves exit the pelvis anteriorly (femoral nerve and obturator nerve), some posteriorly (sciatic nerve and inferior gluteal nerve), and others do not exit the pelvis (superior gluteal nerve).

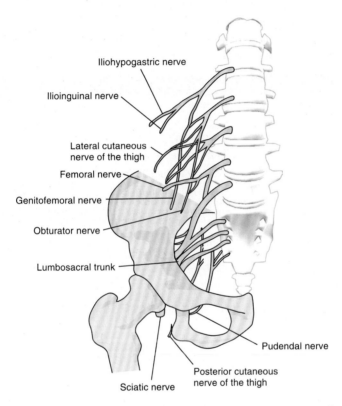

Simplified schematic of the lumbosacral plexus. (Reprinted with permission from Brody T, Hall C. *Therapuetic Exercise: Moving Toward Function*. 4th ed. Philadelphia, PA: Wolters Kluwer; 2017:Figure 19.37.)

A simplified scheme to remember the major functions of the nerves of the legs is as follows: the "anterior nerves" move the thigh "anteriorly"/forward (femoral nerve) and medially/inward (obturator nerve), while the "posterior nerves" pull the hip posteriorly/backward (inferior gluteal nerve). The sciatic nerve is a "posterior" nerve, which innervates all muscles below the knee. The tibial nerve, a continuation of the sciatic nerve, runs posteriorly and supplies muscles in the posterior leg compartment. The peroneal nerve swings around the fibular head and divides into deep and superficial branches that supply the anterior compartment leg muscles. To better remember where which branch goes, consider the following mnemonic: the tib-**I**-al nerve runs on the **I**nside of the leg (posteriorly) and is responsible for "ankle **In**" movement (inversion), while the per-**O**-neal nerve runs on the **O**utside of the leg (anteriorly) is responsible for "ankle **O**ut" movement (eversion). The functions of the tibial and peroneal nerves regarding up and down movements of the ankle can be remembered as follows: the anterior branch (peroneal nerve) contracts anterior muscles of the leg causing the foot to go UP, while the posterior branch (tibial nerve) contracts the posterior muscles of the leg, causing the foot to go DOWN as if pushing down on the **GAS** pedal (**GAS**trocnemius-soleus muscle complex).

We offer here a simplified scheme for associating appropriate lumbosacral nerve roots with their major nerves and muscles:

Root	Nerve	Muscle	Function
L1 (L2)	L1, L2 roots and femoral nerve	Iliopsoas	Hip flexion (hip up)
L3 (L4)	Femoral	Quadriceps	Knee extension (knee out)
L4 (L5)	Deep peroneal	Tibialis anterior	Ankle dorsiflexion (foot up)
L5	Deep peroneal	Extensor hallucis longus	Toe dorsiflexion (toe up)
S1, S2	Tibial	Flexor hallucis longus	Toe plantar flexion (toe down)
S1, S2	Tibial	Gastrocnemius	Ankle plantar flexion (foot down)
S1, S2	Sciatic	Hamstrings	Knee flexion

A practical, simplified guide to testing leg muscles is shown below:

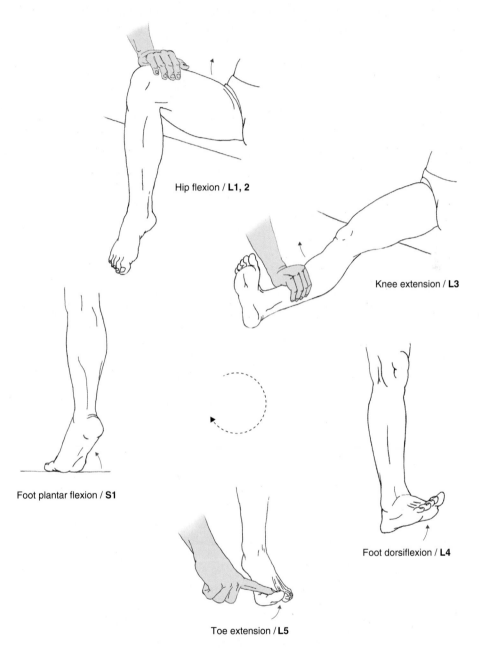

Hip flexion / **L1, 2**

Knee extension / **L3**

Foot plantar flexion / **S1**

Foot dorsiflexion / **L4**

Toe extension / **L5**

Practical guide to lower extremity strength testing.

In this section, we discuss disorders affecting leg nerves (lateral femoral cutaneous neuropathy, Chapter 6), plexuses (lumbosacral plexopathy in a cancer patient, Chapter 8), roots (common lumbosacral radiculopathies, Chapter 9), or a combination thereof (peripheral foot drop, Chapter 7; diabetic amyotrophy, Chapter 10). Logically, the cauda equina syndrome belongs in the section on peripheral nervous system disorders of the leg, but because of the frequent overlap with the conus medullaris syndrome, is relegated to the section on spinal cord disorders.

6 Meralgia Paresthetica

Compression of the lateral femoral cutaneous nerve (LFCN)

CORE FEATURES

1. History of spine or pelvic surgery, pregnancy, rapid weight loss or weight gain, use of tight belts or tight pants at the time of symptom onset or symptom worsening.
2. Tingling and burning over the lateral thigh.
   Sensory loss is always limited to a discrete area of the anterolateral thigh, but pain radiation may involve a larger area.
3. No motor deficits on examination.
   The LFCN is a pure sensory nerve.
4. Normal muscle stretch reflexes.
   No testable muscle stretch reflex is mediated via the LFCN.
5. Symptoms exacerbated with the pelvic compression test.
   In a pelvic compression test, the patient is placed on the lateral recumbent position and downward pressure is applied by the examiner for 45 s on the lateral aspect of the anterior superior iliac spine.

SYNOPSIS

The LFCN derives from the L2 and L3 nerve roots. The LFCN is susceptible to compression along its course through the psoas muscle, within the abdominal cavity, under the inguinal ligament, and in the anterior thigh. The most common site of impingement of the LFCN—under the inguinal ligament—is referred to as meralgia paresthetica (MP) (from Greek "meros"—thigh and "algos"—pain). MP is usually the result of increased pressure on the nerve due to intra-abdominal pressure, weight gain, or external causes such as wearing tight pants. Being a small nerve with a variable anatomical course, LCFN may also be damaged during surgery of the spine or pelvis.

Diagnosis of MP is made on clinical grounds, and no testing is required. In atypical cases, imaging may be pursued to rule out pelvic metastases or upper lumbar disk herniation that may mimic MP. Excellent outcomes are expected with conservative management. Local anesthetic creams or neuropathic pain medications may be helpful when pain is significant. In the rare treatment-recalcitrant MP cases, local nerve injections, pulsed radiofrequency therapy, or surgery may be considered.

FIGURE

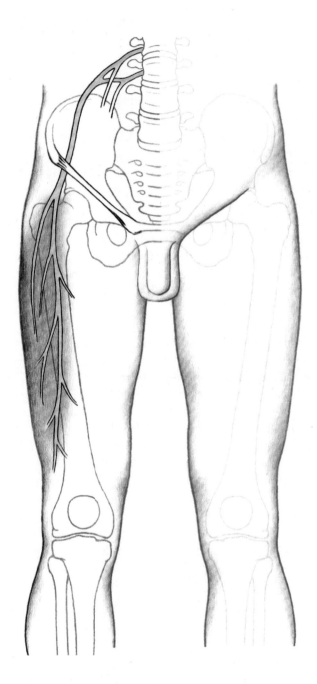

Lateral femoral cutaneous nerve, which derives from the L2 and L3 nerve roots, is highlighted in yellow. Its sensory area of innervation is shown in blue.

QUESTIONS FOR SELF-STUDY

1. How would you differentiate an L2 or L3 radiculopathy from MP on neurologic examination?
2. What nonpharmacological recommendations should be offered to a patient with MP?
3. What medications are commonly used to alleviate the burning and tingling sensations of MP?
4. Provide a clinical scenario of the LFCN could be injured within the psoas; under the inguinal ligaments; and in the thigh region.
5. The femoral nerve passes under the inguinal ligament more medially than the LFCN. The femoral nerve passes through and innervates the psoas muscle, before entering the thigh where it innervates the quadriceps. The femoral nerve is a mixed motor and sensory nerve which may be injured during surgery by deep retractors or inappropriate lithotomy positioning. Review the neuroanatomy of the femoral nerve and work out the motor, sensory, and reflex abnormalities caused by injuries to the femoral nerve at the level of the inguinal canal.

CHALLENGE

Other than the LCFN and the femoral nerve, which other nerves may be injured, in the inguinal region? What are the symptoms and signs associated with these injuries?

REFERENCES

Cheatham SW, Kolber MJ, Salamh PA. Meralgia paresthetica: a review of the literature. *Int J Sports Phys Ther.* 2013;8(6):883-893. [free online resource]

Kuponiyi O, Alleemudder DI, Latunde-Dada A, Eedarapalli P. Nerve injuries associated with gynaecological surgery. *The Obstetrician & Gynaecologist.* 2014;16:29-36.

Patijn J, Mekhail N, Hayek S, Lataster A, van Kleef M, Van Zundert J. Meralgia paresthetica. *Pain Pract.* 2011;11(3):302-308.

Peripheral Foot Drop

The most common peripheral causes of foot drop are L5 radiculopathy and common peroneal neuropathy

CORE FEATURES

	L5 Radiculopathy	Common Peroneal Nerve Palsy
1. Sensory	Anterior, lower two-thirds of the leg; part of the dorsum of foot	Dorsum of the foot and lateral leg
2. The main motor deficit that differentiates two entities	Hip abduction	Ankle eversion (tested with the foot at 90° angle)
3. Pain	Common, usually radiating from the back into the buttock and leg	Rare; if present, is usually dull and ill-defined around the knee
4. Provocative test	Pain reproduced with straight leg test (with the patient supine, raise leg gently to 30°-60°)	Tinel sign at the fibular head
5. Common mechanism of injury	Disk herniation; spinal stenosis	Fibular fracture; knee dislocation; knee surgery; compression at the fibular head due to habitual leg crossing; prolonged squatting; plaster cast

SYNOPSIS

The sciatic nerve, the largest and longest peripheral nerve in the body, originates from the L4, L5, S1, and S2 nerve roots. The sciatic nerve leaves the pelvis posteriorly via the sciatic notch, travels through the piriformis muscle, enters the posterior thigh, where it innervates the hamstring muscles, and splits into tibial and common peroneal branches at the level of the popliteal fossa. The common peroneal nerve swings around the fibular head to enter the anterior leg compartment and is responsible for innervating the muscles that lift the foot ("dorsiflexion"). The common peroneal nerve is relatively unprotected as it passes over the head of the fibula. Hence, common peroneal nerve injury at the fibular head is the most common leg mononeuropathy and the most common cause of foot drop.

In addition to a common peroneal neuropathy and L5 radiculopathy, which are contrasted in the *Core Features* Table, isolated foot drop can be caused by lesions anywhere along the pathway from the lumbosacral nerve roots to the tibialis anterior muscle. Thus, the differential diagnosis of peripheral foot drop includes lumbar plexopathy, sciatic neuropathy, and deep peroneal nerve injury. Moreover, because the term "foot drop" is applied to any condition in which foot dorsiflexion is affected more than foot plantar flexion, central nervous system (CNS) lesions (stroke, multiple sclerosis), motor neuron disease (eg, ALS), polyneuropathies (Charcot-Marie-Tooth), and myopathies can also present with foot drop. In these cases, the examination will demonstrate a pattern of muscle weakness not restricted to sciatic nerve–innervated muscles.

FIGURE

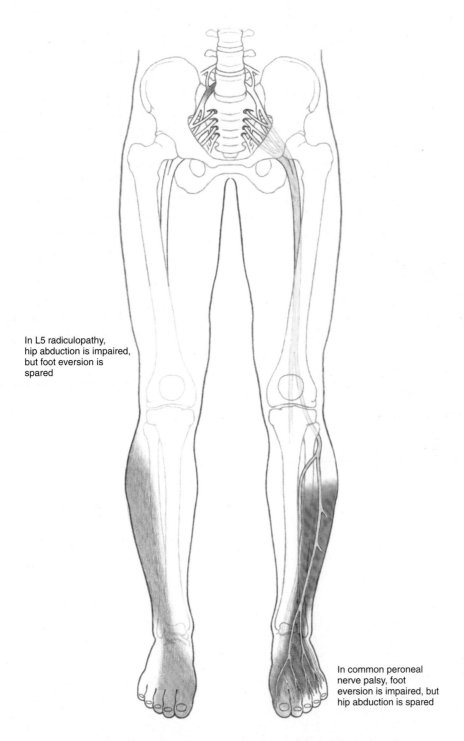

In L5 radiculopathy, hip abduction is impaired, but foot eversion is spared

In common peroneal nerve palsy, foot eversion is impaired, but hip abduction is spared

Sensory loss in peripheral foot drop due to L5 root injury (blue, right leg) and common peroneal nerve injury (red/orange, left leg). The L5 nerve root is in blue; sciatic nerve and its tibial and peroneal branches are in yellow.

QUESTIONS FOR SELF-STUDY

1. Which neurologic findings help differentiate foot drop due to stroke from a foot drop due to peroneal nerve palsy?
2. Explain how motor examination of the ankle helps to differentiate foot drop due to sciatic nerve injury (hip surgery or improper placement of intramuscular injection) from foot drop due to peroneal nerve palsy.
3. Which sensory finding helps to differentiate a foot drop from a common peroneal nerve palsy from a foot drop due to a deep peroneal nerve palsy?
4. What advice would you give to a patient with a common peroneal nerve neuropathy to avoid further exacerbating nerve damage?
5. A 40-year-old man with a history of a recent left tibial fracture presents with leg pain and foot drop. On examination, there is tenderness over the anterior left leg compartment, weakness in ankle, and toe dorsiflexion and sensory loss in the first dorsal web space on the left side. The dorsalis pedis pulse is absent on the left. What condition must be emergently evaluated in this clinical setting to prevent irreversible neurologic injury?

CHALLENGE

"Peroneal nerve stimulator" is a commercially available device for patients with foot drop. The nerve stimulator is wrapped around the leg above the knee and sends discharges along the peroneal nerve as the patient swings their leg to make a step. Describe the expected sensory and motor effects of peroneal nerve stimulation in a patient with foot drop due to stroke. Which causes of foot drop are not amenable to treatment with a peroneal nerve stimulator?

REFERENCES

Baima J, Krivickas L. Evaluation and treatment of peroneal neuropathy. *Curr Rev Musculoskelet Med.* 2008;1(2): 147-153. [free online resource]

Humphreys DB, Novak CB, Mackinnon SE. Patient outcome after common peroneal nerve decompression. *J Neurosurg.* 2007;107(2):314-318.

Stewart JD. Foot drop: where, why and what to do? *Pract Neurol.* 2008;8(3):158-169.

8 Neoplastic Lumbosacral Plexopathy

Compression or invasion of the lumbar plexus by neoplasm

CORE FEATURES

1. Unilateral leg pain.
   Pain is a near-universal manifestation of cancer-related lumbosacral plexopathy. Leg pain may precede other neurologic symptoms by weeks or months. Lower back pain is common.
2. Leg weakness.
   The pattern of leg weakness will depend on where the lumbosacral plexus is involved: lumbar plexopathy (L1-L4 nerve roots) may be confused with a femoral neuropathy, while sacral plexopathy (L5-S4 nerve roots) may be confused with sciatic neuropathy.
3. Leg edema.
   Compromise of venous outflow of the legs by tumor causes asymmetric leg edema.
4. Rectal mass palpated on rectal examination.
   In the modern era, a pelvic or retroperitoneal mass is much more likely to be identified on magnetic resonance imaging (MRI) or computed tomography (CT) than on physical examination. The absence of a mass lesion does not rule out a neoplastic etiology as plexopathy may be due to neural invasion rather than compression of the plexus.
5. Hydronephrosis occurs when a tumor compresses renal outflow pathways.
   Hydronephrosis can be detected with CT or MRI of abdomen and pelvis, or with renal ultrasound.

SYNOPSIS

In a patient with a history of malignancy, especially an abdominal or pelvic neoplasm, who presents with symptoms and signs of lumbar plexopathy, a neoplastic etiology is the likely culprit and is indicative of cancer progression. However, the differential diagnosis of lumbosacral plexopathy is broad and includes psoas abscess; retroperitoneal hematoma; aneurysms of the abdominal aorta or common iliac artery; trauma to spine, pelvis, or hips; surgical injury; obstetric complications; radiation plexopathy; and diabetic amyotrophy.

FIGURE

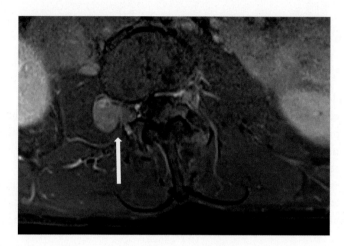

Ganglioneuroma, a rare tumor arising from the sympathetic ganglia, is invading the right psoas muscle (arrow) and exerting pressure on the lumbosacral plexus.

QUESTIONS FOR SELF-STUDY

1. What muscles should be tested to distinguish a lumbar plexopathy from a femoral neuropathy?
2. What muscles should be tested to distinguish a sacral plexopathy from a sciatic neuropathy?
3. A 70-year-old woman with deep vein thrombosis (DVT), on anticoagulant therapy, acutely develops lower back and left thigh pain. Examination shows left suprainguinal tenderness, a left groin mass, and weakness on left hip flexion. What diagnosis must be considered in this patient? What laboratory and imaging studies should be performed urgently?
4. Propose a mechanism whereby lumbosacral plexopathy is caused by (a) an infection, (b) surgery, and (c) pregnancy.
5. Nerves of the lumbosacral plexus carry autonomic fibers as well as motor and sensory fibers. Describe the autonomic manifestations to be expected if the autonomic outflow via the lower sacral nerve roots is disrupted. What skin changes in the legs may be expected due to the loss of autonomic function?

CHALLENGE

When a cancer patient with a history of radiation therapy presents with symptoms of possible lumbosacral plexopathy, clinicians are faced with the challenging task of differentiating neoplastic from radiation causes of plexopathy. Which clinical, electromyography (EMG) and MRI findings favor radiation-induced over neoplastic etiology?

REFERENCES

Brejt N, Berry J, Nisbet A, Bloomfield D, Burkill G. Pelvic radiculopathies, lumbosacral plexopathies, and neuropathies in oncologic disease: a multidisciplinary approach to a diagnostic challenge. *Cancer Imaging.* 2013;13(4):591-601. [free online resource]

Jaeckle KA, Young DF, Foley KM. The natural history of lumbosacral plexopathy in cancer. *Neurology.* 1985;35(1):8-15.

Jaeckle KA. Neurologic manifestations of neoplastic and radiation-induced plexopathies. *Semin Neurol.* 2010;30(3):254-262.

9 Acute Lumbosacral Radiculopathies: L5 and S1 ∎

Compression of lumbosacral nerve roots is most commonly due to degenerative lumbosacral spine disease

CORE FEATURES

	L4/L5 Radiculopathy (L5 Nerve Root Affected)	L5/S1 Radiculopathy (S1 Nerve Root Affected)
1. Main motor deficit	Weakness of foot and toe dorsiflexion and hip abduction	Weakness of foot plantar flexion and hip extension
2. Sensory deficits	Anterior leg and anterolateral dorsum of the foot	Posterior leg and plantar aspect of the foot
3. Ankle reflex	Usually normal and never absent	Usually depressed or absent
4. Pain	Radiating from the lower back or buttock to the lateral aspect of the thigh, lower leg, and dorsum of the foot	Radiating from the lower back or buttock to the posterior aspect of the thigh, calf, and heel
5. MRI lumbosacral spine	L4/5 disk herniation (common in younger patients) or lumbar spine arthropathy—facet joint hypertrophy, osteophyte formation (common in older patients)	L5/S1 disk herniation (common in younger patients) or lumbar spine arthropathy (common in older patients)

SYNOPSIS

In the general population, the lifetime prevalence of significant low-back pain is approximately 80%. Degenerative causes such as spinal stenosis, spondylotic disease, facet joint hypertrophy, and disk herniation are the most common. Acute lumbosacral radiculopathy due to disk herniation accounts for a small minority of cases of low-back pain but is still quite prevalent, with an estimated lifetime prevalence of 3%. The L4-L5 and L5-S1 articulations have the greatest motion in the lumbar spine, and 90% of lumbosacral disk herniations occur at these two levels.

Lumbar spine MRI is not indicated for the typical cases of lumbosacral radiculopathy, where there are no significant motor or autonomic deficits and radicular pain is reproducible with straight leg test. Conservative measures and passage of time lead to symptom resolution within days to weeks. In rare cases where there is weakness or bowel or bladder incontinence or retention, urgent imaging of the lower spine is mandatory. Other "red flags" that may prompt imaging even in the absence of focal neurologic deficits include a history of malignancy, immunodeficient state, back trauma, systemic symptoms, intractable pain or pain that is worse at rest.

FIGURE

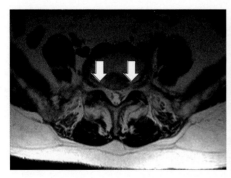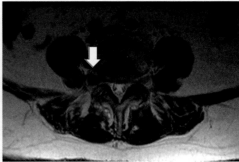

Normal disk and patent foramen (arrows) are shown on the left. Right lateral extraforamenal disk herniation (arrow) causing severe sciatic pain is shown on the right.

QUESTIONS FOR SELF-STUDY

1. What are the nonneurologic causes of apparent hip flexion weakness and knee extension weakness?
2. What are the major motor, sensory, and reflex findings in patients with L2/3 (compression of L3 nerve root) and L3/4 (L4 nerve root) radiculopathies?
3. A patient with a history of lumbar disk herniation complains of radiating pain and cramping in both legs when walking. Symptoms abate when leaning forward on the shopping cart ("shopping cart sign"). What diagnosis do you suspect?
4. A patient with typical radicular symptoms who does not have an obvious disk herniation within the spinal canal may have what kind of disk herniation that is often missed on MRI?
5. Name the common causes of noncompressive radiculopathy.

CHALLENGE

What is the clinical implication of "testicular ptosis," whereby a markedly lower testicle is observed on the side of the pain? Explain how this condition can be due to a radiculopathy. (Compare your answer with Bartleson JD, et al. Neurol Clin Pract. 2015;5(2):178-181.)

REFERENCES

Tarulli AW, Raynor EM. Lumbosacral radiculopathy. *Neurol Clin.* 2007;25(2):387-405.
Tavee JO, Levin KH. Low back pain. *Continuum (Minneap Minn).* 2017;23(2, Selected Topics in Outpatient Neurology):467-486.
Tawa N, Rhoda A, Diener I. Accuracy of clinical neurological examination in diagnosing lumbo-sacral radiculopathy: a systematic literature review. *BMC Musculoskelet Disord.* 2017;18(1):93. [free online resource]

10 Diabetic Amyotrophy (Lumbosacral Radiculoplexus Neuropathy)

Painful, acute polyradiculoneuropathy in patients with diabetes mellitus

CORE FEATURES

1. History of type 2 diabetes mellitus (T2DM).
   A typical patient is a middle-aged individual with mild T2DM. In approximately 25% of patients, the diagnosis of diabetes is unknown at the time of presentation.
2. Unexplained weight loss often precedes the onset of symptoms.
3. Acute onset of unilateral and severe leg pain.
   Pain is reported in thigh, hip, buttock, and low back.
4. Subacute onset of unilateral proximal leg weakness.
   Weakness progressively worsens, with half of the patients requiring a wheelchair at nadir, followed by slow and incomplete recovery. Pain and weakness may spread to the other leg within weeks of presentation.
5. Autonomic dysfunction.
   Orthostatic hypotension, tachycardia, urinary and sexual dysfunction, constipation, or diarrhea is common.

SYNOPSIS

Diabetic lumbosacral radiculoplexus neuropathy is a rare monophasic disorder occurring in patients with relatively mild T2DM. In contrast, symmetric axonal sensorimotor polyneuropathy is common, chronic, progressive, and usually associated with long-standing and poorly controlled diabetes mellitus. Diabetic lumbosacral radiculoplexus neuropathy can be conceptualized as microvasculitis of the lumbosacral nerve roots, plexus, and nerves of the leg, including the femoral nerve. Microvasculitis may explain the intense pain (nerve ischemia), pattern, and severity of weakness.

FIGURE

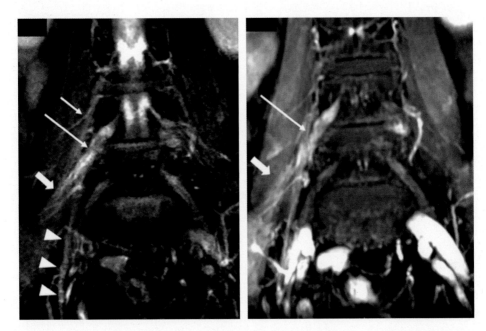

MRI in diabetic lumbosacral radiculoplexus neuropathy (diabetic amytrophy) shows increased caliber and T2 signal (right) and abnormal T1 contrast enhancement (left) of the right L3 nerve (short thin arrow), L4 nerve (long thin arrow), proximal portion of the femoral nerve (short thick arrow), and right obturator nerve (arrowheads). (Reprinted with permission from Cianfoni A, Luigetti M, Madia F, et al. Teaching neuroImage: MRI of diabetic lumbar plexopathy treated with local steroid injection. *Neurology.* 2009;72(6):e32-e33.)

QUESTIONS FOR SELF-STUDY

1. Testing of which muscles help differentiate diabetic lumbosacral radiculoplexus neuropathy from a femoral neuropathy?
2. Explain why EMG testing of paraspinal muscles can help differentiate lumbosacral radiculoplexus neuropathy from a lumbar plexopathy.
3. A 50-year-old man with a history of diabetic lumbosacral radiculoplexus neuropathy develops severe arm pain, numbness, and weakness suggestive of brachial plexopathy. What is the likely explanation of these symptoms?
4. A 60-year-old man presents with symptoms highly suggestive of diabetic radiculoplexus neuropathy, but he has no history of diabetes mellitus, and blood glucose testing is within a normal range. What is the likely diagnosis?
5. Provide examples of focal mononeuropathies in patients with diabetes mellitus.

CHALLENGE

"Amyotrophy" means "muscle (Greek: 'myo') atrophy," the usual sequela of diabetic amyotrophy. Explain why injury to nerves in diabetic amyotrophy results in muscle atrophy.

REFERENCES

Laughlin RS, Dyck PJ. Diabetic radiculoplexus neuropathies. *Handb Clin Neurol.* 2014;126:45-52.
Pasnoor M, Dimachkie MM, Barohn RJ. Diabetic neuropathy part 2: proximal and asymmetric phenotypes. *Neurol Clin.* 2013;31(2):447-462. [free online resource]

Polyneuropathies

A Very Brief Introduction to Polyneuropathies

Nerve is a simple, solid body, the cause of voluntary motion, but difficult to perceive in dissection. According to Erasistratus and Herophilus, there are nerves capable of sensation, but according to Asclepiades, not at all. According to Erasistratus, there are two kinds of nerves, sensory and motor nerves.

Rufus of Ephesus[*]

A peripheral nerve contains motor, sensory, and autonomic fibers. The motor signal starts in the motor neuron in the anterior horn of the spinal cord and travels via the ventral nerve root, plexus, and the nerve to reach the neuromuscular junction. The sensory signal travels in the opposite direction: it originates at the nerve ending near the sensory receptor and travels up the peripheral nerve, plexus, and root to arrive at the neuronal cell bodies within the dorsal root ganglia, which is located in the intervertebral foramina. Myelinated large nerve fibers are the "express lanes"—they carry signal 50 times faster than the unmyelinated nerves. This explains why when touching a scalding object, the sensation of touch conveyed by myelinated fibers precedes by an appreciable time interval the sensation of hotness conveyed via unmyelinated nerve fibers.

Nerve conduction studies (NCS) test the patency of the large myelinated fibers. To test sensory fibers, a nerve is stimulated at point A and a response—"sensory nerve action potential"—is recorded at point B. The time from stimulation to recording divided by distance between point A and point B is the speed of conduction of sensory fibers. To test motor fibers, the nerve is stimulated at two points along its course—at a more proximal point A and at a more distant point B—while muscle response is measured at point C, over a muscle innervated by the respective nerve. The muscle response is called the "compound muscle action potential," CMAP. The time difference between stimulation of points A and B and the response at point C, divided by the distance between points A and B, is the speed of conduction along the motor nerve. The amplitude of the CMAPs corresponds roughly to how much muscle tissue is excited by the nerve. If the nerve is damaged and signal strength is diminished, then it fails to excite as much muscle tissue and CMAPs are smaller. This is seen in axonal neuropathies. The speed of conduction is not much affected in axonal neuropathies since speed does not depend on the number of myelinated axons within the nerve as much as on the presence of at least some myelinated fibers. As long as at least some of the myelinated axons are intact, the speed along the nerve is roughly unchanged. In contrast, when

---

[*]Herophilus and Erasistratus were Greek physicians in the third century BCE who established the first anatomical school in Alexandria where they performed systematic dissection of human cadavers (and possibly vivisection as well). The passage from Rufus of Ephesus, who lived several centuries after Herophilus and Erasistratus, in the first century CE, illustrates the difficulties in anatomical studies of the nervous system. (Cited from Acar F. Herophilus of Chalcedon: a pioneer in neuroscience. *Neurosurgery*. 2005;56(4):861-867.)

myelinated nerve fibers are stripped off their myelin, as in demyelinating neuropathies, the speed of conduction is greatly reduced, but the magnitude of the CMAPs is not very much diminished because roughly the same "quantity" of the electrical signal is transduced to the muscle. When signal decays rapidly between point A and points B, stimulation at point A may not yield any CMAP at all. This is called "conduction block"—an important finding in demyelinating neuropathies and compression mononeuropathies.

NCS allow the classification of neuropathies into primarily axonal or primarily demyelinating. This characterization helps to narrow down the differential diagnosis. NCS also help elucidate the pattern of nerve injury. In radiculopathy, motor nerves deriving from a single nerve root may be affected and others are spared. In a plexopathy, nerves supplied by several nerve roots are involved. In a mononeuropathy, such as radial nerve palsy or common peroneal palsy, NCS can help localize where along the nerve the compression has occured. In polyneuropathies, abnormalities are present in multiple nerves. NCS of motor and sensory fibers can clarify whether a neuropathy is motor, sensory, or—as is usually the case—sensorimotor. Combining historical data with findings on neurologic examination and NCS allows one to elucidate the etiology of polyneuropathy in many patients. This section presents important examples of chronic, acute, axonal, and demyelinating polyneuropathies.

REFERENCES

Bromberg MB. An electrodiagnostic approach to the evaluation of peripheral neuropathies. *Phys Med Rehabil Clin N Am.* 2013;24(1):153-168.

Mallik A, Weir AI. Nerve conduction studies: essentials and pitfalls in practice. *J Neurol Neurosurg Psychiatry.* 2005;76(suppl 2):ii23-ii31. [free online resource]

11 Diabetic Sensorimotor Polyneuropathy

Chronic, sensorimotor polyneuropathy due to diabetes mellitus

CORE FEATURES

1. History of type 1 or type 2 diabetes mellitus (DM).
   Risk factors for developing diabetic sensorimotor polyneuropathy (DPN) are the duration of DM and inadequate blood glucose control.
2. "Stocking-glove" pattern of sensory loss.
   This represents the classic distribution in axonal, length-dependent polyneuropathies: the longer the axons, the more likely it is to be damaged. Vibration is most commonly diminished or lost in the toes.
3. Foot pain.
   Discomfort, cramping, and numbness in the feet are common complaints. A minority of patients will have neuropathic pain characterized by tingly, prickly, achy, burning, and electric sensations.
4. Absent or diminished ankle reflexes.
   Depressed or absent ankle reflexes have the highest sensitivity for DPN of all physical examination signs.
5. NCS are consistent with "sensory-more-than-motor" axonal polyneuropathy.
   Evaluation of NCS may not be necessary in typical cases, as DPN occurs in up to half of patients with long-standing DM.

SYNOPSIS

More than a dozen different types of neuropathies are associated with DM or diabetic treatments—DPN, autonomic, small-fiber, acute painful sensory, hyperglycemic neuropathies, mononeuropathies, diabetic lumbosacral radiculoplexus neuropathy, and others. DPN, by far the most common of the diabetic neuropathies, is a chronic, distal, symmetric, large- and small-fiber, axonal sensorimotor polyneuropathy. DPN is the most common cause of polyneuropathy in Western countries. Because DPN is a "dying back" neuropathy, the longest axons are affected first. Thus, symptoms typically start at the toes and slowly progress to involve the feet and sometimes the fingers, hands, and, very rarely, the trunk. Loss of large sensory nerve fibers results in deficits of vibratory sensation and joint position sense. Motor nerves are usually not as much affected, and frank weakness is uncommon. DPN may coexist with autonomic neuropathy.

Patients with chronic DPN are prone to foot ulceration because they lack protective sensation and have abnormal sweating and poor wound healing. Routine foot examination should, therefore, be part of the evaluation of all patients with DPN.

FIGURES

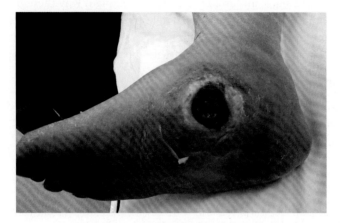

Charcot foot is usually seen in patients with diabetic polyneuropathy (DPN). The foot is deformed, mechanically unstable, and prone to ulcerations. There is collapse of midfoot ("rocker-bottom" deformity). Early recognition and treatment of Charcot foot may prevent fractures, osteomyelitis, and limb amputation. (Reprinted with permission from Wiesel SW. *Operative Techniques in Orthopaedic Surgery*. 2nd ed. Philadelphia, PA: Wolters Kluwer; 2015. Part 8. Figure 42.5.)

QUESTIONS FOR SELF-STUDY

1. A 60-year-old woman with type 2 DM reports painful tingling in both feet. Examination demonstrates normal muscle strength, normal muscle stretch reflexes, and diminished pinprick and temperature discrimination. You suspect diabetic axonal sensorimotor polyneuropathy, but electrodiagnostic studies (electromyography [EMG]/NCS) are normal. What kind of neuropathy is consistent with normal NCS? Which test could confirm your suspicion of a neuropathy?

2. A 70-year-old woman with type 2 DM reports difficulty keeping up with her exercise routine and not sweating as much as she used to. On examination, there is mild tachycardia and orthostatic hypotension. What type of diabetic neuropathy could account for these symptoms? What additional symptoms you would try to elicit to confirm your suspicion? How can you objectively assess the patient's sweating function? What is a reliable bedside test of sweating? (Compare your answer with Khurana RK. *Clin Auton Res.* 2017;27(2):91-95. [free online resource])

3. A 50-year-old man with type 2 DM presents with symptoms and signs of a progressive painful distal symmetric polyneuropathy involving both feet, hands, and trunk over a course of few weeks. He endorses depression and a 20-lb. weight loss. Explain why this history is not consistent with DPN. What other diagnosis needs to be considered especially in view of his recent weight loss? What recommendations would you provide that could potentially reverse his symptoms?

4. A 70-year-old man with type 2 DM presents with symptoms suggestive of a painful distal symmetric polyneuropathy. Examination shows the loss of both ankle reflexes, bilateral Babinski signs, and mildly spastic gait. Explain why these findings are not consistent with DPN. Suggest additional investigations for reversible conditions that could account for the patient's symptoms.

5. What are the first-line medications for treating painful diabetic neuropathy?

CHALLENGE

What is "end-organ" damage due to DM? Compare the prevalence of end-organ damage across different organ systems, including the peripheral nerves. What screening tests are recommended to forestall end-organ damage in DM?

REFERENCES

Russell JW, Zilliox LA. Diabetic neuropathies. *Continuum (Minneap Minn)*. 2014;20(5 Peripheral Nervous System Disorders):1226-1240.

Shehab DK, Al-Jarallah KF, Abraham M, et al. Back to basics: ankle reflex in the evaluation of peripheral neuropathy in type 2 diabetes mellitus. *QJM*. 2012;105(4):315-320. [free online resource]

12 Chronic Inflammatory Demyelinating Polyneuropathy ▭

Chronic immune-mediated demyelinating polyradiculoneuropathy

CORE FEATURES

1. Insidious, progressive, symmetric muscle weakness of proximal and distal muscles.
   By definition, symptoms of chronic inflammatory demyelinating polyneuropathy (CIDP) progress for 2 months or more. The clinical course is slowly progressive or relapsing-remitting.
2. Acral paresthesias.
   Sensory deficits are typically less prominent than motor deficits, though patients may complain of considerable neuropathic pain.
3. Diffuse hypo- or areflexia.
4. NCS show velocity slowing, conduction block, the disappearance of F-waves, and dispersion and reduction of CMAPs.
5. Albuminocytologic dissociation in CSF.
   The cerebrospinal fluid (CSF) protein content is elevated, often >60 mg/dL, while the white blood cell (WBC) count is normal or only slightly elevated (always <10 cells/mm³).

SYNOPSIS

Chronic and acute inflammatory demyelinating polyneuropathies (CIDP and AIDP) are immune-mediated disorders causing demyelination of roots, plexi, and peripheral nerves. The two conditions differ in several important aspects. CIDP is insidious and chronic, while AIDP is acute and monophasic. CIDP rarely causes autonomic dysfunction or neuromuscular respiratory failure, while AIDP can cause both. CIDP responds well to corticosteroids, but AIDP does not.

Diagnosis and subtyping of CIDP require electrodiagnostic studies. The choice of immunomodulatory therapy may depend on the specific subtype, defined clinically and electrodiagnostically, as well as the associated autoantibodies. Magnetic resonance imaging (MRI) of nerve roots and plexuses and nerve biopsy, though not required, support the diagnosis of CIDP if there is contrast enhancement or hypertrophy of spinal nerve roots and plexuses on MRI and evidence of inflammation, demyelination, and remyelination ("onion bulbs") on nerve biopsy.

FIGURE

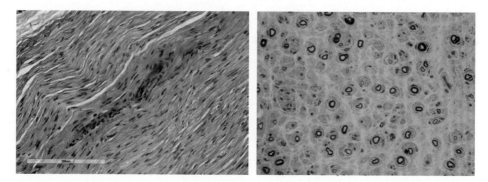

H&E-stained section showing endoneurial edema and scant chronic inflammatory infiltrates, 400× magnification. Toluidine blue–stained sections show loss of myelinated fibers and extensive onion bulb formation, 600× magnification. (Courtesy of Shahad Abdulameer, MD and Ewa Borys, MD, PhD, Department of Pathology, Loyola University Chicago, Stritch School of Medicine.)

QUESTIONS FOR SELF-STUDY

1. CIDP may have similar findings on NCS as genetic demyelinating polyneuropathies (Charcot-Marie-Tooth disease). How would you differentiate acquired from inherited demyelinating polyneuropathies based on physical examination?
2. Which treatments are effective for both CIDP and AIDP, and which treatments are only effective for CIDP, but not for AIDP?
3. An important CIDP variant is a pure motor demyelinating neuropathy, which tends to respond to intravenous immunoglobulin (IVIG). This treatable entity must be differentiated from amyotrophic lateral sclerosis (ALS), a relentlessly progressive and uniformly lethal motor neuron disorder. Explain how EMG would help differentiate between these two conditions.
4. In axonal neuropathies, the distal muscles are preferentially affected and distal muscle stretch reflexes are hypoactive, while proximal muscle strength and proximal muscle stretch reflexes are preserved. In demyelinating polyneuropathies, both proximal and distal muscles are affected, and muscle stretch reflexes are hypoactive or absent diffusely. Provide a plausible explanation for these clinical differences between axonal and demyelinating neuropathies.
5. A subset of CIDP patients exhibit autoantibodies that may be pathogenic. What segments of the myelinated nerves are the antibodies directed at? What is the clinical significance of these autoantibodies?

CHALLENGE

In addition to muscle weakness and sensory findings, patients with CIDP may exhibit ataxia. Explain how ataxia could occur when cerebellar function is normal.

REFERENCES

Mathey EK, Park SB, Hughes RAC, et al. Chronic inflammatory demyelinating polyradiculoneuropathy: from pathology to phenotype. *J Neurol Neurosurg Psychiatry.* 2015;86(9):973-985.

Sander HW, Latov N. Research criteria for defining patients with CIDP. *Neurology.* 2003;60(8 suppl 3):S8-S15.

Vural A, Doppler K, Meinl E. Autoantibodies against the node of ranvier in seropositive chronic inflammatory demyelinating polyneuropathy: diagnostic, pathogenic, and therapeutic relevance. *Front Immunol.* 2018;9:1029. [free online resource]

13   Guillain-Barré Syndrome

Acute, immune-mediated, demyelinating polyradiculoneuropathy

CORE FEATURES

1. Rapidly progressive paralysis.
   Weakness typically starts in the legs ("ascending paralysis") and progresses to involve the arms and often respiratory, bulbar (dysphagia, dysarthria), and facial (facial diplegia) muscles as well. In approximately 20% of patients, paralysis of respiratory muscles leads to respiratory failure, necessitating mechanical ventilation. Nadir occurs within 2 weeks of onset followed by slow and often incomplete recovery.
2. Diffusely decreased or absent muscle stretch reflexes.
   Reflexes are decreased the most in the weaker limbs.
3. Paresthesias and muscle aches present early in the disease.
   Objective sensory deficits emerge later.
4. Autonomic dysfunction.
   Arrhythmias or labile blood pressure are the most serious autonomic symptoms and may necessitate continuous cardiac monitoring. Bowel or bladder dysfunction is common and require monitoring for urinary retention and ileus.
5. CSF albuminocytologic dissociation.
   The combination of normal CSF leukocyte count and high CSF protein content level is highly characteristic of Guillain-Barré syndrome (GBS).

SYNOPSIS

GBS is an umbrella term for acute autoimmune demyelinating disorders of roots, plexi, and peripheral nerves. Variants of GBS include acute inflammatory demyelinating polyradiculoneuropathy (AIDP), acute motor axonal neuropathy (AMAN), and acute motor sensory axonal neuropathy (AMSAN). Miller-Fisher syndrome, characterized by areflexia, ophthalmoparesis, and ataxia, presumably has similar pathogenesis as GBS.

    GBS may be triggered by an infection with *Campylobacter jejuni*, cytomegalovirus, *Mycoplasma pneumoniae*, Epstein-Barr virus, West Nile Virus, Zika virus, and human immune deficiency virus (HIV). Unlike in CIDP, electrodiagnostic studies are not required prior to the start of treatment because signs of diffuse demyelination may not be present on NCV studies early in the disease. One of the early findings on NCS is the prolongation of F-wave latency. F-waves are elicited by suprastimulating a motor nerve. Timing from nerve stimulation to contraction—F-wave latency—is prolonged if there is slow conduction anywhere along the motor nerves or roots. Other electromyographic features of demyelination—conduction blocks, dispersion, and reduction of CMAPs—emerge later in the disease course. Inflammation of the spinal nerve roots may cause leakage of proteins in the CSF, and lack of inflammation in the subarachnoid space may explain the absence of inflammatory cells in the CSF (hence, "albuminocytologic dissociation"). Treatments for GBS include IVIG and plasmapheresis. Supportive management is essential. Even with the best management, fatal outcomes may occur in 5% to 10% of cases, usually due to cardiovascular and respiratory complications.

FIGURE

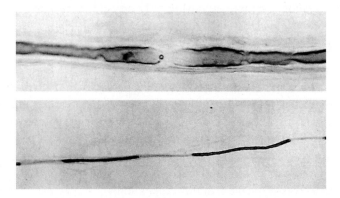

Teased myelin nerve fibers in GBS shows segmental demyelination (bottom panel), which starts at the nodes of Ranvier (upper panel). (Reprinted with permission from Husain AN, Stocker JT, Dehner LP. *Stocker and Dehner's Pediatric Pathology*. 4th ed. Philadelphia, PA: Wolters Kluwer; 2015: Figure 27.12.)

QUESTIONS FOR SELF-STUDY

1. Rapidly progressive quadriparesis is a neurologic emergency. It is essential to quickly differentiate an array of diagnostic possibilities. The neurologic examination to elucidate the pattern of muscle weakness and to assess for cranial nerve involvement and sensory and autonomic deficits will help narrow down the differential (for comprehensive differential diagnosis see (Leonhard SE et al reference below). Explain how the pattern of sensory deficits helps to differentiate GBS from cervical spinal cord injury, an important cause of acute quadriparesis.
2. What are key neurologic findings that help differentiate GBS from the diseases of neuromusjunction diseases that can cause quadriparesis—myasthenia gravis, botulism, hypermagnesemia, tick paralysis, or organophosphate poisoning? Name one key NCS finding that supports the diagnosis of GBS and one key finding that supports the diagnosis of neuromuscular junction disorders.
3. Which simple bedside test predicts whether a patient may require mechanical ventilation? What respiratory parameters predict the need for ventilation?
4. Testing of which reflex may help determine whether a patient is at risk for aspiration?
5. What are the most important indications for admitting patients with GBS to an ICU?

CHALLENGE

A 15-year-old boy has muscle cramping and marked generalized weakness after a strenuous mountain hike. His urine color turned orange. He has had similar symptoms once before. What part of neuroaxis is likely affected? What disease category should be considered?

REFERENCES

Leonhard SE, Mandarakas MR, Gondim FAA, et al. Diagnosis and management of Guillain-Barré syndrome in ten steps. *Nat Rev Neurol.* 2019;15(11):671-683. [free online resource]
Willison HJ, Jacobs BC, van Doorn PA. Guillain-Barré syndrome. *Lancet.* 2016;388(10045):717-727.

14 Critical Illness Polyneuropathy and Critical Illness Myopathy

The most common causes of acquired generalized muscle weakness in critically ill patients

CORE FEATURES

Critical illness polyneuropathy (CIP) and critical illness myopathy (CIM) often coexist. The table provides a simplified, dichotomous view of the two conditions.

	CIP	CIM
Antecedent medical history	Systemic inflammatory response syndrome (SIRS); multiorgan failure	SIRS; use of corticosteroids, neuromuscular blocking agents
Pattern of muscle weakness	Distal more than proximal muscle weakness	Both distal and proximal muscles
Difficulty weaning patients off the ventilator	Yes	Yes
Muscle stretch reflexes	Diminished or absent	Reflexes may be diminished but are not absent
Muscle biopsy	Grouped atrophy mostly affecting type 2 muscle fibers	Selective loss of myosin filaments

SYNOPSIS

CIP and CIM are the most likely causes of acquired quadriparesis and failure to wean off the ventilator in critically ill patients. CIP is an axonal polyneuropathy, so the most distally innervated muscles are affected first, and muscle stretch reflexes are hypoactive or absent. In CIM, both proximal and distal muscles may be affected and muscle stretch reflexes are not absent. Management of CIP/CIM includes aggressive treatment of SIRS; limiting corticosteroid use; avoiding neuromuscular blocking agents; blood glucose control; and early mobilization and rehabilitation. Despite the severity of muscle weakness, most patients with CIP and CIM have either partial or complete recovery within months. Still, approximately 30% of patients do not recover the ability to ambulate independently, and some patients are not able to come off the ventilator.

FIGURE

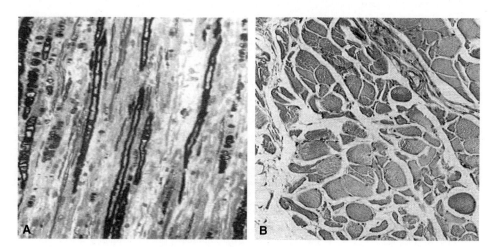

Nerve (left) and muscle (right) biopsies of a patient with severe CIP and failure to wean from a ventilator. (A) shows degenerating and dying axons and myelin collapse. (B) shows small atrophic, angulated muscle fibers secondary to axonal degeneration. (From Zochodne DW, Bolton CF, Wells GA, et al. Critical illness polyneuropathy. A complication of sepsis and multiple organ failure. *Brain*. 1987;110(Pt 4):819-841. Reproduced by permission of Oxford University Press.)

QUESTIONS FOR SELF-STUDY

1. Which key features differentiate CIP from GBS on NCS?
2. What is the likelihood of developing CIP/CIM in a patient with status asthmaticus who requires intubation and intravenous steroids; a patient with SIRS admitted to ICU; and a patient with SIRS and multiorgan failure?
3. Therapeutic neuromuscular blockade causes quadriparesis. The effects of neuromuscular blockade may be prolonged in critically ill patients with renal or liver failure. Explain how "train-of-four testing" could help titrate the depth of neuromuscular blockade and avoiding "over-paralysis."
4. What are the common infectious, vascular, nerve-, joint-, and skin-related complications of prolonged immobilization? What type of intervention could decrease the risk of these complications?
5. Which physical examination findings help to differentiate neuromuscular causes of difficulty weaning from pulmonary and cardiac causes?

CHALLENGE

Explain why "group muscle atrophy" is present on muscle biopsy in CIP but not CIM.

REFERENCES

Heunks LM, van der Hoeven JG. Clinical review: the ABC of weaning failure - a structured approach. *Crit Care*. 2010;14(6):245. [free online resource]

Shepherd S, Batra A, Lerner DP. Review of critical illness myopathy and neuropathy. *Neurohospitalist*. 2017;7(1):41-48.

Stevens RD, Dowdy DW, Michaels RK, et al. Neuromuscular dysfunction acquired in critical illness: a systematic review. *Intensive Care Med*. 2007;33(11):1876-1891.

Disorders of the Neuromuscular Junction

A Very Brief Introduction to Disorders of the Neuromuscular Junction

I have under my charge a prudent and honest Woman, who for many years have been obnoxious to this sort of spurious Palsie, not only in her members but also in her tongue; she for some time can speak freely and readily enough, but after she has spoken long, or hastily, or eagerly, she is not able to speak a word, but becomes mute as a Fish, nor can she recover the use of her voice under an hour or two.

Thomas Willis*

The neuromuscular junction (NMJ) comprises the presynaptic nerve terminal, the neuromuscular synapse, and the postsynaptic skeletal muscle membrane. Signal transduction from nerve to muscle can be conceptualized as a triathlon of "jumping" (saltatory nerve conduction), "swimming" (diffusion of neurotransmitter across the NMJ), and "pulling" (contraction of muscle fibers). When a sufficiently strong electrical signal arrives at the presynaptic membrane, it causes the nerve membrane to depolarize and voltage-gated calcium channels (VGCCs) to open. The influx of calcium into the nerve terminus causes the acetylcholine (ACh)-filled vesicles to fuse with cell membranes and ACh spills out into the synaptic cleft. As ACh molecules diffuse across the synapse, they bind to ACh receptors on the postsynaptic muscle membrane, causing the muscle membrane to depolarize. If the sum total of depolarization is strong enough to set off an action potential along the muscle, then a wave of depolarization sweeps along the muscle membrane leading to muscle contraction. In order for the muscles to contract again, ACh needs to be removed from the receptor. This function is accomplished by the acetylcholinesterase enzyme within the NMJ.

---

*Thomas Willis (1621-1675), a brilliant English anatomist, physician, and founding member of the Royal Society coined the term "neurology" for the study of the nervous system. Willis' manifold contributions to neurology include description of the cerebral circulation—the eponymous "circle of Willis;" naming of the cranial nerves; discovery that hemiplegia may be due to lesions in the internal capsule; early description of the autonomic nervous system; discovery that lesions of the vagus nerve cause cardiac arrhythmia; and the first known description of myasthenia gravis cited in the epigraph (Hughes T. The early history of myasthenia gravis. Neuromuscul Disord. 2005 Dec;15(12):878-86).

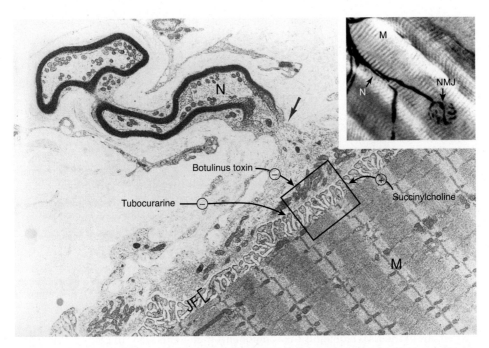

Electron micrograph shows nerve terminus (N), neuromuscular junction (NMJ), and skeletal myofiber (M). (Reprinted with permission from Dudek RW. *High-Yield Histopathology*. 2nd ed. Philadelphia, PA: Wolters Kluwer Health/Lippincott Williams & Wilkins; 2011: Figure 8-4B.)

Dysfunction of the NMJ could be due to presynaptic deficits (Lambert-Eaton myasthenic syndrome [LEMS] [Chapter 16], botulism [Chapter 17], and ciguatoxin poisoning), or postsynaptic deficits (myasthenia gravis [Chapter 15] and organophosphate poisoning). The schematic picture below shows which of the NMJ components are affected in the various NMJ disorders.

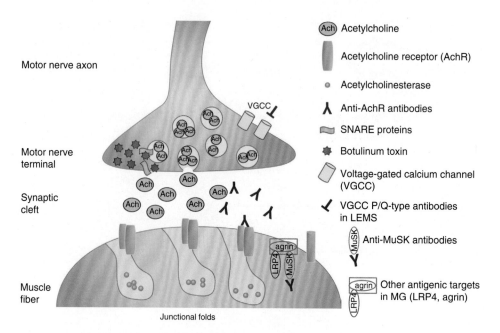

A schematic of the NMJ highlights the components that are relevant to pathophysiology of NMJ disorders. (Reprinted with permission from Louis ED, Mayer SA, Rowland LP. *Merritt's Neurology*. 13th ed. Philadelphia, PA: Wolters Kluwer; 2016: Figure 89.1.)

REFERENCE

Verschuuren J, Strijbos E, Vincent A. Neuromuscular junction disorders. *Handb Clin Neurol*. 2016;133:447-466.

15 Myasthenia Gravis

Autoimmune disorder of the postsynaptic neuromuscular junction

CORE FEATURES

1. Muscle fatigability.
   Muscle weakness is worse following exertion and overheating and better after rest and cooling.
2. Extraocular muscle (EOM) weakness.
   Asymmetric and variable ptosis and diplopia are the most common symptoms. The EOMs are involved in 90% of patients with MG, and are the only muscles involved in 15% of patients ("ocular MG").
3. Acetylcholine receptor antibodies (AChR Abs) in serum.
   Present in 80% to 90% of patients with generalized MG and 60% of patients with ocular MG. AChR-seronegative cases should be tested for muscle-specific kinase (MuSK) autoantibodies and anti–low-density lipoprotein receptor–related protein (LRP4) autoantibodies. Some cases remain "triple seronegative."
4. On electrodiagnostic studies, the width of the compound muscle action potentials (CMAPs) waveform decreases by 10% to 15% with repetitive nerve stimulation.
5. Single-fiber electromicrography (EMG) shows increased "jitter."
   Single-fiber EMG is a technically difficult test but can be diagnostically helpful in mild or purely ocular cases.

SYNOPSIS

AChR autoantibodies target the nicotinic acetylcholine receptors on the muscle (post-synaptic) side of the NMJ and cause receptor blockade and destruction of AChR via complement-mediated and other autoimmune mechanisms. The net result is that the postsynaptic membrane becomes less responsive to ACh, especially if the nerve is stimulated repeatedly, which explains the worsening of weakness after exercise. Since nicotinic AChR is found in only in NMJ in skeletal muscles, but not in smooth muscles or glands, MG manifests with skeletal muscle weakness but not autonomic dysfunction. Predominant involvement of EOMs has been attributed to the presence of embryonic isoform of ACHRs in the EOMs that are particularly well-suited targets of AChR auto-antibodies. AChR-seronegative patients may harbor antibodies to other protein constituents of the AChR complex—MUSK and LRP4—and their disease may be clinically indistinguishable from AChR-seropositive MG.

   The similarity between MG and poisoning with curare—a plant toxin that blocks the ACh receptor that was long used by natives of South and Central America for hunting and warfare—suggested to Mary Walker and others the idea of treating MG patients with physostigmine, a cholinesterase inhibitor. This treatment produced dramatic yet short-lived improvement ("The miracle of St. Alfege's"; see https://www.jameslindlibrary.org/walker-mb-1934/. [free online resource]). A related compound, pyridostigmine (Mestinon), is still used symptomatically for MG alongside with disease-modifying immunomodulatory therapies and thymectomy.

FIGURES

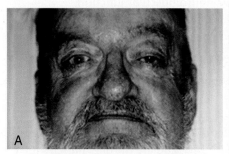 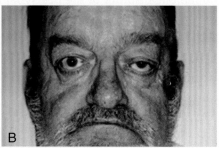

Ice pack test. Right-sided ptosis (left panel) in a patient with myasthenia gravis (MG) largely resolves after application of ice compress (right panel). (Reprinted with permission from Campbell WW. *Clinical Signs in Neurology: A Compendium*. Philadelphia, PA: Wolters Kluwer; 2015: Figure 1.1.)

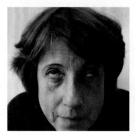 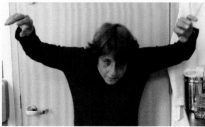 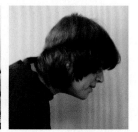

A patient with generalized myasthenia gravis (MG) exhibits bilateral ptosis and facial weakness (left), bilateral proximal arm weakness (middle), and head drop (right). (Reprinted with permission from Louis ED, Mayer SA, Rowland LP. *Merritt's Neurology*. 13th ed. Philadelphia, PA: Wolters Kluwer; 2016: Figure 89.2 B,C,D.)

QUESTIONS FOR SELF-STUDY

1. How would you test for extraocular muscle (EOM) fatigability at the bedside?
2. Respiratory failure, the dreaded complication of MG, was responsible for a 20% to 30% mortality rate in historic cohorts within 3 years of MG onset. What are the warning signs of impending respiratory crisis in MG? Which advances in the management of myasthenic crisis contributed to the decrease in mortality rate in MG to less than 5% in the contemporary cohorts?
3. What precautions must be given to every patient with MG regarding prescription medications, over-the-counter medications, supplements, and anesthesia?
4. What are the immunomodulatory therapies used for MG? What are their presumed mechanisms of action?
5. A mother with MG can pass AChR antibodies to the fetus via the placenta. What symptoms should be monitored for in the newborn of a mother with MG?

CHALLENGE

A 65-year-old man with MG experiences worsening muscle weakness despite a significant increase in pyridostigmine dose. He is admitted to an ICU in respiratory crisis. In addition to worsening MG, what is the other major diagnostic consideration to explain worsening muscle weakness in this patient? How does pupillary examination assist in differentiating between these two major possibilities? Why pupillary responses are not impaired in MG?

REFERENCES

Gilhus NE. Myasthenia gravis. *N Engl J Med.* 2017;376(13):e25.

Pevzner A, Schoser B, Peters K. Anti-LRP4 autoantibodies in AChR- and MuSK-antibody-negative myasthenia gravis. *J Neurol.* 2012;259(3):427-435.

Porter JD, Baker RS. Muscles of a different 'color': the unusual properties of the extraocular muscles may predispose or protect them in neurogenic and myogenic disease. *Neurology.* 1996;46(1):30-37.

16 | Lambert-Eaton Myasthenic Syndrome

A paraneoplastic or autoimmune disorder of the presynaptic neuromuscular junction

CORE FEATURES

1. Fluctuating weakness.
   Muscle weakness typically begins in the legs and proceeds to the arms and then to the ocular and bulbar musculature.
2. Autonomic symptoms.
   The autonomic symptoms are of the kind seen in the anticholinergic syndrome: dry mouth, constipation, micturition difficulties, erectile dysfunction, and orthostatic hypotension.
3. Antibodies against voltage-gated calcium channel (VGCC).
   These autoantibodies are present in up to 95% of patients with LEMS.
4. Repetitive nerve stimulation shows an increase in the CMAPs.
   A brief increase in CMAP amplitude after exercise or after high-frequency repetitive stimulation is considered abnormal.
5. Small-cell lung cancer.
   In a small minority of patients, LEMS is associated with non–lung cancer or not associated with cancer.

SYNOPSIS

The autoantibodies in LEMS bind to VGCC on the presynaptic membranes and cross-link VGCC leading to the reduced entry of calcium during depolarization and decreased ACh release into the synapse. The decrement in ACh release from the motor and autonomic—especially parasympathetic—nerve endings explains skeletal muscle weakness and anticholinergic symptoms. Treatment with the potassium channel blocker, 3,4-diaminopyridine, ameliorates symptoms of LEMS, presumably by prolonging the action potentials at the NMJ terminal. Complex immunomodulatory and tumor therapies are best deferred to a specialist.

FIGURE

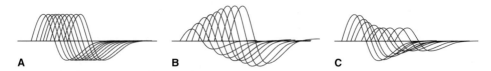

Repetitive nerve stimulation test does not cause any changes in the amplitude of compound muscle action potentials (CMAPs) in a normal person (A) but causes an incremental (increased) response in a patient with Lambert-Eaton myasthenic syndrome (B) and a decremental response in a patient with myasthenia gravis (C). (Reprinted with permission from Louis ED, Mayer SA, Rowland LP. *Merritt's Neurology*. 13th ed. Philadelphia, PA: Wolters Kluwer; 2016: Figures 6.5 and 5.8.)

QUESTIONS FOR SELF-STUDY

1. Contrast the typical pattern of muscle weakness in LEMS and MG.
2. Define "paraneoplastic syndrome." Could MG ever be considered a paraneoplastic syndrome?
3. What imaging studies are required for a previously healthy patient who develops LEMS?
4. 3,4-Diaminopyridine provides symptomatic relief in LEMS but has a dose-limiting side effect. Predict the side effect based on the drug's mechanism of action.
5. Explain why monotherapy with acetylcholinesterase inhibitors, such as pyridostigmine, works in MG but not in LEMS.

CHALLENGE

What are the Witebsky postulates for establishing the autoimmune nature of disease? Does LEMS satisfy Witebsky criteria for autoimmunity? (Compare your answer with Rose and Bona reference below.)

REFERENCES

Rose NR, Bona C. Defining criteria for autoimmune diseases (Witebsky's postulates revisited). *Immunol Today.* 1993;14(9):426-430. [free online resource]

Titulaer MJ, Lang B, Verschuuren JJ. Lambert-Eaton myasthenic syndrome: from clinical characteristics to therapeutic strategies. *Lancet Neurol.* 2011;10(12):1098-1107.

17 Botulism

Flaccid paralysis due to toxin produced by *Clostridium botulinum*

CORE FEATURES

1. Facial, extraocular, bulbar, and pharyngeal muscles affected first.
   Early symptoms are double vision, dysarthria, dysphagia, dysphonia, "expressionless face," eyelid ptosis, poor suck, weak cry.
2. Descending, symmetric flaccid paralysis may lead to neuromuscular respiratory failure.
   The tempo of illness is generally faster in botulism compared to Guillain-Barré syndrome (GBS).
3. Prominent autonomic symptoms.
   Anhidrosis, dry mouth, postural hypotension, urinary retention, and constipation are characteristic symptoms.
4. Pupils are large (mydriatic) and poorly reactive.
5. History of potential exposure to botulism toxin.
   Feeding infants possibly contaminated foods such as home-canned food or honey. Among adults, injection drug use is a risk factor for botulism.

SYNOPSIS

Botulinum toxins are among the most powerful toxins. They are lethal to humans in doses of 1/10,000 of a microgram. Botulinum toxins are produced by the ubiquitous *Clostridium botulinum (C. botulinum)*. *C. botulinum* spores are ingested by humans, but because they do not germinate in the gut, they are excreted without harm. Infants may be susceptible to botulism because their guts have not been as yet colonized with normal gut flora, thus allowing *C. botulinum* spores to germinate and release the toxin into the bloodstream. Adults almost never develop foodborne botulism, unless they have structural gut problems. Rather, contamination of wounds with botulin toxin or self-injection of botulism in "black tar" heroin is the more common mode of entry of *C. botulinum* in adults. When the diagnosis is suspected on clinical grounds, testing for *C. botulinum* or botulinum toxin in consumed food or body fluids may help confirm it, but the sensitivity and specificity of these tests are low.

Botulin toxins cause paralysis by breaking down soluble N-ethylmaleimide-sensitive factor attachment protein receptors (SNAREs) in the presynaptic terminal, thereby preventing vesicles containing ACh from fusing with the nerve membranes and releasing ACh into the neuromuscular cleft. Both muscle and autonomic fibers are affected, hence paralysis and autonomic symptoms are cardinal features of botulism. Botulinum toxin binding is irreversible, but because the nerve terminals regenerate, full or near-full recovery is achievable within weeks to months if the patient survives the acute phase of the illness. Supportive care has reduced mortality from botulism from 60% in the 1950s, to less than 5% today. Botulism-specific treatments for foodborne and infantile botulism are available and should be administered rapidly before irreversible binding of botulism is completed. Botulism is a public health emergency that must be immediately reported to local health authorities.

FIGURE

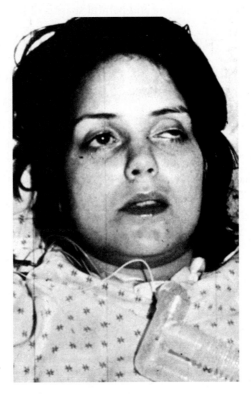

Young woman with botulism. Cranial nerve findings include bilateral ptosis (worse on the left), left exotropia and facial paresis. (Reprinted with permission from Fisher GR, Boyce TG, Correa AG. *Moffet's Pediatric Infectious Diseases: A Problem-Oriented Approach.* 5th ed. Philadelphia, PA: Wolters Kluwer; 2017: Figure 9.9.)

QUESTIONS FOR SELF-STUDY

1. Explain why pupils are large and poorly reactive in botulism but normal in size and reactivity in MG.
2. Patients with botulism may not exhibit typical signs of respiratory failure such as thrashing and agitation because of motor paralysis. What kind of monitoring should be implemented to avoid missing early signs of respiratory failure in patients with botulism?
3. Explain why botulism does not cause altered mental status (unless patient develops hypoxia).
4. In addition to supportive care, botulism-specific treatment is available in infantile botulism that cuts in half the duration of hospital stay. What is the treatment and what is its mechanism of action?

5. Another *Clostridium* species that produces a notoriously powerful neurotoxin is *Clostridium tetani*. Tetanus is very rare in countries with effective vaccination programs but causes thousands of deaths in countries where vaccination programs are suboptimal. The tetanus toxin interferes with neurotransmission by cleaving membrane proteins involved in neuroexocytosis. Compare the site of action of tetanus and botulin toxins, and explain how these differences account for different symptomatology: increased muscle tone and painful spasms of tetanus versus the flaccid paralysis of botulism.

CHALLENGE

Repetitive nerve stimulation elicits a larger CMAP in botulism and a smaller CMAP in MG. Explain why.

REFERENCES

Rao AK, Lin NH, Griese SE, Chatham-Stephens K, Badell ML, Sobel J. Clinical criteria to trigger suspicion for botulism: an evidence-based tool to facilitate timely recognition of suspected cases during sporadic events and outbreaks. *Clin Infect Dis.* 2017;66(suppl_1):S38-S42. [free online resource]

Rosow LK, Strober JB. Infant botulism: review and clinical update. *Pediatr Neurol.* 2015;52(5):487-492.

https://www.cdc.gov/botulism/health-professional.html. [free online resource]

Disorders of the Skeletal Muscle

A Very Brief Introduction to Disorders of the Skeletal Muscle

> If, as we have shown, animal electricity produces muscular contractions once set in action by external artifices, it is a requirement of reason that it should produce them also when induced to action also by internal and natural causes; the contractions are indeed the same in both cases for what concerns their essence, and differ only in degree and force.
>
> **Luigi Galvani[*]**

The essential function of skeletal muscles is to contract. Muscle contraction is accomplished by myofibrils—long chains of myosin, actin, and other proteins. When myofibrils are "turned on," myosin slides on actin, reducing the length of the myofibers and causing the muscle to contract. Myofibrils are packed within multinucleated muscle cells—"muscle fibers"—that could span the entire length of the muscles. Each muscle fiber is covered by a thin layer of reticular fibers called the endomysium. A group of muscle fibers forms a muscle fascicle which is covered with the perimysium. Muscle fascicles come together to form a muscle bundle covered by the epimysium, which is contiguous with tendons. The relationship between myofibrils, muscle fibers, muscle fascicles, and muscles is illustrated in the schematic below.

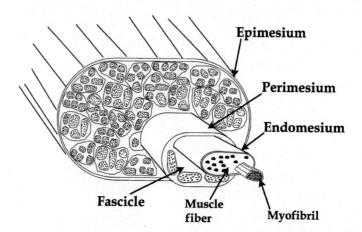

A schematic shows the relation between myofibril, muscle fiber (myofiber), muscle fascicle, and muscle. (Reprinted with permission from Chila A. American Osteopathic Association. Foundations of Osteopathic Medicine. 3rd ed. Philadelphia, PA: Wolters Kluwer Health/Lippincott Williams & Wilkins; 2010: Figure 8.11.)

---

[*]Luigi Galvani (1737-1798), an Italian physician-scientist, discovered that muscle contraction is the result of an electrical discharge. The debate between Galvani and Alessandro Volta on the origin of electric discharge culminated in the latter's discovery of a battery. Galvani holds a rare distinction of having his name turned into a verb, an appropriate homage to the man who galvanized the study of electromagnetism. (Citation is from Piccolino M. Luigi Galvani's path to animal electricity. C R Biol. 2006;329(5-6):303-318.)

Each motor neuron, located in the anterior horn of the spinal cord, innervates a variable number of muscle cells. The motor neuron and the muscle fibers it innervates are called the "motor unit." All muscle fibers within the motor unit are of the same metabolic type. There are two basic metabolic muscle fiber types. Type 1, or "slow-

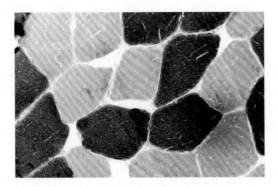

Intermixture of type I (pale) and type II (dark) muscle fibers on ATPase stain in normal skeletal muscle. (Reprinted with permission from Rubin R, Strayer DS. *Rubin's Pathology: Clinicopathologic Foundations of Medicine*. 5th ed. Philadelphia, PA: Wolters Kluwer Health/Lippincott Williams & Wilkins; 2008: Figure 27.21)

twitch," muscle fibers rely mainly on oxidative mechanisms for energy production and are used mainly in slow and steady contraction. Type 2, or "fast-twitch," muscle fibers rely mainly on glycolysis for energy production and are used mainly fast and explosive muscle contraction. Each muscle fiber type can be easily determined with ATPase stains. In a normal muscle, there is a patchwork of type 1 and type 2 muscle fibers as shown below:

In diseases of the motor neurons and nerves—when the motor neurons or axons degenerate—the neighboring motor neurons take over and "convert" the newly acquired muscle fibers into their metabolic type. As a result, instead of the usual patchwork of type 1 and 2 muscle fibers, one finds groupings of fibers of a single type. This "fiber grouping" is a hallmark of neurogenic diseases and is not found in myopathies. Myopathies, on other hand, often affect predominantly either type 1 or type 2 muscle fibers. For example, steroid-induced myopathy or chronic alcoholic myopathy (Chapter 23) is predominantly type 2 myopathy. In addition to ATPase, a variety of other diagnostic muscle stains are available. These stains can be used to quantitate a specific protein constituent of muscle fibers (dystrophin stain for muscular dystrophies), to identify mitochondrial abnormalities (toxic myopathies), to determine glycogen and lipid content (may be decreased or increased in metabolic myopathies), and to characterize inflammatory reaction (polymyositis and dermatomyositis).

REFERENCE

Joyce NC, Oskarsson B, Jin L-W. Muscle biopsy evaluation in neuromuscular disorders. *Phys Med Rehabil Clin N Am.* 2012;23(3):609-631. [free online resource]

18 Duchenne Muscular Dystrophy

Childhood-onset, progressive proximal myopathy due to a mutation in the dystrophin gene (X-linked).

CORE FEATURES

1. Progressive, proximal ("limb-girdle") myopathy with onset before the age of 5 years. Duchenne muscular dystrophy (DMD) should be suspected in a previously ambulatory child who is exhibiting delays in reaching motor milestones. Toe walking and waddling gait are characteristic. Progression is relentless, and by adolescence, patients are wheelchair-bound.
2. Calf pseudohypertrophy
   Calves appear hypertrophic due to the deposition of fat and connective tissue in the calf muscles.
3. Progressive dilated cardiomyopathy
   Develops in childhood, and regular cardiac screening is recommended. Heart failure is the main reason why the average lifespan of patients is only 25 years.
4. Serum creatine kinase (CK) is elevated more than 10-fold
5. Mutation in the dystrophin gene
   DMD is usually the result of an "out-of-frame" mutation, which leads to very little functional dystrophin. Genetic testing has replaced muscle biopsy as the gold standard for diagnosis.

SYNOPSIS

The dystrophinopathies are caused by mutations in the very large *DMD* gene located on the X-chromosome. Dystrophin, the product of *DMD* gene, is part of a large complex that connects the cytoskeleton within the muscle fiber to the extracellular matrix. DMD is the most severe on the spectrum of dystrophinopathies that includes Becker muscular dystrophy (onset at 6 years of age, ambulatory in adolescence, near-normal lifespan); isolated quadriceps myopathy; asymptomatic hyper-CKemia; young-onset dilated cardiomyopathy; and intellectual disability (dystrophin is found in the brain as well as muscle, and patient with DMD usually have some degree of intellectual impairment). Pathologically, DMD is characterized by loss of dystrophin in the muscle on dystrophin stain, necrosis, endomysial fibrosis, and inflammation. Chronic administrations of corticosteroids slow down disease progression.

FIGURES

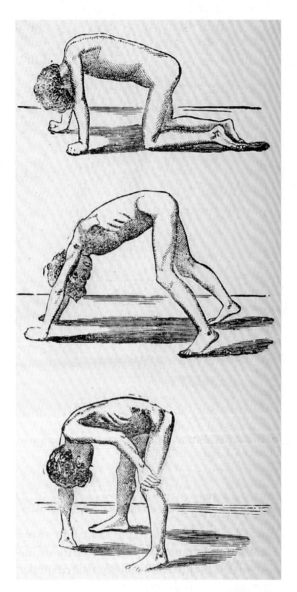

Gowers sign shows typical pattern of rising from floor in a child with proximal leg weakness. (From Gowers WR. *A Manual of Diseases of the Nervous System*. London: Churchill; 1886.)

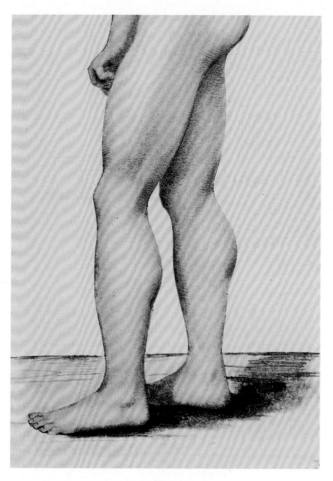

Pseudohypertrophy of the calves. (From Koplik H. *The Diseases of Infancy and Childhood*. 4th ed. Philadelphia, PA: Lea & Febiger; 1918.)

QUESTIONS FOR SELF-STUDY

1. What is an "in-frame" and an "out-of-frame" mutation? Are dystrophinopathies more clinically severe with "in-frame" or with "out-of-frame" mutations? Why?
2. Up to 40% of female carriers of the DMD mutation may experience skeletal and cardiac muscle compromise. What is the presumed mechanism of weakness in women who have one functional copy of dystrophin?
3. What are the risks of DMD to a male and female child if the mother is a carrier of the mutation? What are the risks of DMD to a male and female child if the father carries the mutation?
4. Healthy parents have two sons with genetically proven DMD. Yet, maternal leukocyte testing is negative for DMD mutation. What genetic phenomenon could explain this clinical scenario? Is there a risk of DMD to subsequent male children?

5. A child presents with delayed motor milestones and a progressive proximal myopathy. DMD is suspected on clinical grounds, but muscle biopsy shows a normal pattern of dystrophin staining. What other genetic mutations involving the same membrane-associated protein complex as dystrophin may result in a clinical picture similar to DMD?

CHALLENGE

Understanding the genetic mechanisms of diseases guides rational drug development that is targeted to the specific mutation. Devise a drug that may be effective if DMD is due to nonsense "stop" mutation. Devise a drug that could be effective if DMD is due to mutation in an exon that leads to a "wrong start" of RNA transcription of dystrophin. (Compare your responses to the mechanisms of action of two drugs conditionally approved for DMD—eteplirsen and ataluren.)

REFERENCES

Darras BT, Urion DK, Ghosh PS, et al. Dystrophinopathies. In: Adam MP, Ardinger HH, Pagon RA, et al, eds. *GeneReviews® [Internet].* Seattle, WA: University of Washington; 2000:1993-2018. [updated April 26, 2018]. [free online resource]

Wicklund MP. The muscular dystrophies. *Continuum (Minneap Minn).* 2013;19(6, Muscle Disease):1535-1570.

An autosomal-dominant, multisystem disorder that causes a progressive distal myopathy in adults.

CORE FEATURES

1. Distal more than proximal muscle weakness
   Foot drop and dexterity problems occur early in the course of the disease.
2. Elongated ("Hatchet") face
   Facial weakness with bilateral eyelid ptosis, temporalis muscle atrophy, and premature frontal baldness.
3. Myotonia—impaired ability to relax the muscles
   Myotonia usually precedes overt muscle weakness.
4. Early cataracts
   Posterior subcapsular cataracts develop in the second or third decades of life.
5. Family history of muscle weakness and myotonia
   Even clinically asymptomatic parent who carries the mutant gene will often exhibit myotonia on examination.

SYNOPSIS

DM1, the most common inherited muscle disorder in adults, is due to a pathologic number of GTC repeats in the *DMPK* gene. As most trinucleotide repeat disorders, DM1 is inherited in an autosomal dominant pattern and exhibits the phenomenon of anticipation—children have more repeats than their parents and more severe disease course. The *DMPK* gene mutation leads to missplicing of mRNA and cellular toxicity in skeletal muscles, heart, muscle, brain, eyes, gastrointestinal, and endocrine organs. Hence, DM1 is a multisystem disorder. In muscles, the transcribed mutant *DMPK* mRNA causes the missplicing of the chloride channels resulting in myotonia. The weakness of facial and levator palpebrae muscles leads to the characteristic elongated facial appearance. Patients with clinical features of DM1, but negative genetic testing, should be tested for myotonic dystrophy type 2 - proximal myotonic myopathy (PROMM), a clinically similar disorder with milder symptomatology that is due to pathogenic repeats in *CNBP* gene.

FIGURE

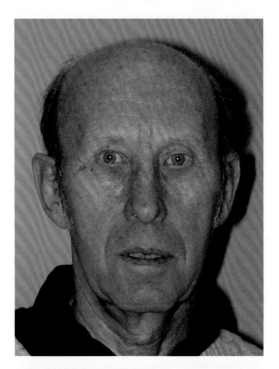

Long and narrow face, receding hairline, and wasting temporalis muscles are the typical features of myotonic dystrophy type 1 (DM1). (Reprinted by permission from Springer: Schaaf CP, Zschocke J. Mutations and genetic variability. In: Schaaf CP, Zschocke J, eds. *Basic Knowledge of Human Genetics*. 2nd ed. Dordrecht: Springer Berlin Heidelberg; 2013:31-50:Figure 3-7. Copyright © 2013 Springer-Verlag Berlin Heidelberg.)

QUESTIONS FOR SELF-STUDY

1. What questions would you ask patients to elicit a history of myotonia? (Compare your answers with Trivedi et al, referenced below.)
2. How would you test for action and percussion myotonia?
3. What is the risk of disease transmission to male and female children if one parent is affected with DM1? What is the expected disease severity if the mother or father carries the mutation? What strategies at the preconception stage can prevent passing on the mutation to offspring?
4. DM1 also causes myotonia of smooth muscles in the GI tract, gallbladder, and uterus. What are the clinical consequences of myotonia involving these organs?
5. DM1 is currently incurable, but correct diagnosis is essential because many complications can be prevented. For each of the major organ systems, list the main complication associated with DM1 and strategies available to minimize the risk to the patients: Compare your answers with Bird et al. reference below.

Organ System	Main Complication	Recommended Testing	Strategies to Prevent Complication
Cardiac			
Pulmonary			
Endocrine			
Ophthalmic			
Gastrointestinal			

CHALLENGE

A 20-year-old otherwise healthy man complains of painless "muscle stiffness" of face and arms whenever he is out in the cold. His father has similar symptoms. On examination, he has grip and eye closure myotonia, but no weakness. Electromyograph (EMG) shows spontaneous, waxing and waning discharges of muscle fibers, whose duration increases with cold exposure. What rare group of disorders should to be considered? What is the underlying genetic defect?

REFERENCES

Bird TD. Myotonic dystrophy type 1. In: Adam MP, Ardinger HH, Pagon RA, et al, eds. *GeneReviews® [Internet]*. Seattle, WA: University of Washington; 1999:1993-2018. [free online resource]

Trivedi JR, Bundy B, Statland J, et al. Non-dystrophic myotonia: prospective study of objective and patient reported outcomes. *Brain*. 2013;136(pt 7):2189-2200.

Turner C, Hilton-Jones D. Myotonic dystrophy: diagnosis, management and new therapies. *Curr Opin Neurol*. 2014;27(5):599-606.

20 Polymyositis and dermatomyositis

Immune-mediated, inflammatory myopathies.

CORE FEATURES

Polymyositis and dermatomyositis are autoimmune muscle disorders presenting with subacute (weeks-to-months) symmetric proximal muscle weakness and marked CK elevation in serum (up to ×50 of the upper limit of normal). The main features that assist in differentiating these two disorders are shown in the table below:

	Polymyositis	Dermatomyositis
1. Skin manifestations	None	"Heliotrope rash," nail-fold dilated capillaries, Gottron papules, photosensitivity rash
2. Myositis-specific autoantibodies	Rare	Common (anti-Jo1, Mi-2 MDA-5, TIF-1, NXP-2, others)
3. Association with underlying malignancy	None	Risk of cancer ~30%
4. Association with interstitial lung disease	Rare	Common
5. Muscle biopsy	No vasculopathy or immune complex deposition; inflammatory infiltrate in endomysial region; mostly CD8 T-cells	Complement-mediated micro-angiopathy; inflammatory infiltrate in perimysial region; mostly CD4 cells

SYNOPSIS

Traditional differentiation of inflammatory myopathies into polymyositis and dermatomyositis is evolving into a classification based on autoantibodies, which correlate with cutaneous and lung manifestations, cancer risk, and histological differences on muscle biopsy. Histidyl-tRNA synthetase (Jo-1) and other aminoacyl-tRNA synthetases are markers for the "antisynthetase syndrome": myositis, interstitial lung disease, mechanic's hands, arthritis, and Raynaud phenomenon. "Overlap syndrome" refers to an inflammatory myopathy in the context of systemic connective tissue diseases, such as systemic sclerosis, systemic lupus erythematosus (SLE), or rheumatoid arthritis (RA). "Immune-mediated necrotizing myopathy," previously subsumed under polymyositis, is now considered a stand-alone entity associated with signal recognition particle (SRP) or 3-hydroxy-3-methylglutaryl coenzyme A (HMG-CoA) reductase autoantibodies and necrotic muscle pathology. Future modifications to the classifications of inflammatory myopathies are to be expected.

Overdiagnosis of inflammatory myopathies is a common problem. It is essential to consider and rule out alternative explanations for progressive muscle weakness in adults—inclusion body myositis; toxic and endocrine causes; adult-onset muscular dystrophies; metabolic or mitochondrial myopathies—before embarking on long-term therapy with steroids, immunosuppressants, and biologicals, which carry a significant risk of serious side effects.

FIGURES

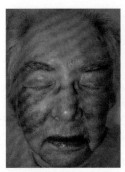 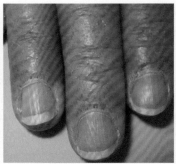 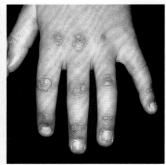

Classic dermatologic findings in dermatomyositis: heliotrope rash (left); nail-fold dilated capillary loops (middle); violaceous, flat-topped papules on the knuckles of the fingers (Gottron papules, right). (From Dr. Barankin Dermatology Collection.)

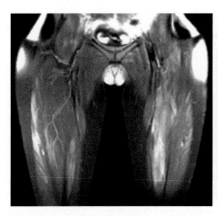 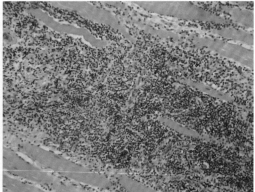

T1-weighted, fat-suppressed, contrast-enhanced MRI of pelvis and thighs of a 23-year-old woman with polymyositis shows enhancement (hyperintense signal) in several groups of thigh muscles. Muscle biopsy of another patient with polymyositis shows extensive mononuclear inflammatory cells chiefly infiltrating the endomysium. (A, Reprinted with permission from Greenspan A, Gershwin ME. *Imaging in Rheumatology: A Clinical Approach.* Philadelphia, PA: Wolters Kluwer; 2017:Figure 8.16c. B, Reprinted with permission from Rubin E, Reisner HM. *Essentials of Rubin's Pathology.* 6th ed. Philadelphia, PA: Wolters Kluwer Health/Lippincott Williams & Wilkins; 2013: Figure 27.10.)

QUESTIONS FOR SELF-STUDY

1. What activities of daily living are most commonly affected in patients with proximal myopathies? What questions would you ask to elicit symptoms of proximal muscle weakness?
2. How would you differentiate muscle weakness due to a myopathy from nonneurologic weakness? What is "break-away" or collapsing weakness?
3. What is the practical importance of differentiating DM from PM since both conditions are typically treated with steroids?

4. A 50-year-old patient with muscle biopsy-proven inflammatory myopathy experiences clinical worsening after a period of improvement on oral corticosteroids. What reversible myopathy should be considered in this context?

5. A 70-year-old man presents with slowly progressive proximal myopathy of approximately 1-year duration associated with elevated serum CK. He reports that ever since he was a teenager, he would always have muscle cramps at the start of exercise, which would usually improve within a few minutes. What type of myopathy does this history suggest? What is the explanation for the resolution of muscle cramps after exercise?

CHALLENGE

Explain why elevations of aspartate aminotransferase (AST) and alanine aminotransferase (ALT) are observed among patients with myopathies, while elevation of glutamyltransferase (GGT) is not. Explain how to differentiate skeletal from cardiac muscle breakdown with a serum test.

REFERENCES

Dalakas MC. Inflammatory muscle diseases. *N Engl J Med.* 2015;372(18):1734-1747.
Mammen AL. Autoimmune myopathies. *Continuum (Minneap Minn).* 2016;22(6, Muscle and Neuromuscular Junction Disorders):1852-1870.
Mammen AL. Which nonautoimmune myopathies are most frequently misdiagnosed as myositis? *Curr Opin Rheumatol.* 2017;29(6):618-622. [free online resource]

21 Inclusion Body Myositis

Inflammatory, slowly progressive myopathy in older patients.

CORE FEATURES

1. Onset after 50 years of age
   The mean age of onset is around 60 years; the disease is more common in men.
2. Insidious onset and slow progression of muscle weakness
   The mean time from symptom onset to diagnosis is 5 years.
3. Early and asymmetric weakness in knee extension, foot extension (plantar flexion), and finger flexion
   This peculiar pattern is not observed in other myopathies.
4. Muscle biopsy shows inflammation and muscle degeneration
   Fulminant endomysial inflammation with lymphocytes around individual muscle fibers may suggest polymyositis, but degenerative changes—rimmed vacuoles, inclusion bodies, misfolded proteins, and mitochondrial changes—help differentiate inflammatory bowel disease (IBD) from polymyositis.
5. Myopathy is refractory to corticosteroids or immunosuppression

SYNOPSIS

Lack of response to corticosteroids and immunosuppression in patients with inclusion body myositis (IBM) is puzzling as inflammatory changes on muscle biopsy are even more extensive than in steroid-responsive inflammatory myositides. It is possible that an inflammation-independent myodegenerative process drives disease progression, or that current immunomodulatory approaches do not target relevant immunopathogenic pathways. Clinically, IBM differs from inflammatory myopathies by the slower course and peculiar and often asymmetric pattern of proximal and distal muscle involvement. IBM progresses slowly but inexorably and leads to loss of ambulation within 2 decades of onset. The weakness of facial muscles and swallowing problems due to cricopharyngeal muscle weakness occur in half of the patients.

FIGURE

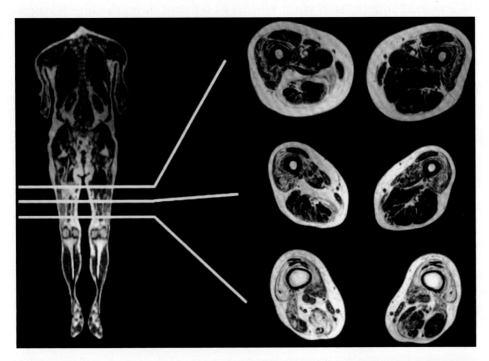

Whole body T1-weighted MRI of muscles with three axial cross-sections through the thigh (yellow lines) in a patient with IBM. Note the fatty replacement of muscles predominantly in the anterior thigh compartment, with a greater severity in the more distal part of muscles. (Reprinted with permission from Lilleker JB. Advances in the early diagnosis and therapy of inclusion body myositis. *Curr Opin Rheumatol.* 2018;30(6):644-649.)

QUESTIONS FOR SELF-STUDY

1. IBM is often misdiagnosed as polymyositis, but the two diseases usually have different patterns of weakness. Fill in the name of the disease that causes the respective pattern of weakness:
   Knee extension is weaker than hip flexion in _____.
   Finger flexion is stronger than shoulder abduction in _____.
2. Another neuromuscular condition with an asymmetric pattern of muscle weakness and atrophy in amyotrophic lateral sclerosis (ALS). What clinical features help differentiate ALS from IBM? What are the main electromyographic differences in these two disorders?
3. What common activities of daily living would be challenging for patients with IBM given the pattern of muscle weakness?
4. What supportive therapies should be recommended to patients with IBM?
5. What autoantibody is associated with IBM?

CHALLENGE

Test yourself as you go from a sitting to a standing position. Which are the main muscles activated during this task? Which muscles are activated during standing? (Compare your answer with Cuesta-Vargas et al. *Biomed Res Int.* 2013;2013:173148 and Joseph J. *Clin Orthop.* 1962;25:92-97. [free online resource]). Explain why patients with IBM may not be able to stand up from a chair but are able to stand unassisted.

REFERENCES

Greenberg SA. Inclusion body myositis. *Continuum (Minneap Minn).* 2016;22(6, Muscle and Neuromuscular Junction Disorders):1871-1888.

Naddaf E, Barohn RJ, Dimachkie MM. Inclusion body myositis: update on pathogenesis and treatment. *Neurotherapeutics.* 2018;15(4):995-1005. [free online resource]

22 | Toxic myopathies ◼▭

Myopathies resulting from external exposure, usually medication-induced.

CORE FEATURES

1. Temporal association between toxic exposure and onset of muscle weakness
   The onset of myopathy is typically within weeks of starting the offending agent.
2. Subacute course of proximal muscle weakness
   Acute muscle weakness is rare (some chemotherapy agents and snake envenomation).
3. Serum CK is elevated
4. Myalgias and muscle cramps are more common than with other myopathies
5. No further progression or improvement once the offending agent is removed

SYNOPSIS

Hundreds of substances have been implicated as causes of toxic myopathy. Alcohol is probably the most common and is discussed in the next chapter. Among commonly prescribed medications are corticosteroids, HMG-CoA reductase inhibitors (statins), colchicine, amiodarone, some antiretrovirals, vincristine, and hydroxychloroquine and others. The presumptive mechanisms of injury include direct myotoxicity, mitochondrial inhibition, interference with microtubule formation, loss of myosin, and inflammation. The mainstay of treatment is the discontinuation of the offending agent.

FIGURE

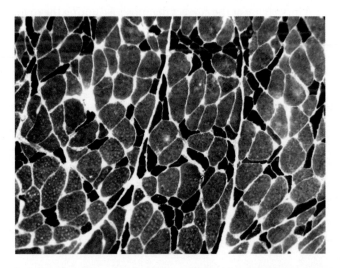

Profound atrophy of type 2 fibers (dark cells) in muscle biopsy from a patient with steroid myopathy (adenosine triphosphatase [ATPase] stain at pH 9.4). (Courtesy of Andrea M. Corse, MD. Mammen AL. Toxic myopathies. *Continuum (Minneap Minn).* 2013;19(6, Muscle Disease):1634-1649.)

QUESTIONS FOR SELF-STUDY

1. A 60-year-old man who was recently started on a statin presents to the ED with myalgias, diffuse muscle weakness, CK elevated to ×15,000 upper limit and dark "tea-colored" appearance of urine. Which very rare complication of statin therapy should you suspect? Explain why kidney failure is a concern in this clinical context. What are the essential steps of management to prevent kidney failure?

2. You are evaluating a 40-year-old man with a new-onset proximal muscle weakness. The patient reports considerable weight gain, especially in the truncal area, height loss, easy bruising, new-onset diabetes mellitus, and new-onset hypertension. Can you explain all these features with a single diagnosis?

3. A 60-year-old patient on dexamethasone for brain metastases presents with proximal leg weakness. You suspect steroid-induced myopathy. Serum CK and EMG/NCS studies are normal. Are these data consistent with the proposed diagnosis?

4. What is a plausible mechanism by which the antiretroviral agent azidothymidine (AZT) causes myopathy? What category of genetic disorders does this myopathy resemble clinically and histopathologically?

5. Rhabdomyolysis is characterized by acute onset of muscle necrosis typically in the context of drug exposure, crush injuries, strenuous physical exertion, prolonged immobilization, and infections. What conditions need to be considered in individuals with recurrent rhabdomyolysis triggered by exercise?

CHALLENGE

A 50-year-old woman started on a statin and develops myalgias, proximal muscle weakness, and serum CK elevation. Statin-induced myopathy is suspected and the statin is discontinued. However, muscle weakness continues to progress. What additional testing may be helpful in arriving at the correct diagnosis assuming the myopathy is related to statin use? (In this chapter, we highlight very rare complications of statin therapy. Statins are generally very safe and currently used by tens of millions of individuals.)

REFERENCES

Dalakas MC. Toxic and drug-induced myopathies. *J Neurol Neurosurg Psychiatry*. 2009;80(8):832-838.
Pasnoor M, Barohn RJ, Dimachkie MM. Toxic myopathies. *Neurol Clin*. 2014;32(3):647-670. [free online resource]

23 Chronic Alcoholic myopathy

Myopathy associated with long-standing and excessive alcohol consumption.

CORE FEATURES

1. History of chronic alcohol use disorder
   Consumption of more than 100 g of ethanol daily (seven 12-oz. cans of beer) for more than 3 years leads to chronic alcohol myopathy in the majority of patients.
2. Insidious progression of proximal muscle weakness
   Symptoms develop over many months.
3. Proximal more than distal muscle wasting
   Patients with alcohol use disorder may exhibit up to 30% of muscle mass loss, likely the result of myopathy being comorbid with neuropathy and malnutrition.
4. Painless
   There are no myalgias, muscle tenderness, or muscle cramping.
5. Atrophy of predominantly type II muscle fibers on muscle biopsy

SYNOPSIS

Alcohol use disorder is highly prevalent in the general population. Annual economic cost related to alcohol use in the United States is estimated to be over $250 billion, and roughly 1 in 10 deaths among working-age adults are related to excessive alcohol consumption. Numerous neurologic complications are associated with chronic alcohol use: cerebellar degeneration (approximately 25% of patient with chronic use); Wernicke-Korsakoff encephalopathy (10% of chronic users); alcoholic dementia; chronic alcoholic myopathy (50% of patients with alcohol use disorder), and sensorimotor axonal polyneuropathy effects (up to 90%). Alcoholic myopathy is likely due to the toxic effects of alcohol, malnutrition, and liver disease. The condition tends to progress with continued alcohol abuse, but some degree of recovery is possible if patients successfully refrain from alcohol. Acute alcoholic myopathy is a rarer form of myopathy and estimated to affect 1% of patients with alcohol use disorder. Acute alcoholic myopathy is almost the inverse of chronic alcoholic myopathy: its mode of onset is rapid; it usually follows a period of binge drinking; muscles are swollen and tender; serum CK is elevated; myoglobin is present in the urine; type 1 muscle fibers are affected; prognosis is generally favorable with rapid and complete recovery.

QUESTIONS FOR SELF-STUDY

1. Which features on neurologic examination would allow you to determine whether a patient suffers from alcoholic myopathy or alcoholic polyneuropathy?
2. Cardiomyopathy is another myopathic complication of alcohol use disorder. What clinical features help differentiate exercise intolerance due to cardiomyopathy from weakness due to skeletal myopathy?
3. What are the current guidelines for maximum daily alcohol consumption for men and nonpregnant women? (Compare your response with https://www.rethinkingdrinking.niaaa.nih.gov/How-much-is-too-much/Default.aspx. [free online resource])

4. Acute alcoholic myopathy is one of the more common causes of rhabdomyolysis. How would you diagnose rhabdomyolysis in a patient presenting with acute alcoholic myopathy?
5. Which electrolytes need to be monitored in a patient with acute alcoholic myopathy? Why?

CHALLENGE

Gait instability is common in patients with long-standing alcohol use disorder and may result from restrictive (anterosuperior vermis) alcoholic cerebellar degeneration, neuropathy, myopathy, or any combination of the above. What are the main features of cerebellar, neuropathic, and myopathic gait that may help you decide what areas of the nervous system is affected? (For an excellent video summary of basic gait patterns, see http://stanfordmedicine25.stanford.edu/the25/gait.html. [free online resource])

REFERENCES

De la Monte SM, Kril JJ. Human alcohol-related neuropathology. *Acta Neuropathol.* 2014;127(1):71-90.

Noble JM, Weimer LH. Neurologic complications of alcoholism. *Continuum (Minneap Minn).* 2014;20(3, Neurology of Systemic Disease):624-641.

Preedy VR, Adachi J, Ueno Y, et al. Alcoholic skeletal muscle myopathy: definitions, features, the contribution of neuropathy, impact and diagnosis. *Eur J Neurol.* 2001;8(6):677-687. [free online resource]

24 Hypothyroid myopathy

Myopathy associated with hypothyroidism.

CORE FEATURES

1. Slowly progressive, mild proximal myopathy
2. Muscle pain
   Myalgias, muscle cramps, and muscle stiffness associated with hypothyroidism may occur even in the absence of overt myopathy. Myoedema and "hung-up" muscle stretch reflexes are nonsensitive but suggestive findings for hypothyroidism.
3. Systemic symptoms and signs of hypothyroidism
   Weight gain, cold intolerance, somnolence, depression, bradycardia, constipation, and dry skin are common, but their absence does not exclude the diagnosis. Patients with otherwise unexplained myopathy and serum CK elevation warrant thyroid function studies.
4. Laboratory findings of hypothyroidism
   Elevated thyroid-stimulating hormone (TSH) levels, low free triiodothyronine/T3 and thyroxine/T4 levels.
5. Myopathy resolves with thyroid hormone replacement therapy

SYNOPSIS

Hypothyroidism induces global inhibition of the oxidative pathways and dysfunction of the respiratory chain in myocytes. This leads to the upregulation of the anaerobic metabolism (the breakdown of glycogen into pyruvate) and a decrease in intracellular pH. The clinical consequences of these metabolic changes are muscle cramping and fatigue following trivial exertion. Pathologic consequences include an increase in the number of mitochondria in myocytes and glycogen accumulation.

FIGURE

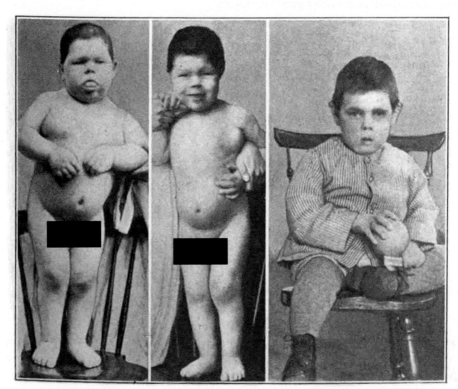

August 3, 1914.   August 17, 1914.   November 27, 1914.

FIG. 76.—Infantile myxedema. Ten years old. Treated by large doses of thyroid tablets. (A. Josefson.)

The historic figure shows the dramatic effect of thyroid therapy in untreated hypothyroidism ("cretinism"). Discovery of thyroid replacement therapy is one of the triumphs of modern medicine. (From Jelliffe SE, White WA. *Diseases of the Nervous System: A Text-Book of Neurology and Psychiatry*. 2nd ed. Philadelphia, PA: Lea & Febiger; 1917.)

QUESTIONS FOR SELF-STUDY

1. Define myoedema. How do you test for myoedema? Define "hung-up" reflex? What phase of the muscle stretch reflex would you look for to determine if a patient has "hung-up" reflex?
2. Hypothyroidism can involve the central nervous system (CNS) and the peripheral nervous system (PNS). Provide examples of hypothyroidism's effect on CNS and the PNS.
3. Provide a clinical scenario in which hypothyroidism can impair the NMJ function.
4. Myopathy is a common feature of hyperthyroidism as well as hypothyroidism. Describe the systemic and neurologic signs that point toward a diagnosis of hyperthyroidism.

5. A 40-year-old man with a history of hyperthyroidism presents to the ED with acute onset of generalized muscle weakness. While waiting for a hospital bed, the weakness self-resolves. He recalls a similar, but a milder, episode in prior weeks. What is the likely diagnosis?

CHALLENGE

Describe a clinical scenario when hypothyroid myopathy occurs in the setting of normal serum TSH levels.

REFERENCES

Katzberg HD, Kassardjian CD. Toxic and endocrine myopathies. *Continuum (Minneap Minn)*. 2016;22(6, Muscle and Neuromuscular Junction Disorders):1815-1828.

Sindoni A, Rodolico C, Pappalardo MA, Portaro S, Benvenga S. Hypothyroid myopathy: a peculiar clinical presentation of thyroid failure. Review of the literature. *Rev Endocr Metab Disord*. 2016;17(4):499-519. [free online resource]

Disorders of the Spinal Cord

A Very Brief Introduction to Disorders of the Spinal Cord

All the nerves manifestly arise from the spinal cord … and the spinal cord consists of the same substance as the brain from which it is derived.

Leonardo da Vinci*

The spinal cord lies within the vertebral canal where it is enveloped by the dura mater, the arachnoid mater, and the pia mater. About 45 cm in length and less than a thumb size in width, the spinal cord is the cable that connects the brain to the body.

The spinal cord is a highly organized anatomical structure. It can be conceptualized as a series of "slabs" of uneven width. Each "slab" corresponds to a spinal cord level connecting the spinal cord to the peripheral nerves via a pair of ventral (motor) roots and dorsal (sensory) nerve roots. Complete spinal cord transection results in paralysis of all muscles below the level of injury, loss of sensation to all modalities below the level of injury, and loss of bladder and bowel control.

---

*Leonardo da Vinci (1452-1519), the quintessential Renaissance man, made a number of highly original neurologic observations and neuroanatomical illustrations that remained unknown until publication of his notebooks 300 years after his death. Among his discoveries is the frog pithing experiment: "The frog instantly dies when the medulla of the spine is perforated; and previously it lived without head, without heart or internal (organs) intestines or skin. Here, therefore, appears to lay the foundation of movement and life." This discovery makes Leonardo the originator of the brain death concept, which only entered scientific consciousness in the second part of the 20th century. The citations are from Pevsner J. Leonardo da Vinci's contributions to neuroscience. Trends Neurosci. 2002;25(4):217-220.

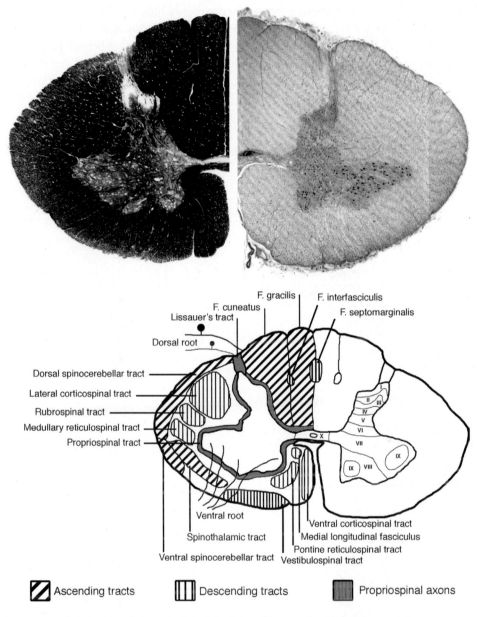

Upper panel, Left side of the spinal cord is stained for myelin (Luxol blue stain) and highlights the white matter (dark blue), while the right side is stained for neuronal cell bodies (Nissl stain) and highlights anterior horn motor neurons (pale blue). Lower panel, Schematic of spinal cord transection. The spinal cord is shown in anatomical convention (ventral surface is at the bottom). (Reprinted with permission from Schwartz ED, Flanders AE. *Spinal Trauma: Imaging, Diagnosis, and Management.* Philadelphia, PA: Wolters Kluwer Health/Lippincott Williams & Wilkins; 2007: Figure 1.4.)

The spinal cord is traditionally divided into 8 cervical levels (C1 nerve roots exit above C1 vertebra and C8 root exits below the C7 vertebra); 12 thoracic levels (thoracic nerve roots exit below the their respective thoracic vertebrae); 5 lumbar levels, whose nerve roots exit below the L1 to L5 vertebrae; 5 sacral levels, whose nerve roots exit below S1 to S5; and the vestigial coccygeal nerve root of little clinical significance. The spinal cord of an adult takes up only the upper two-thirds of the vertebral canal, ending at the L1/L2 vertebral levels. The figure below shows the relationship between the spinal cord level and nerve root level in an embryo when spinal cord level and spinal nerve root levels are still aligned, and in an adult, where the spinal cord level lies above the respective nerve root exit.

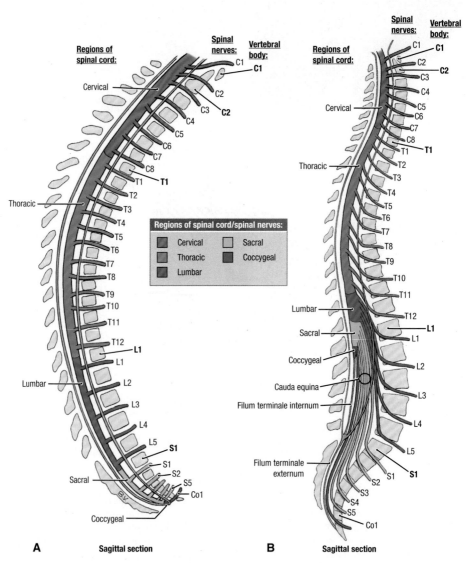

Relationship between the spinal cord level and the vertebral level (root exit) in an embryo (A) and an adult (B). Note that the vertebral canal is roughly same length as spinal cord in embryo but considerably longer than spinal cord in an adult. Cervical, thoracic, lumbar, and sacral segments are shown in red, blue, purple, and green, respectively. (Reprinted with permission from Agur AMR, Dalley AF. *Grant's Atlas of Anatomy*. 15th ed. Philadelphia, PA: Wolters Kluwer; 2020: Figure 1.46A-B.)

As C1 does not have a sensory nerve root, there are altogether 29 sensory nerve roots, which supply 29 distinct dermatomes. Muscles supplied by a single motor nerve root are referred to as myotomes. Although there are 30 motor nerve roots, there are only a handful of myotomes—those of the arms and legs—that can be tested clinically (see "Introduction to Innervation of Upper Extremities" and the "Introduction to Innervation of Lower Extremities").

When the spinal cord is examined in cross section, one can appreciate that the myelinated white matter is spread around the peripheral aspect of the spinal cord, while the butterfly-like gray matter lies at its center. Cell bodies of the motor neuron bodies lie within the ventral horns of gray matter. Second-order cell bodies of sensory neurons lie in the dorsal horns; the first-order sensory neuron cell bodies are in the dorsal root ganglia, just outside the spinal cord. Cell bodies of autonomic nerves are located within the intermediolateral spinal cord column extending from T1 to L3 for sympathetic nerves and from S2 to S4 for parasympathetic nerves.

The spinal cord white matter is organized into three funiculi or columns: anterior/ventral; lateral; and posterior/dorsal. These funiculi are traversed by multiple ascending and descending tracts. The anterior funiculus contains the descending uncrossed corticospinal tract. The lateral funiculus carries the lateral corticospinal tract, as well as the ascending spinothalamic sensory pathway for pain and temperature. The posterior (dorsal) funiculus contains ascending sensory pathways for position/proprioception/touch. Because the spinothalamic tract fibers cross shortly after their point of entry into the spinal cord, while the other major tracts cross at a lower medullary level, transection of the RIGHT half of the spinal cord will cause upper motor neuron paresis and impaired joint position/vibration sense on the RIGHT side of the body below the level of the transection, and loss of pain and temperature on the LEFT side of the body below the level transection. This constellation of findings defines the Brown-Séquard syndrome. Examples of other classic spinal cord syndromes will be discussed in the chapters that follow.

REFERENCES

Kirshblum SC, Burns SP, Biering-Sorensen F, et al. International standards for neurological classification of spinal cord injury (revised 2011). *J Spinal Cord Med.* 2011;34(6):535-546.

Nógrádi A, Vrbová G. *Anatomy and physiology of the spinal cord.* In: *Madame Curie Bioscience Database* [Internet]. Austin, TX: Landes Bioscience; 2000-2013. Available at https://www.ncbi.nlm.nih.gov/books/NBK6229/.

25 Amyotrophic Lateral Sclerosis

A progressive neurodegenerative disease of the upper and lower motor neurons

CORE FEATURES

1. Inexorably progressive quadriparesis.
   Muscle weakness typically starts in one limb ("flail hand" syndrome) and progresses to quadriparesis and respiratory failure.
2. Bulbar symptoms and signs.
   Amyotrophic lateral sclerosis (ALS) affects motor nuclei of cranial nerves leading to dysphagia, dysphonia, dysarthria, and facial diplegia. Bulbar-onset presentations portend a worse prognosis.
3. Diffuse fasciculations and atrophy.
   Fasciculations are irregular, fast, fine, spontaneous muscle twitches. Fasciculations are a sign of muscle denervation. They can be seen in any affected muscle—in the tongue, limbs, chest, and abdomen.
4. Pathologic hyperreflexia.
   A brisk gag reflex and a brisk jaw jerk imply bulbar involvement. A Babinski sign is usually present alongside limb hyperreflexia.
5. Electromyography (EMG) shows evidence of denervation at three or more different bulbar and spinal cord segments.
   Denervation is characterized by abnormally large polyphasic motor units, fibrillations, and fasciculations. Sensory nerve conduction studies are normal.

SYNOPSIS

ALS is a purely motor disease, like the myopathies and some of the neuromuscular junction (NMJ) disorders previously discussed. The most important distinguishing feature of ALS is that it affects both the upper motor neurons in the motor cortex as well as the lower motor neurons in the anterior horns of the spinal cord and in the brainstem. Lower motor neuron involvement manifests as muscle weakness with decreased muscle tone, hyporefexia or areflexia, muscle atrophy, and fasciculations. Upper motor neuron involvement manifests as weakness, increased muscle tone, and hyperreflexia. ALS affects both upper and lower motor neurons and therefore presents both lower and upper motor neuron signs—an unusual constellation. Rarely, ALS can present with only upper motor neurons findings (primary lateral sclerosis) or only lower motor neuron manifestations (progressive muscular atrophy). Progression of ALS is relentless with an estimated median survival of 30 months, though survival for longer than 10 years can occur.

FIGURE

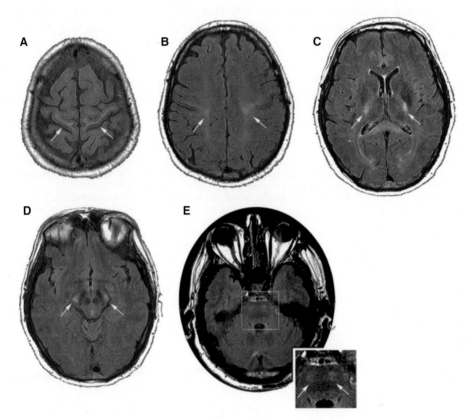

Axial brain FLAIR magnetic resonance imaging (MRI) in amyotrophic lateral sclerosis (ALS) shows symmetric hyperintensities in the precentral gyri (A), corona radiata (B), posterior limbs of the internal capsules (C), cerebral peduncles in the midbrain (D), and ventral pons (E) corresponding to the degenerating corticospinal tracts (white arrows). (Reprinted with permission from Kuo SH, Kwan JY. Teaching neuroImage: corticospinal tract. *Neurology*. 2008;71(6):e10.)

QUESTIONS FOR SELF-STUDY

1. Fasciculations are characteristic but not specific to ALS. In what other conditions can fasciculations be seen?
2. ALS patients may exhibit symptoms of pseudobulbar and bulbar palsies. What are the symptoms of pseudobulbar and bulbar palsies? How can you distinguish one from the other?
3. Explain the importance of testing the gag and jaw reflexes when trying to differentiate ALS from other causes of quadriparesis, such as upper cervical spinal cord injuries.
4. A 50-year-old man presents with upper motor neuron signs involving the legs and lower motor neuron signs involving the arms. What treatable disorder must be considered?

5. Like with many complex and disabling neurologic disorders, better outcomes are achieved in multidisciplinary patient care settings. Which interventions regarding swallowing, verbal communication, nutrition, and avoidance of early respiratory failure have been associated with prolonged survival among patients with ALS?

CHALLENGE

A 60-year-old man with ALS develops impulsivity, impaired judgment, and word-finding difficulties. What area of the nervous system is likely affected? What is the probable diagnosis?

REFERENCES

Kinsley L, Siddique T. Amyotrophic lateral sclerosis overview. In: Adam MP, Ardinger HH, Pagon RA, et al, eds. *GeneReviews*® [Internet]. Seattle, WA: University of Washington, Seattle; 2001. Available at https://www.ncbi.nlm.nih.gov/books/NBK1450/. [Updated February 12, 2015]. [free online resource]

Kiernan MC, Vucic S, Cheah BC, et al. Amyotrophic lateral sclerosis. *Lancet*. 2011;377(9769):942-955.

26 Vitamin B12 Deficiency (Subacute Combined degeneration) ▰

Vitamin B12 deficiency leads to demyelination and axonal loss in the peripheral and central nervous system

CORE FEATURES

1. Painful acral paresthesias are early symptoms.
   Paresthesias (tingling) typically start symmetrically in the hands and then spread to the feet.
2. Spastic-ataxic gait.
   This type of gait disorder results from demyelination of the dorsal columns (impaired vibration and position sense) and lateral corticospinal tracts (spasticity of the lower extremities).
3. Low serum B12 levels.
   Other hematologic abnormalities include megaloblastic anemia, hypersegmented neutrophils on peripheral smear, and high levels of homocysteine and methylmalonic acid in serum. The neurologic manifestations of B12 deficiency can occur in the absence of anemia and even with "low-normal" serum B12 levels.
4. MRI of the spinal cord may show abnormal linear T2-bright signal abnormalities in the dorsal columns and in the lateral columns.
   MRI signal abnormalities may resolve after B12 supplementation.
5. Nerve conduction studies (NCS) are consistent with a sensory-motor axonopathy.

SYNOPSIS

Autoimmune B12 deficiency—pernicious anemia—results from the destruction of gastric parietal cells and loss of the intrinsic factor, which is required for B12 absorption. Vitamin B12 is necessary for the production of long-chain fatty acids and DNA synthesis. Deficiency of vitamin B12 manifests as demyelination of large myelinated tracts (myelopathy), peripheral nerves (neuropathy), and bone marrow suppression (megaloblastic anemia). Pathological studies demonstrate early myelin degeneration involving the dorsal aspect of the cervical and upper thoracic segments of the cord; with the subsequent compromise of the lateral and anterior funiculi. Pernicious anemia was a fatal disorder until the landmark discovery that liver extract reverses this condition (see G. Minot's Nobel Prize acceptance speech referenced below). B12 deficiency is a treatable condition and, as such, must always be considered in the differential diagnosis of patients with subacute onset myelopathy, neuropathy, and cognitive decline. Treatment with B12 supplementation arrests disease progression and may reverse symptoms.

FIGURES

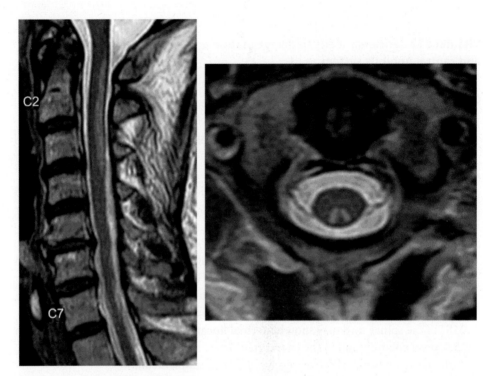

Sagittal T2-weighted magnetic resonance (MR) image of the cervical spinal cord in B12 deficiency shows hyperintense signal in the dorsal aspect of the cord from C1 to C4. Axial T2 shows abnormal signal in posterior columns of the cord. (Reprinted with permission from Kumar A, Singh AK. Teaching neuroimage: inverted V sign in subacute combined degeneration of spinal cord. *Neurology*. 2009;72(1):e4.)

QUESTIONS FOR SELF-STUDY

1. Neurologic examination of a patient with B12 deficiency may show the presence of a Babinski sign and depressed or absent ankle reflexes. How could you explain this combination of upper and lower motor neuron signs?
2. What is the neuroanatomic basis for the selective loss of vibration and position sense with relative preservation of pain and temperature sensation in patients with B12 deficiency?
3. In addition to symptoms attributable to the spinal cord and peripheral nerves, what neuropsychiatric manifestations should be further inquired when evaluating patients with B12 deficiency?
4. Which foods are high in vitamin B12? Which popular diet is associated with B12 deficiency?
5. A 40-year-old woman who underwent gastric bypass presents with megaloblastic anemia thought to be due to nutritional causes. Serum B12 level is in the low-normal range (215 pg/mg), and serum folate level is below the lower limit of normal. Supplementation with folate corrects the anemia, but the patient develops acral paresthesias and stiff gait. How do you explain this turn of events?

CHALLENGE

A 50-year-old man with a history of gastric bypass is noncompliant with vitamin supplementation. He presents with vibratory loss of the lower limbs and spastic ataxia. Serum B12 level is below the lower limit of normal. Despite intramuscular B12 injections, his condition continues to deteriorate. What other reversible nutritional deficiency must not be overlooked in this setting?

REFERENCES

Green R, Allen LH, Bjørke-Monsen AL, et al. Vitamin B12 deficiency. *Nat Rev Dis Primers.* 2017;3:17040.

Minot GR. *Nobel Lecture: The Development of Liver Therapy in Pernicious Anemia.* Nobelprize.org. Available at http://www.nobelprize.org/nobel_prizes/medicine/laureates/1934/minot-lecture.html. [free online resource]

Compression of the cervical spinal cord and nerve roots due to degenerative changes in the cervical spine

CORE FEATURES

1. Insidious onset of symptoms.
   The clinical course may be slowly progressive or stepwise with periods of stability. The myelopathy may not progress beyond the initial stages.
2. Spastic-ataxic gait pattern.
   Increased muscle tone in the legs and loss of vibration accounts for this distinctive gait pattern.
3. Impaired dexterity.
   Patients complain of numbness and clumsiness of hands.
4. Neck stiffness and pain.
   Patients may report neck pain or pain in the arms and/or shoulders. Lhermitte sign may be present. The range of motion in the neck may be decreased.
5. MRI of the cervical spine shows multilevel degenerative cervical spine disease and cord compression.
   Intrinsic cervical spinal cord signal abnormalities and "pancake enhancement" are sometimes seen at or above the level of compression.

SYNOPSIS

Degenerative spine changes represent "wear and tear" that comes with advancing age. Cervical spondylotic myelopathy is rarely seen among patients younger than 50 years. Spinal cord compression results from a combination of protrusion and ossification of cervical disks into the spinal canal, thickening of the ligamentum flavum and other ligaments, and a congenitally narrow spinal canal. Whether patients with cervical spondylotic myelopathy require decompression surgery is not always easy to determine. Degenerative changes and "soft" myelopathic signs (muscle stretch hyperreflexia) are commonly seen as part of aging and in most instances do not lead to overt disability. On the other hand, cervical spondylotic myelopathy may cause permanent neurologic deficits and place patients at risk for quadriparesis after falls or other accidents associated with neck hyperextension.

FIGURE

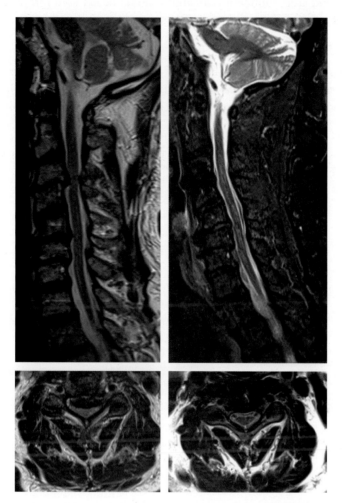

A 71-year-old man with cervical spondylosis and myelomalacia at the level of C3-C4 due to cord compression. The figure shows T2 sagittal and axial T2 view at the level of maximal compression before the surgery (left panel) and after cervical decompression (right panel).

QUESTIONS FOR SELF-STUDY

1. What is Lhermitte sign? Where does it localize the lesion to?
2. A patient with suspected cervical spondylotic myelopathy has normal pectoralis and biceps reflexes but exaggerated triceps reflexes. At what vertebral level would you expect to find the spinal cord compression on the MRI?
3. Abnormal gait in elderly individuals is seen in many conditions including normal-pressure hydrocephalus. Describe the differences in gait patterns in "frontal" and myelopathic disorders.
4. What are the congenital and acquired medical conditions associated with increased risk of compressive myelopathies?

5. In a patient with chronic myelopathy without spinal cord compression on MRI, what infectious and autoimmune myelopathies should be assessed for? Which ancillary tests may be necessary to evaluate for these conditions?

CHALLENGE

Cervical decompression is the treatment of choice in patients with worsening neurologic deficits secondary to cervical spondylotic myelopathy. Explain how intraoperative neurophysiological monitoring can forestall complications of cervical spine surgery.

REFERENCES

Young WF. Cervical spondylotic myelopathy: a common cause of spinal cord dysfunction in older persons. *Am Fam Physician.* 2000;62(5):1064-1070; 1073. [free online resource]

Zhovtis Ryerson L, Herbert J, Howard J, et al. Adult-onset spastic paraparesis: an approach to diagnostic work-up. *J Neurol Sci.* 2014;346(1-2):43-50.

28   Syringomyelia (Syrinx)

Expanding cavitation of the central aspect of the spinal cord; often associated with congenital cranial malformations

CORE FEATURES

1. Dissociated sensory loss in a "cape" or "hemicape" distribution.
   Loss of pain and temperature over the shoulders and arms with preservation of touch, joint position, and vibration sense is the hallmark of syringomyelia.
2. Slowly progressive, bilateral, usually asymmetric, loss of dexterity.
3. Atrophy of intrinsic hand muscles.
   Due to anterior expansion of the syrinx and loss of anterior horn motor neurons.
4. Asymmetric loss of muscle stretch reflexes in the upper extremities.
   Lower extremity reflexes may be exaggerated.
5. MRI of the spine shows central cavitation usually involving the cervical spinal cord.
   The signal within the cavity has similar characteristics to cerebrospinal fluid (CSF)- bright white on T2-weighted sequences, and dark on T1-weighted sequences.

SYNOPSIS

"Dissociated sensory loss"—the most characteristic feature of a syrinx—is the result of interruptions of the spinothalamic tracts from the arms as they cross within the central cervical cord. Patients may have painless burns and cuts on their hands. Ventral extension of the syrinx leads to loss of anterior horn motor neurons with subsequent atrophy of intrinsic hand muscles and loss of hand and finger dexterity. The dorsal columns are spared, so the vibration and joint position sense are preserved. Because a syrinx is a CSF-filled cavity, it has similar signal characteristics as CSF in all MRI sequences. Syringomyelia is associated with Chiari type I malformation, Klippel-Feil anomaly, or scoliosis. Less commonly, a syrinx may be the result of trauma, spinal cord neoplasm, and spinal arachnoiditis.

FIGURE

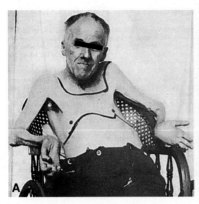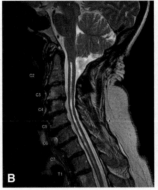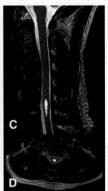

A, Cape distribution of sensory loss and atrophy of intrinsic hand muscles in a patient with long-standing syrinx. B, MRI of a 55-year-old woman with a syrinx status post decompressive suboccipital craniectomy shows residual syrinx from C2 to upper thoracic spine. Patient had residual hoarseness and spinothalamic pattern of dissociated sensory loss in upper extremities. C and D, Sagittal and axial views of a smaller syrinx in a different patient who did not undergo surgery. (A, Reprinted with permission from Cadwalader WB. *Diseases of the Spinal Cord.* Baltimore, MD: The Williams and Wilkins Company; 1932:103:Figure 49.)

QUESTIONS FOR SELF-STUDY

1. Explain why a syrinx can cause lower motor neuron signs in the hands and upper motor neuron signs in the legs.
2. A 30-year-old patient presents with dissociated sensory loss and intrinsic hand muscle atrophy. A syrinx is suspected. The neurologic examination also demonstrates nystagmus, loss of facial pain sensation, tongue atrophy, and dysphagia. What findings would you expect to find on the MRI of the brain?
3. What is Chiari type I and what is Chiari type II malformation?
4. What is a "Charcot joint"? What is the relevance of a Charcot joint to syringomyelia?
5. A 30-year-old woman presents with loss of dexterity and atrophy of her hands. The sensation is preserved and MRI of the cervical spine is reported as "normal." In addition to ALS, what other conditions should you consider in this clinical context? Explain how the flexion/extension MRI of the cervical spine may help clarify the diagnosis.

CHALLENGE

A syrinx extending to the upper thoracic spine may be associated with a Horner syndrome due to the involvement of the descending oculosympathetic pathway. Name some of the other neurologic findings in the cranium that are due to lesions below the level of the foramen magnum.

REFERENCES

Goetz LL, McAvoy SM. *Posttraumatic syringomyelia.* In: *StatPearls* [Internet]. Treasure Island, FL: StatPearls Publishing; 2019. Available at https://www.ncbi.nlm.nih.gov/books/NBK470405/. [free online resource]

Hidalgo JA, Dulebohn SC. *Arnold Chiari malformation.* In: *StatPearls* [Internet]. Treasure Island, FL: StatPearls Publishing; 2018. Available at https://www.ncbi.nlm.nih.gov/books/NBK431076/. [free online resource]

Acute Transverse Myelitis

Inflammatory spinal cord disorder

CORE FEATURES

1. Subacute clinical course.
   Acute transverse myelitis (ATM) takes several days to maximal symptoms followed by stabilization and slow but usually incomplete recovery. Progression of symptoms to nadir over less than 4 hours or more than 3 weeks should prompt a search for an alternative diagnosis.
2. Asymmetric ascending sensory loss.
   A sensory level is helpful to localize the lesion to the spinal cord, but is only present in about half of patients with ATM.
3. Bilateral asymmetric muscle weakness.
   Weakness usually starts in the legs and may involve the arms if the lesion is in the cervical spinal cord.
4. Bowel and bladder symptoms.
   Early urinary retention and constipation are common.
5. MRI of the spinal cord shows T2-hyperintense cord lesion that may expand the cord and may show enhancement on T1-contrast-enhanced sequences.
   The absence of a cord lesion at some point in the course of the disease should call into question the diagnosis of ATM.

SYNOPSIS

Inflammation of the spinal cord in ATM typically involves most of the cross section of the cord and, therefore, impairs the transmission along most of the major motor, sensory, and autonomic pathways. Evolution over the course of days is typical of inflammatory disorders. In contrast, a spinal cord infarction causes severe disability within minutes to hours, while progression over months to years favor toxic-metabolic-genetic causes, spondylotic myelopathy, or spinal cord vascular malformations such as a dural arteriovenous fistula (DAVFs). Inflammatory spinal cord disorders usually show CSF pleocytosis with elevated protein content, but this is not specific for ATM. Similarly, contrast enhancement on MRI, which signifies the breakdown of the blood-spinal cord barrier, while typical of inflammatory etiologies, can also be seen with other conditions and even in spinal cord compression.

FIGURE

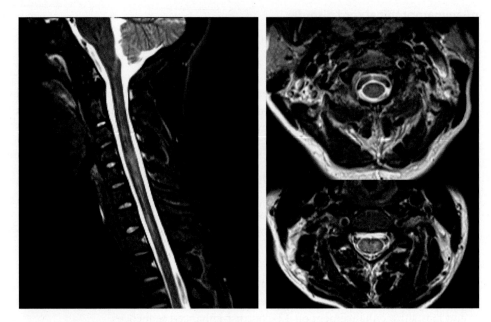

A 27-year-old woman who became paralyzed from the neck down within several hours. Magnetic resonance imaging (MRI) of the cord shows an extensive T2-hyperintense lesion involving most of the cervical cord with mild cord expansion at C3-4 level. She was diagnosed with acute transverse myelitis (ATM) and treated with IV methylprednisolone and plasmapheresis. She was eventually able to walk with a cane.

QUESTIONS FOR SELF-STUDY

1. Guillain-Barré syndrome (GBS) and ATM may present with ascending numbness. Define "thoracic sensory level" and explain why the findings of a sensory level help distinguish these two conditions.
2. What is the initial test for patients presenting with acute myelopathy? What causes must be urgently ruled out before proceeding with workup for possible ATM?
3. Name treatable infectious etiologies of infectious myelitis.
4. What is the standard treatment approach for autoimmune-mediated ATM?
5. ATM may be a monophasic disorder or the first manifestation of a relapsing-remitting disorder. Name the most important conditions associated with short-segment and with "longitudinally extensive" (>3 vertebral segments long) myelitis. What testing is necessary to stratify the patient's risk of disease recurrence?

CHALLENGE

Explain why the loss of temperature/pain sensation on one side of the body and decreased strength and proprioception on the contralateral side is not observed in peripheral nerve disorders such as GBS. Explain the neuroanatomic basis for these findings.

REFERENCES

Barreras P, Fitzgerald KC, Mealy MA, et al. Clinical biomarkers differentiate myelitis from vascular and other causes of myelopathy. *Neurology*. 2018;90(1):e12-e21.
Schmalstieg WF, Weinshenker BG. Approach to acute or subacute myelopathy. *Neurology*. 2010;75(18 suppl 1):S2-S8. [free online resource]

30 Conus Medullaris Syndrome and Cauda Equina Syndrome

Conus medullaris syndrome (CMS) results from injury to the caudal spinal cord (conus medullaris) and lumbosacral nerve roots. Cauda equina syndrome (CES) is the result of injury to the lumbosacral nerve roots within the spinal canal below the termination of the spinal cord (very rare, emergency).

CORE FEATURES

The conus medullaris and cauda equina are often affected by the same pathologic process, and clinical differentiation between the two syndromes is seldom clear-cut. For didactic purposes, the characteristic features of the two syndromes are juxtaposed in the table below.

	Conus Medullaris Syndrome	Cauda Equina Syndrome
1. Saddle anesthesia (sensory loss in the perianal and genital area)	Usually more symmetric distribution of sensory loss	Asymmetric sensory loss and dermatomal distribution more common
2. Muscle stretch reflexes	Patellar—often preserved Ankle—hypoactive	Patellar—hypoactive Ankle—hypoactive or lost
3. Loss of rectal tone and loss of "anal wink" reflex	Yes	Yes
4. Bladder/sexual dysfunction	Early urinary retention, overflow incontinence, erectile dysfunction	Usually not as prominent as in CMS
5. Back pain	Usually not as severe as in CES	Usually severe, with radicular pattern of radiation

SYNOPSIS

The conus medullaris refers to the caudal end of the spinal cord, opposite to the L1-L2 vertebral bodies in most adults. The conus medullaris is part of the central nervous system (CNS). The cauda equina refers to the lumbar and sacral spinal nerve roots in the spinal canal distal to the conus medullaris. The cauda equina is part of the peripheral nervous system (PNS). CMS and CES usually overlap. Findings of upper motor neuron signs point to the involvement of the conus medullaris. Low-back pain, saddle anesthesia pattern, and loss of rectal tone are the most consistently reported symptoms, while leg weakness is variable and may not be present. The causes of CMS and CES are highly diverse and include central disk herniations, lumbar spinal canal stenosis, spine trauma, spinal cord infarction, intramedullary tumors, granulomatous disease, arteriovenous malformations, hematomas, and infections of lumbosacral spinal nerve roots such as Elsberg syndrome, due to reactivation of HSV2 infection. CMS/CES due to compressive causes should be treated as neurosurgical emergencies.

FIGURE

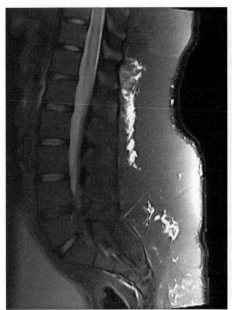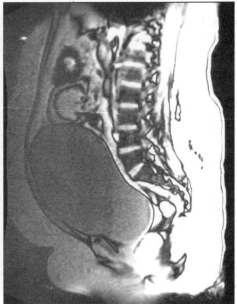

Diffusely abnormal T2-hyperintense signal in the lower thoracic cord and conus medullaris of an 18-year-old woman with myelin oligodendrocyte glycoprotein (MOG) antibody–associated meningoencephalitis (left panel). The patient had a very distended bladder due to urinary retention (right) and required catheterization.

QUESTIONS FOR SELF-STUDY

1. Mechanical low-back pain is highly prevalent in the general population and very rarely leads to any neurologic disability. Back pain of CMS/CES is an exception to this generalization. Describe the triad of symptoms—"red flags" of back pain—that suggest CMS/CES.
2. What is the initial test recommended in the evaluation of patients with acute CMS/CES?
3. Explain why the patellar reflexes are usually preserved when the conus medullaris is damaged, but absent when only the cauda equina is affected.
4. "Sacral sparing" is a positive prognostic feature in spinal cord injury. Name one motor, one sensory, and one reflex finding that attests to the patency of sacral nerve roots.
5. What are the treatable causes of CMS/CES?

CHALLENGE

What developmental pathology related to the failure of the neural tube to close should be considered in a young adolescent with progressive spastic paraparesis and bowel-bladder dysfunction?

REFERENCES

Brouwers E, van de Meent H, Curt A, et al. Definitions of traumatic conus medullaris and cauda equina syndrome: a systematic literature review. *Spinal Cord*. 2017;55(10):886-890.

Fraser S. Cauda equina syndrome: a literature review of its definition and clinical presentation. *Arch Phys Med Rehabil*. 2009;90:1964-1968. [free online resource]

Savoldi F. Kaufmann TJ, Flanagan EP, et al. Elsberg syndrome: a rarely recognized cause of cauda equina syndrome and lower thoracic myelitis. *Neurol Neuroimmunol Neuroinflamm*. 2017;4(4):e355.

Disorders of the Brainstem and Cranial Nerves

A Very Brief Introduction to Disorders of the Brainstem and the Cranial Nerves

An ass being tied and thrown, the superior maxillary branch of the fifth nerve was exposed. Touching this nerve gave acute pain. It was divided, but no change took place in the motion of the nostril… In the ass, where the [facial] nerve of the face had been cut, the most remarkable contrast was exhibited in the two sides of its face: for whilst the one side was in universal and powerful contraction, the other, where the nerve was divided, remained quite placid.

Charles Bell*

The brainstem begins at the cervico-medullary junction where the spinal cord ends. The brainstem is a more complex anatomical structure than the spinal cord, but the two share some anatomical features. Like the spinal cord—and unlike cerebrum and cerebellum—the brainstem contains the gray matter nuclei on the inside and the white matter on the outside. Like the spinal cord, the brainstem motor nuclei and pathways lie ventrally, and the sensory nuclei and sensory pathways—dorsally. The spinal cord connects to the peripheral nervous system (PNS) via pairs of motor and sensory nerve roots, while the brainstem outputs and inputs are mediated via pairs of cranial nerves that connect to multiple motor, sensory, and autonomic (parasympathetic) nuclei located throughout the brainstem. The brainstem also contains a number of structures involved in higher-order integration—the diffusely distributed reticular formation involved in sustaining awareness; the substantia nigra, which is part of basal ganglia network regulating movements; and the rostral interstitial nucleus of Cajal that controls conjugate vertical eye movements. The brainstem connects dorsally to the cerebellum, via the three pairs of cerebellar peduncles. Cerebellum is a major brain structure involved in motor planning, learning, and coordination.

A unique feature of brainstem anatomy is that nuclei of cranial nerves III to XII—with few exceptions—regulate ipsilateral cranial functions, while most of the long-tract pathways traversing the brainstem control contralateral half of the body. This neuroanatomic arrangement explains the unique "brainstem crossed syndromes," whereby a lesion involving the RIGHT side of the brainstem produces symptoms on the RIGHT side of the head and the LEFT half of the body. Crossed-syndromes will be discussed in the section on Vascular Disorders (Chapter 61). This section focuses on important syndromes involving cranial nerves and ocular motility.

---

*Charles Bell (1774-1842), a Scottish surgeon, anatomist, and anatomic illustrator, is best known for his work on the facial nerve and the eponymous Bell Palsy. The description of the experiments that distinguish between motor and sensory nerves of the face is taken from Bell's treatise "On the Nerves; Giving an Account of Some Experiments on Their Structure and Functions, Which Lead to a New Arrangement of the System." Bell's explanation on the distinction between motor and sensory functions is somewhat unclear, and this gave rise to a prolonged dispute on the priority of the discovery. (Bradley J. Matters of priority: Herbert Mayo, Charles Bell and discoveries in the nervous system. Med Hist. 2014;58(4):564-584.)

31 Bell Palsy

Facial nerve paralysis, possibly of viral etiology

CORE FEATURES

1. Acute onset of unilateral facial weakness.
   The nadir of facial muscle weakness is reached within days, followed by slow improvement over weeks.
2. Weakness involves both upper and lower facial muscles.
   Patients are unable to wrinkle the forehead, tightly close their eye, smile, or puff out the cheek on the affected side.
3. Sensation over the face is preserved.
   Patients may report unilateral muscle tightness or fullness, but objective sensory testing does not disclose any sensory deficits.
4. Loss of taste on the anterior two-thirds of the tongue ipsilateral to the weakness.
   The taste sensation is tested by asking the patient to protrude the tongue and applying a cotton tip dipped in sugar or saltwater to the sides of the tongue, and asking the patient to identify the taste.
5. Hyperacusis.
   The patient is sensitive to loud noises in the ipsilateral ear.

SYNOPSIS

The facial nerve (CN VII) has a complex anatomical course and contains multiple fiber types. Its functions are summed up in a ditty: "tears, tastes and salivates; moves the face, dampens sound waves" (adapted from Biller J, Gruener G, Brazis PW. *DeMyer's. The Neurologic Examination. A Programmed Text.* 7th ed. New York: McGraw-Hill Education; 2017:194-200). In peripheral facial nerve palsy, one observes not only ipsilateral facial muscle weakness but also hyperacusis (if the lesion is proximal to branch to the stapedius muscle), impaired taste in the anterior two-thirds of tongue (if the lesion is proximal to the chorda tympani branch), and absent tearing due to loss of parasympathetic input to the lacrimal gland. The presence of all of these symptoms allows one to precisely localize the lesion within the facial nerve between brainstem exit (as proximal to this point the facial nerve fascicles do not carry either taste or parasympathetic fibers) and the branch to chorda tympani (as distal to this point the facial nerve only carries motor fibers). Consistent with this prediction, MRI of the brain during the acute phase of Bell palsy discloses enhancement within the temporal bone portion of the facial nerve. (MRI of the brain is not required to confirm Bell palsy as the constellation of symptoms and signs reliably rules out brainstem pathology.) The facial sensation is not affected in Bell palsy as facial sensation is conveyed by the trigeminal nerve. The etiology of Bell palsy is presumed to be viral (herpes simplex virus type 1). Steroids modestly shorten symptoms, while the role of antivirals is less clear. Patients with Bell palsy are susceptible to corneal damage if they are not able to fully close the eye and have impaired tearing. Application of artificial tears during daytime and eye patch at nighttime help prevent this complication.

Several months after Bell palsy, patients may develop facial synkinesis. This phenomenon is a result of aberrant nerve regeneration wherein nerve twigs that normally supply a particular muscle or gland are rerouted to a different muscle group or gland during nerve regeneration. Clinical manifestations include eyelid narrowing when smiling, lifting of cheek when closing the eye, or tearing after salivation is stimulated (parasympathetic fibers that supply the salivary glands are rerouted to the lacrimal glands).

FIGURES

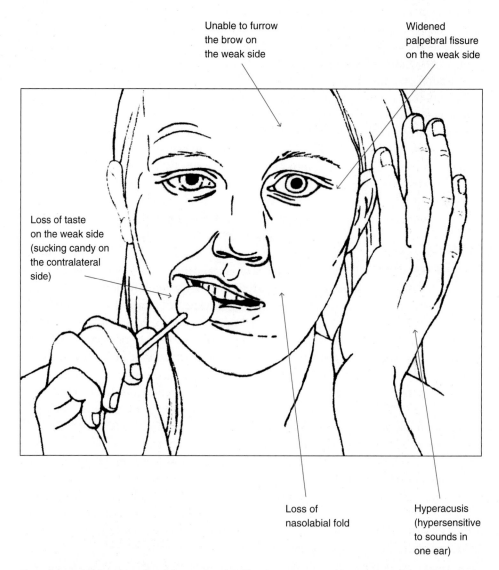

Unable to furrow the brow on the weak side

Widened palpebral fissure on the weak side

Loss of taste on the weak side (sucking candy on the contralateral side)

Loss of nasolabial fold

Hyperacusis (hypersensitive to sounds in one ear)

The schematic shows cardinal features of Bell palsy: upper and lower facial weakness (loss of furrows over left forehead and nasolabial fold flattening on the left side); hyperacusis (patient protecting left ear against loud sounds with her hand); loss of taste on the left side causes the patient to suck the candy on the right side.

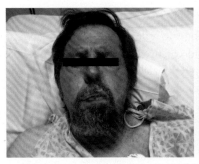 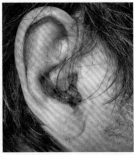

A patient with Ramsay Hunt syndrome presented with facial palsy. Left panel: facial asymmetry and inability to puff up his right cheek when trying to whistle. Right panel: pathognomonic herpetic vesicles in the external ear.

QUESTIONS FOR SELF-STUDY

1. Cerebral lesions cause lower more than upper facial muscle weakness: Frowning produces near-symmetric creasing of the forehead, while smiling causes the weak side to deviate to the unaffected side. In contrast, facial nerve palsy due to a peripheral or brainstem injury causes a similar degree of weakness in the upper and lower facial muscles. Explain why.

2. In evaluating a patient with acute onset of unilateral peripheral facial nerve palsy, you notice fluid-filled vesicles within the external ear canal. What symptoms in addition to facial palsy can be expected in this condition?

3. Match clinical findings with the probable location of the lesion causing unilateral facial weakness:

Symptoms	Location of Lesion
a. Facial weakness + abducens nerve palsy on the same side	Contralateral cerebral hemisphere
b. Facial weakness + weakness in arm and leg on the same side	Ipsilateral brainstem
c. Facial weakness + meningismus	Mastoid portion of the temporal bone
d. Facial weakness + decreased hearing on the same side	Subarachnoid space

4. Bilateral peripheral facial nerve paralysis is unusual. Name systemic conditions associated with bilateral facial nerve paralysis.

5. The great Persian physician, Abu Bakr Muhammad ibn Zakariya Razi (865-925 CE), popularly known as al Razi, provided a detailed description of facial palsy and commented that the "source of facial distortion is either spasm or paralysis, and these two can be differentiated by pain, as the paralytic type is without pain." (Sajadi MM, Sajadi MRM, Tabatabaie SM. The history of facial palsy and spasm: Hippocrates to Razi. *Neurology.* 2011;77(2):174-178.) In addition to pain, what other clinical features help differentiate (ipsilateral) facial palsy from (contralateral) hemifacial spasm?

CHALLENGE

Bell phenomenon (the palpebral oculogyric reflex) refers to a reflexive upward movement of the eye upon attempted eyelid closure. This phenomenon is easy to observe when eyelid closure is impaired during Bell palsy as shown in the figure above. Explain why Bell phenomenon with upward deviation is present in progressive supranuclear palsy even though voluntary upward eye movements are impaired.

REFERENCES

Gilden DH. Clinical practice. Bell's palsy. *N Engl J Med*. 2004;351(13):1323-1331.
Loomis C, Mullen MT. Differentiating facial weakness caused by Bell's palsy vs. acute stroke: can you tell the difference? *J Emerg Med Serv*. 2014;39:5. [free online resource]
Zandian A, Osiro S, Hudson R, et al. The neurologist's dilemma: a comprehensive clinical review of Bell's palsy, with emphasis on current management trends. *Med Sci Monit*. 2014;20:83-90. [free online resource]

32 Trigeminal Neuralgia (Tic Douloureux)

Paroxysmal pain in the distribution of the trigeminal nerve

CORE FEATURES

1. Paroxysms of unilateral pain in an area supplied by a division of the trigeminal nerve
   V2 division (maxillary) is the most commonly affected. Pain typically lasts a few seconds and is so severe as to cause the patient to interrupt their activities and grimace. Pain may be infrequent or recur up to hundreds of times daily.
2. Pain precipitated by touching "trigger points" in the trigeminal nerve distribution.
   Touching, kissing, chewing, tooth brushing, the wind blowing on the face, and even talking and smiling can trigger paroxysms of trigeminal neuralgia.
3. Neurologic examination is normal.
   There are no sensory or motor trigeminal nerve deficits.
4. No autonomic dysfunction (lacrimation, ptosis, nasal congestion) during the attack.
   This feature helps to distinguish trigeminal neuralgia from trigeminal autonomic cephalgias.
5. Pain is alleviated, and may be completely relieved, with antiseizure medications
   Sodium channel blockers such as carbamazepine, oxcarbazepine, and lamotrigine are used most commonly. Dose-limiting side effects may preclude full pain control.

SYNOPSIS

The trigeminal (Latin for "threefold") nerve conveys sensory information from the face, mouth, nose, nasal sinuses, and parts of the dura matter via ophthalmic (V1), maxillary (V2) and mandibular (V3) branches. These three branches come together at Gasserian ganglion that lies within a dural recess at the apex of the middle cranial fossa ("Meckel cave"). Gasserian ganglion to the trigeminal nerve is what dorsal root ganglion is to the peripheral nerve. Upon entering the pons, the sensory axons are relayed to the main nucleus (part of the dorsal column/medial lemniscus pathway) or the spinal nuclei of the trigeminal nerve, which are widely distributed throughout the lengths of the brainstem and upper cervical spinal cord. The trigeminal nerve also carries motor fibers from the motor nucleus of the trigeminal nerve in the pons to the muscles of mastication.

Classic trigeminal neuralgia is a result of compression of the trigeminal nerve by a vascular loop in the subarachnoid space. The loop can be visualized with a dedicated MRI, as shown in the figure below. The vascular compression is not sufficient to cause permanent sensory or motor deficits. If sensory deficit or impaired corneal or jaw reflexes are present, this suggests that the trigeminal neuralgia may be secondary to a demyelinating or neoplastic process. The pain of trigeminal neuralgia is of such severity as to cause involuntarily grimace, which explains the original French designation tic douloureux—a "painful tic." Because the pain often radiates to the jaw, patients not uncommonly undergo unnecessary dental procedures before the neurologic cause of pain is discovered.

FIGURE

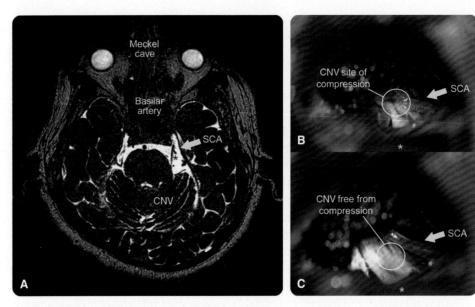

Trigeminal neuralgia due to aberrant vascular loop. A, MRI demonstrates compression of the left trigeminal nerve compression (red asterisk) by the superior cerebellar artery (SCA) (yellow arrow). B, Left retrosigmoid craniotomy with microsurgical dissection revealed the trigeminal nerve adherent to the left SCA (yellow arrow). C, The nerve was freed from the pulsating artery (yellow arrow). (Reprinted with permission from Bakhsheshian J, Goshtasbi K, Strickland BA, Pham MH. Teaching video neuroimages: Trigeminal neuralgia due to compression by the superior cerebellar artery. *Neurology.* 2017;89(24):e290.)

QUESTIONS FOR SELF-STUDY

1. A 35-year-old woman presents with trigeminal neuralgia. Examination shows ipsilateral facial hyperesthesia, optic nerve pallor, and diffuse muscle stretch hyperreflexia. What is the unifying diagnosis that may explain these findings?
2. A 60-year-old woman with trigeminal neuralgia is successfully treated with carbamazepine, but reports feeling "drunk"—drowsy, tremulous, unsteady on her feet. What is the likely explanation?
3. A 50-year-old man reports few-second paroxysms of severe pain in the ophthalmic (V1) distribution associated with ipsilateral tearing and eyelid ptosis. What is the likely diagnosis?
4. Varicella-zoster virus (VZV) can cause chronic pain in the trigeminal distribution (herpes zoster ophthalmicus). Explain why it is important to determine whether zoster vesicles are present on the external or internal surface of the tip of the nose ("Hutchinson sign").
5. A 20-year-old woman presents with hemifacial numbness to all modalities that extends up to her hairline and involves the external ear. Explain why these findings are not consistent with an neurologic etiology. What is the likely diagnosis?

CHALLENGE

A 40-year-old man reports paroxysmal pain involving the right posterior aspect of the mouth and ear triggered by yawning. Pain is severe and sometimes causes him to faint. What is the diagnosis? What is the likely mechanism of syncope?

REFERENCES

Cruccu G, Finnerup NB, Jensen TS, et al. Trigeminal neuralgia: new classification and diagnostic grading for practice and research. *Neurology*. 2016;87(2):220-228. [free online resource]

Pierce JMS. Glossopharyngeal neuralgia. *Eur Neurol*. 2006;55:49-52.

33 Third Nerve Palsy

Isolated third nerve palsy may be due to nerve compression, microvascular ischemia, or trauma

CORE FEATURES

1. Unilateral periorbital pain.
   Pain is almost invariably present in acute third nerve palsy, but slowly growing tumors may be painless.
2. Diplopia.
   Patients may complain of horizontal, vertical, or oblique binocular diplopia depending on which extraocular muscles are affected by the third nerve palsy.
3. Extraocular motility impaired.
   In complete third nerve palsy, the involved eye is "down and out" in the primary gaze. In partial third nerve palsy, there may be a limitation in elevation, ADduction, and depression of the affected eye.
4. Eyelid ptosis.
   Eyelid ptosis may be complete or incomplete.
5. Dilated pupil.
   A dilated pupil is a hallmark of a compressive etiology and may antecede diplopia and eyelid ptosis. When you see a "blown" pupil, think "blown" blood vessel (cerebral aneurysm). Urgent angiographic evaluation is mandatory: early treatment may prevent a catastrophic subarachnoid hemorrhage.

SYNOPSIS

The third cranial nerve (CN III) exits from the ventral midbrain, traverses the subarachnoid space in the interpeduncular cistern, pierces the dura matter, enters the cavernous sinus, exits the skull via the superior orbital fissure, and innervates the levator palpebrae and all extraocular muscles except for the lateral rectus (eye ABductor/CN VI) and the superior oblique (depressor and internal rotator/CN IV). CN III also carries parasympathetic fibers to the dilator pupillary muscles of the iris mediating pupillary constriction.

CN III can be damaged anywhere along its pathway: within the brainstem (tumor, stroke); subarachnoid space (aneurysm, tumor, infection, uncal herniation); cavernous sinus (pituitary apoplexy, cavernous sinus thrombosis, cavernous-carotid fistula, aneurysm); and orbit (tumor or pseudotumor of the orbit). The constellation of findings that accompany a third nerve palsy often allows precise lesion localization. Other, less readily localizable etiologies include diabetic mononeuropathy (diabetic microangiopathic third), giant cell arteritis, Miller-Fisher syndrome, ophthalmoplegic migraine, and trauma.

An important feature of CN III anatomy is that fibers that innervate the pupils are located peripherally and are the first to be impaired by external compression. Fibers that innervate the extraocular muscles are located within the nerve fascicle and are the first to be involved in diabetic microangiopathic third nerve palsy (ischemia predominantly affects the inner core of the nerve). Thus, classically, "pupil-sparing third nerve palsy" suggests ischemic overcompressive etiology. In practice, even pupil-sparing third nerve palsies should be considered a potential neurologic emergency as the "pupil rule" is not absolute, especially if third nerve palsy is incomplete.

FIGURES

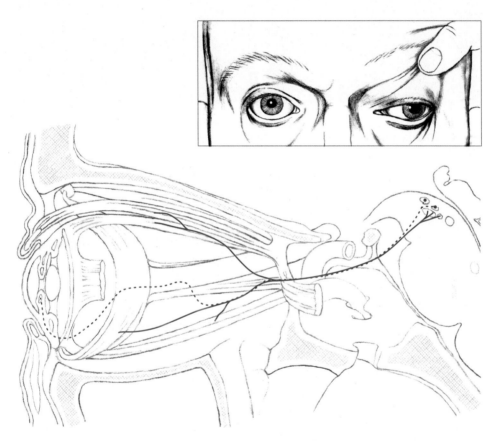

Schematic of CN III. The dotted line corresponds to autonomic fibers that take their origin in the Edinger-Westphal nucleus, while the solid line corresponds to motor fibers that originate in the motor nuclei of CN III. The insert shows complete left eyelid ptosis, dilated left pupil, and "down and out" eye position in complete CN III palsy.

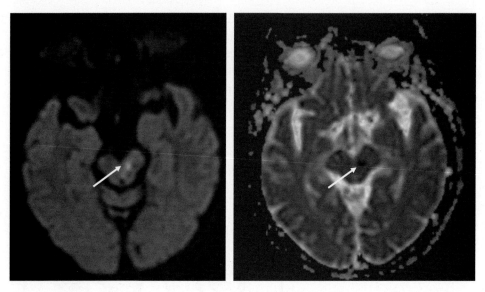

Fascicular third nerve palsy due to a small ischemic stroke (bright on diffusion weighted imaging [DWI] on the left and dark on apparent diffusion coefficient [ADC] sequence on the right).

QUESTIONS FOR SELF-STUDY

1. In a patient with diplopia, one identifies which eye is affected by applying these two rules: (1) diplopia is more pronounced in the direction in which the eye movement is impaired and (2) the image formed by the affected eye ("false image") is on the outside, and the image formed by the unimpaired eye ("true image") is on the inside. Using these two rules, draw the location of a "false" and a "true" image as seen by the patient with (a) complete right third nerve palsy and (b) right sixth nerve palsy.
2. What is internuclear ophthalmoplegia (INO)? How would you differentiate a partial third nerve palsy that causes ADduction deficit from an INO, which also causes an ADduction deficit?
3. An 80-year old-woman is hospitalized in the intensive care unit (ICU) with a large intracerebral hematoma. During a routine neurologic examination, you notice that she appears more drowsy and has a new third nerve palsy. What is the likely mechanism of CNIII palsy in this setting? What is the next urgent step in management?
4. Match symptoms with probable location/etiology of CN III palsy plus…

A. CN V_1, CN VI involvement and proptosis	Uncal herniation due to expanding subdural hematoma
B. Contralateral hemiparesis in an alert and oriented patient	Ruptured posterior communicating artery aneurysm
C. Contralateral hemiparesis in a comatose patient	Midbrain infarction (Weber syndrome)
D. Contralateral tremor and ataxia in an alert and oriented patient	Midbrain infarction (Benedikt syndrome)
E. Nuchal rigidity in a drowsy, disoriented patient	Carotid-cavernous fistula

5. A 70-year-old woman presents with a new onset of temporal and retrobulbar headaches and third nerve palsy. After excluding compressive and structural causes, what important etiology must be considered, which, if missed, can lead to a visual loss?

CHALLENGE

On examining a 70-year-old patient who complains of worsening headaches, you notice that when looking down, the patient's eyelid goes up, and when looking in, his pupil constricts. Explain the pathophysiology of these findings and why you should urgently image his cerebral arteries.

REFERENCES

Keane JR. Third nerve palsy: analysis of 1400 personally examined inpatients. *Can J Neurol Sci.* 2010;37(5):662-670.
Fang C, Leavitt JA, Hodge DO, et al. Incidence and etiologies of acquired third nerve palsy using a population-based method. *JAMA Ophthalmol.* 2017;135(1):23-28. [free online resource]
Bruce BB, Biousse V, Newman NJ. Third nerve palsies. *Semin Neurol.* 2007;27(3):257-268.

34 Cavernous Sinus Syndrome

Painful ophthalmoparesis due to lesion within the cavernous sinus

CORE FEATURES

1. Retroorbital and frontal headaches.
   An increase in pressure within the cavernous sinus causes pain, presumably due to stretching of the dura, a pain-sensitive structure. Cavernous sinus syndrome (CSS) due to a hyperacute event, such as a ruptured brain aneurysm or pituitary apoplexy, presents with vomiting and a thunderclap headache.
2. Blurry vision.
   Upward pressure exerted on the optic chiasm may interfere with the visual input from the bilateral temporal visual fields. The resulting visual field defect—bitemporal hemianopia—is highly characteristic of a chiasmatic lesion. Blurry vision may also be a result of pressure on optic nerves within the cavernous sinus.
3. Unilateral
   CN III and CN VI are more commonly affected than CN IV. Rarely, CSS may cause bilateral ophthalmoparesis (septic cavernous sinus thrombosis).
4. Facial numbness.
   There may be numbness in the V1 and V2 distributions, and the corneal reflex, whose afferent arc is mediated via V1 and V2, may be absent or depressed. Note that V3 is spared in CSS because the mandibular branch does not enter the cavernous sinus.
5. Proptosis and chemosis.
   An example of a red (chemosis), bulging (proptosis) eye due to CSS is shown in the figure below. These symptoms are due to increased cavernous sinus pressure and obstruction of venous outflow from the orbit.

SYNOPSIS

The mnemonic for remembering the structures of the cavernous sinus is (medial-to-lateral) "Oh P-O-T-O-M-A-C"—Optic chiasm and nerves (wall of the sinus), Pituitary, Ophthalmic division of CN V (V1), Trochlearnerve, Oculomotornerve,- Maxillary division of CN V (V2), Abducensnerve, Carotid artery. All the cranial nerves that control ocular motility (CN III, IV, and VI) pass through the cavernous sinus so CSS can cause partial or complete ophthalmoparesis. Pupillary findings are variable. If parasympathetic fibers are primarily affected within CN III, the pupil will be large and poorly reactive. If the sympathetic fibers are predominantly affected as they travel along the carotid arteries within the cavernous sinus, the pupil will be small and there may be other features of Horner syndrome. Brain MRI and MRI of the pituitary gland with and without contrast is helpful for the identification of compressive lesion, infection, hemorrhage, thrombosis, inflammation, or stigmata of head trauma.

FIGURES

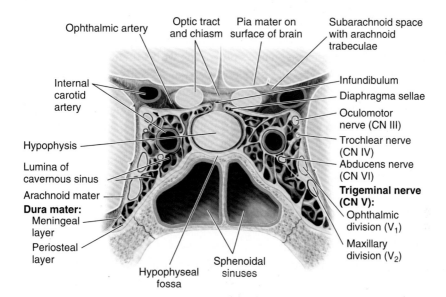

A schematic of the sphenoid sinus. (Reprinted with permission from Harell KM, Dudek RW. *Lippincott® Illustrated Reviews: Anatomy*. Philadelphia, PA: Wolters Kluwer; 2019: Chap 8:UNFig 5.)

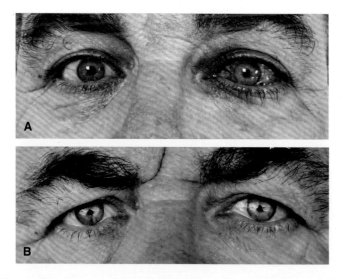

A patient with carotid-cavernous fistula (CCF) has a swollen, red left eye, with marked conjunctival inflammation and ipsilateral sixth nerve palsy (A). All symptoms resolved after embolization of the fistula (B). (Reprinted with permission from Parrilla G, Zamarro J, Díaz-Pérez J. Teaching neuroimages: complex transverse sinus fistula and cavernous sinus syndrome. *Neurology.* 2018;91(16):e1551-e1552.)

QUESTIONS FOR SELF-STUDY

1. Explain how evaluation of sensory loss in the V1 and V2 distributions helps localize the lesion to the cavernous sinus or superior orbital fissure.
2. Explain how the examination of the corneal and pupillary light reflexes helps differentiate CSS from ophthalmoparesis due to myasthenia gravis.
3. A thunderclap headache should be regarded as an emergency until proven otherwise. List the neurologic emergencies presenting with a thunderclap headache.
4. A 30-year-old woman who is 2 days post-partum presents with acute-onset headache, ophthalmoparesis, and hypotension. Serum sodium is low, but routine tests are otherwise unremarkable. Her blood pressure remains dangerously low despite aggressive fluid resuscitation. What neuro-endocrine emergency could account for these symptoms? What therapy must be emergently instituted to avoid hemodynamic collapse? What other endocrine abnormalities may be seen in this patient?
5. A 60-year-old woman with uncontrolled diabetes mellitus presents to the emergency department (ED) with fever, headache, and rapidly progressive ophthalmoparesis. She has a black eschar in the palate. What rare infection must be considered?

CHALLENGE

Explain how CSS may produce a pupil that fails to constrict in the light or dilate in the dark.

REFERENCES

Briet C, Salenave S, Bonneville JF, Laws ER, Chanson P. Pituitary apoplexy. *Endocr Rev*. 2015;36(6):622-645. [free online resource]
Keane JR. Cavernous sinus syndrome. Analysis of 151 cases. *Arch Neurol*. 1996;53(10):967-971.

35   Wernicke Encephalopathy

Severe, potentially fatal central nervous system (CNS) disorder due to thiamine deficiency

CORE FEATURES

1. History of a condition that may result in thiamine deficiency.
   Conditions associated with thiamine deficiency include, among others, alcohol use disorder, hyperemesis gravidarum, bariatric surgery, and malabsorption syndromes.
2. Mental status changes.
   Level of arousal may be slightly impaired (inattention, disorientation) or profoundly depressed (coma).
3. Extraocular movement abnormalities.
   The spectrum of neuro-ophthalmologic findings includes diplopia, nystagmus, conjugate gaze palsies, and ophthalmoparesis.
4. Ataxia.
   Both truncal and gait ataxia may be present.
5. MRI brain shows diffusion restriction and high T2 signal in the hypothalamus (mammillary bodies), thalamus (paraventricular), midbrain (periaqueductal gray), and pons (around the fourth ventricle).
   These lesions may disappear on subsequent imaging after thiamine supplementation.

SYNOPSIS

Wernicke encephalopathy (WE) is due to deficiency of thiamine intake, loss of thiamine, or failure to absorb thiamine in the small intestine. The human body stores only a few weeks' worth of thiamine, and thiamine depletion first affects organs and tissues within high thiamine content and turnover: thalamus and hypothalamus (inattention, impairment of memory and consciousness), brainstem (abnormal eye movements), vestibular nuclei and cerebellum (gait and truncal ataxia), peripheral nerves (neuropathy), and cardiac muscle (heart failure).

The diagnosis of WE is clinical. The classic triad of confusion, ophthalmoplegia, and ataxia is observed in only a minority of cases. WE should be considered in any patient susceptible to thiamine deficiency even if only one feature of the classic triad is present. If WE is suspected, thiamine supplementation should be given without delay and always *before* the administration of intravenous glucose. Characteristic findings on MRI and low level of whole blood thiamine levels retroactively confirm the diagnosis, but one should not wait for these results to implement urgent treatment. Although symptoms of WE often reverse after vitamin supplementation, many survivors go on to develop a severe amnestic disorder (Korsakoff syndrome).

FIGURE

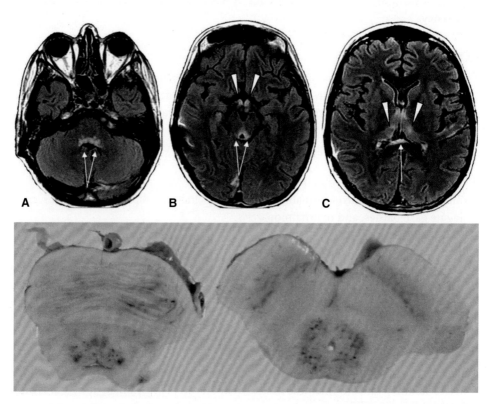

Top panel: Brain MRI Axial T2–fluid-attenuated inversion recovery (FLAIR) images in severe Wernicke encephalopathy show symmetric, abnormal high signal involving the floor of the fourth ventricle (arrows on A), periaqueductal gray matter and colliculi (arrows on B), hypothalamus and mammillary bodies (arrowheads on B), splenium of the corpus callosum (arrow on C), and mesial aspect of the thalami (arrowheads on C). Bottom panel: Autopsy images from a different patient show necrosis and small hemorrhages in central pons and periaqueductal gray matter in fatal case of Wernicke encephalopathy. (Top panel, Reprinted with permission from Luigetti M, De Paulis S, Spinelli P, et al. Teaching NeuroImages: the full-blown neuroimaging of Wernicke encephalopathy. *Neurology*. 2009;72(22):e115.)

QUESTIONS FOR SELF-STUDY

1. Are there any neurologic findings that can unambiguously differentiate WE from acute alcohol intoxication?
2. Explain what complication occurs if one administers intravenous glucose *before* thiamine in a patient with WE? What is the biochemical basis for this complication?
3. Differentiate WE from Korsakoff syndrome based on (1) acuteness of presentation, (2) presence of extraocular abnormalities, and (3) mental status examination findings (presence or absence of anterograde amnesia, retrograde amnesia, confabulation, encephalopathy).

4. A 50-year-old man with severe alcohol use disorder presents with cognitive deficits, ataxia, and dysarthria that persist beyond the period of intoxication. You suspect WE and initiate thiamine injections. The patient's condition fails to improve. MRI shows diffusion restriction in and around the corpus callosum, but not the diencephalon or in the brainstem. What is the likely diagnosis?

5. A 40-year-old homeless man with active alcohol use disorder presents with burning paresthesias and sensory ataxia. The general examination is significant for bibasilar rales, distended jugular veins, and swelling of both feet. He is mentally intact and has normal extraocular movements and no cerebellar findings. What unifying diagnosis could account for the neuropathic and cardiac findings?

CHALLENGE

Korsakoff syndrome illustrates the modular nature of memory: procedural memory is preserved in Korsakoff syndrome, while working memory is grossly impaired. Thus, a patient can be taught how to operate machinery, but is unable to memorize simple instructions. Describe what neuroanatomical structures underlie procedural memory versus working (declarative) memory, and explain why procedural memory is spared in Korsakoff syndrome.

REFERENCES

Day GS, del Campo CM. Wernicke encephalopathy: a medical emergency. *CMAJ.* 2014;186(8):E295. [free online resource]

Noble JM, Weimer LH. Neurologic complications of alcoholism. *Continuum (Minneap Minn).* 2014; 20(3, Neurology of Systemic Disease):624-641.

Neurologic Disorders of Vision

A Very Brief Introduction to Neurological Disorders of Vision

...while he traces the vessels in the direction of their larger trunks, he comes at length to the place of entrance of the optic nerve. This distinguishes itself from the rest of the eye-ground by its white color, for it is not covered with pigment ... the appearance of the sharply penciled red vessels on the clear white is of surprising elegance.

Hermann von Helmholtz[*]

As far as neurologists are concerned, the visual pathway starts at the retina. Photoreceptors in the outer retinal layer perceive light signals and transmit the signal via the various intermediate retinal cells to the ganglion cells of the retina, the first-order neurons of the visual pathway. Ganglion cell axons, of which there are more than one million in each eye, join together to form the optic nerves. The optic nerve travels through the orbit into the cavernous sinus region to join the other optic nerve at the optic chiasm, which is located between the hypothalamus (superiorly) and the pituitary gland (inferiorly). At the optic chiasm, axons from both optic nerves decussate—"chiasm" means "cross-over" in Greek—and form the optic tracts. The decussation allows for all the visual input from right of the visual field to be funneled to the left hemisphere (and vice versa). The first-order axons synapse on second-order neurons within the lateral geniculate nucleus of the thalamus. From the lateral geniculate nucleus, second-order axons project via the optic radiations to the primary visual area in the occipital cortex, where they synapse on the third-order neurons. Visual input and motor output relevant to the same side lateralize to the same cerebral hemisphere. This arrangement may be advantageous for eye-hand coordination. The figure below illustrates how visual information from the right side of the visual field (in red) ends up in the left visual cortex, while the visual information from the left side of the visual field (in blue) ends up in the right visual cortex.

Pre-chiasmatic optic nerve lesions affect the vision of the ipsilateral eye only and are included in the differential diagnosis of monocular visual loss along with an array of ophthalmologic causes—acute glaucoma, vitreous hemorrhage, retinal detachment, uveitis, etc. Important neurologic causes of monocular visual loss include optic neuritis (Chapter 36), giant cell arteritis (Chapter 37), and amaurosis fugax (Chapter 56). Lesions at, or distal to, the optic chiasm affect bilateral vision and cause characteristic field defect—bitemporal visual loss (cavernous sinus syndrome) and homonymous hemianopia (due to posterior cerebral artery strokes).

---

[*]Hermann Ludwig Ferdinand von Helmholtz (1821-1894), a German physician-turned-physicist, left a profound mark on medicine, physiology, psychology, thermodynamics, electromagnetism, and philosophy of science. Helmholtz's invention of the ophthalmoscope, described in the monograph from which the above citation is taken (reproduced in 'Description of an ophthalmoscope'. Optom Wkly. 1963;54:519-23), made it possible to visualize retina and optic nerve in a living person and inaugurated a new era of ophthalmology. Helmholtz was also the first to measure the speed of signal transduction along the sciatic nerves of frogs using a pendulum myograph of his own invention, and could thus be regarded as a forerunner of electrophysiology. (For more on Helmholtz's contribution to neurology, see Haas LF. Hermann von Helmholtz (1821-94). *J Neurol Neurosurg Psychiatry*. 1998 Jun;64(6):787)

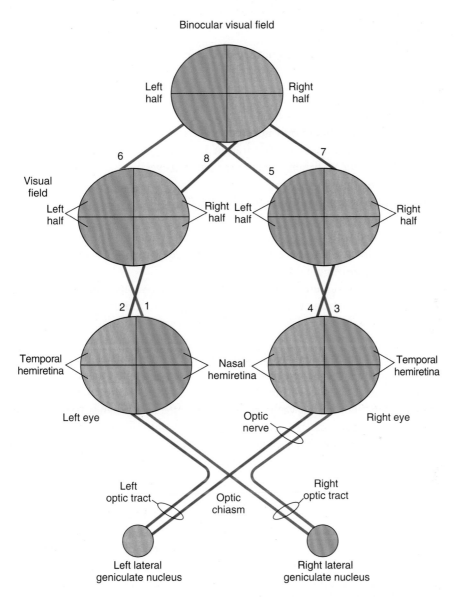

Binocular visual field

Schematic shows how visual information from the right visual hemifield (red) is projected to the nasal portion of the left eye and temporal portion of the right eye (red lines). Axons from the right and left optic nerves regroup within the optic chiasm such that all visual information from the right visual field is carried within the left optic tract to the left lateral geniculate nucleus. (Reprinted with permission from Siegel A, Sapru HN. *Essential Neruoscience*. 4th ed. Philadelphia, PA: Wolters Kluwer; 2018:Figure 15.8.)

REFERENCES

Bagheri N, Mehta S. Acute vision loss. *Prim Care.* 2015;42(3):347-361.
Ireland AC, Carter IB. *Neuroanatomy, optic chiasm.* In: *StatPearls* [Internet]. Treasure Island, FL: StatPearls Publishing; 2019. Available from https://www.ncbi.nlm.nih.gov/books/NBK542287/. [free online resource]

36 Optic Neuritis

Monophasic, optic nerve inflammatory disorder

CORE FINDINGS

1. Monocular impairment of vision.
   Central vision is predominantly affected.
2. Loss of color perception ("red desaturation").
   There is "bleaching" of bright colors in the affected eye.
3. Pain on moving the affected eye.
   There may also be temporal and retroorbital pain.
4. Relative afferent pupillary defect (RAPD).
   RAPD is elicited with the "swinging flashlight test" ("Marcus-Gunn pupil"). RAPD may not be evident when there is only a mild decrease in visual acuity.
5. Optic nerve enhancement on MRI.
   Gadolinium enhancement is best seen on orbital fat-suppressed coronal images. Another common finding is an increase in T2 signal within the optic nerve.

SYNOPSIS

Impaired conduction of visual signals via optic nerve manifests as blurry vision and color desaturation. Pain with eye movements has been attributed to irritation of pain-sensitive meningeal fibers covering the optic nerve. RAPD occurs with any disorder in which one of the optic nerves is preferentially affected. When a beam of light is initially shined in the unaffected eye and subsequently into the affected eye ("swinging flashlight test"), the brain receives relatively less visual stimulation than when the light was shining in the unaffected eye. As a result, there is pupillary dilation ("Marcus-Gunn pupil"), which appears "paradoxical", since a normal pupil constricts when light is shined into it.

During optic neuritis (ON), the blood-nerve barrier is perturbed, resulting in optic nerve enhancement on MRI. As the inflammatory process subsides, vision improves, the pain resolves, and the MRI enhancement dissipates. Most patients regain a visual acuity better than 20/40 in the affected eye within 6 months following the onset of ON. High-dose corticosteroids fasten recovery in immune-mediated ON, but do not have any significant effect on long-term prognosis. The most important question in a previously healthy patient presenting with ON is to stratify the risk of developing multiple sclerosis (MS), or, much less commonly, neuromyelitis optica spectrum disorder, myelin oligodendrocyte glycoprotein antibody–associated disorder, or neurosarcoidosis.

FIGURE

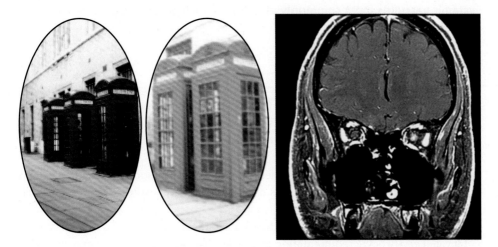

Red desaturation in optic neuritis: bright red color of UK telephone booth as seen with the unaffected eye (left) vs the affected eye (right). Coronal, fat-suppressed MRI of the orbits shows avid enhancement in the left optic nerve. (Reprinted with permission from Preziosa P, Comi G, Filippi M. Optic neuritis in multiple sclerosis: Looking from a patient's eyes. *Neurology*. 2016;87(3):338-339.)

QUESTIONS FOR SELF-STUDY

1. Worsening visual blurring in the eye affected by ON when the patient's body temperature increases is known as "Uhthoff phenomenon". What is the basis of this phenomenon?
2. It has been said, exaggeratedly, that during ON "the patient does not see, and the doctor does not see [what the problem is]". Explain why the funduscopic examination is usually normal in ON.
3. What is the single most important predictor of developing MS after the first attack of ON?
4. What prophylactic treatments should be considered in a patient with ON who is at high risk of developing MS?
5. What demographic, clinical, and MRI features help to differentiate inflammatory ON from ischemic optic neuropathy?

CHALLENGE

Explain why RAPD would not be possible without consensual pupillary reflex.

REFERENCES

Biousse V, Newman NJ. Diagnosis and clinical features of common optic neuropathies. *Lancet Neurol*. 2016;15(13):1355-1367.

Galetta SL, Villoslada P, Levin N, et al. Acute optic neuritis: unmet clinical needs and model for new therapies. *Neurol Neuroimmunol Neuroinflamm*. 2015;2(4):e135. [free online resource]

37 Giant Cell Arteritis

Systemic vasculitis most commonly affecting branches of the extracranial arteries

CORE FEATURES

1. New-onset headache or a new pattern of headache in a patient older than 50 years.
   Peak incidence of giant cell arteritis (GCA) is in the 70 to 80 age group.
2. The temporal artery on the affected side is tender on palpation.
   Pulsation in the temporal artery on the affected may be decreased or absent.
3. Painless monocular visual loss.
   In approximately 30% of patients, there are antecedent episodes of amaurosis fugax within a few days of permanent loss of vision. A timely institution of steroids may preempt permanent loss of vision.
4. Pain in the jaw muscles when chewing (jaw claudication).
5. Elevated erythrocyte sedimentation rate (ESR>50 mm/h).
   ESR is an excellent screening tool for giant cell arteritis (GCA): normal ESR makes GCA highly unlikely. However, ESR elevation is nonspecific—it may be present in many infectious, neoplastic, and inflammatory conditions. Other inflammatory markers commonly elevated in GCA are C-reactive protein and platelet count (thrombocytosis).

SYNOPSIS

GCA is a systemic vasculitis mostly affecting medium-to-large extracranial arteries and accompanied by markers of systemic inflammation and systemic and rheumatologic symptoms. Superficial temporal artery biopsy shows granulomatous inflammation with predominance of monocytes and multinucleated giant cells within the arterial wall. The vasculitis may be patchy ("skip lesions"), making it necessary to obtain 1 to 3 cm in length biopsy specimens of the temporal artery, and to finely section them to detect intramural inflammation. Biopsy shows inflammation of vessel wall in over 85% of GCA cases; rarely, a biopsy of the contralateral temporal artery may be required to confirm the diagnosis.

The vasculitic process causes occlusion of blood vessels and consequent ischemia of the optic nerves and retina. Infarction of the optic nerve (arteritic anterior ischemic optic neuropathy) leads to permanent loss of vision in up to 20% of patients. Vasculitic involvement of other extracranial arteries may manifest as jaw or tongue claudication, or diplopia. Thus, any patient with suspected GCA must be specifically queried as to whether they have experienced transient vision loss, double vision, or jaw pain upon chewing. Infrequently, GCA may involve arteries supplying the brain or limbs, in which case ischemic strokes or limb claudication may ensue.

Corticosteroids are the first line of therapy. They must be initiated right away whenever GCA is strongly suspected. Prompt treatment decreases the risk of vision loss and permanent neurologic damage, but it does not help the recovery of vision in the affected eye. Anti-IL-6 therapy with tocilizumab is highly effective and has been recently FDA-approved for GCA.

FIGURE

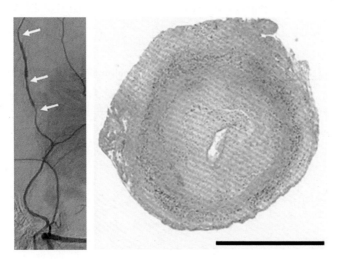

Digital subtraction angiography demonstrates irregularities with "beading" of the distal superficial temporal artery (arrows). Pathologic evaluation of the artery demonstrates concentric intimal hyperplasia with evidence of inflammatory infiltrate within the vessel wall. (Reprinted with permission from Rinaldo L, Arnold Fiebelkorn CE, Chen JJ, et al. Clinical reasoning: headaches and double vision in a 68-year-old woman. *Neurology.* 2018;91(8):e785-e789.)

QUESTIONS FOR SELF-STUDY

1. A patient with acute-onset of painless monocular visual loss shows marked optic disk edema and a splinter hemorrhage. Explain why these funduscopic findings are supportive of anterior ischemic optic neuropathy rather than autoimmune ON.
2. A 70-year-old woman with GCA has been gradually tapering off her steroid dose. Her vision is stable, but she reports new-onset difficulty lifting her arms due to pain and stiffness in muscles of neck, shoulders, and upper arms bilaterally. What is the likely diagnosis?
3. What is the characteristic finding of GCA on color Doppler ultrasonography of the temporal arteries?
4. A 60-year-old man wakes up with a visual loss in the right eye. He has no headache, eye pain, jaw claudication, or systemic symptoms. ESR is 30 mm/h. Funduscopy shows marked right optic nerve swelling and a "crowded" left optic disk. What is the likely diagnosis?
5. A 70-year-old near-sighted woman presents with loss of vision in the left eye. She describes multiple light flashes and floaters prior to the onset of visual loss. Funduscopy is normal. What reversible ophthalmologic cause of vision loss must be considered in this patient?

CHALLENGE

A 70-year-old patient with biopsy-proven GCA develops new-onset blurry vision. Funduscopy is normal. What could be the potential mechanisms of GCA-related vision loss in this patient?

REFERENCES

Salvarani C, Pipitone N, Versari A, Hunder GG. Clinical features of polymyalgia rheumatica and giant cell arteritis. *Nat Rev Rheumatol.* 2012;8(9):509-521.

Stone JH, Klearman M, Collinson N. Trial of tocilizumab in giant-cell arteritis. *N Engl J Med.* 2017;377(4):317-328.

Weyand CM, Goronzy JJ. Giant-cell arteritis and polymyalgia rheumatica. *N Engl J Med.* 2014;371(1):50-57. [free online resource]

38 Idiopathic Intracranial Hypertension

Syndrome of raised intracranial pressure of unknown etiology predominantly affecting overweight or obese women

CORE FEATURES

1. Headache in an overweight woman of childbearing age.
   Although idiopathic intracranial hypertension (IIH) can affect any gender and age, there is a strong predilection for women of childbearing age. Headache may be tensionlike or migrainous in quality; may occur daily; is usually more severe upon awakening or with the Valsalva maneuver. The headache tends not to respond to analgesics but improves promptly with cerebrospinal fluid (CSF) removal. Neck and back pain are common.
2. Transient visual obscurations.
   Less-than-a-minute-long episodes of blurry vision are often triggered by postural changes. Permanent blurry vision due to constricted visual fields and even blindness may ensue.
3. Bilateral papilledema.
   Swelling of the optic nerve disks manifests as blurring of optic disk margins, optic disk hyperemia, and obscuration of major vessels (for examples of papilledema see http://eyewiki.aao.org/Papilledema. [free online resource]). The enlarged blind spot is an early finding in papilledema.
4. Pulsatile tinnitus.
   The bilateral, swooshing sound sensation at the frequency of heartbeat.
5. Increased opening pressure on lumbar puncture (LP).
   To measure intracranial pressure (ICP), always place the patient in the lateral decubitus position. CSF opening pressures of >25 cm H_2O is abnormally high.

SYNOPSIS

Symptoms of increased ICP are not specific as to etiology. The secondary causes of increased ICP must be excluded before a diagnosis of IIH can be made. The most important secondary cause is an intracranial space-occupying lesion. Therefore, the first step in evaluating patients with suspected increased ICP is brain imaging. LP can only be done only after a space-occupying lesion has been excluded. Other secondary causes include cerebral venous sinus thrombosis; meningitis; malignant systemic hypertension; and drug-induced (tetracycline antibiotics; vitamin A; hormonal treatments; withdrawal from corticosteroids). In IIH, brain MRI is often reported as normal, but closer examination may demonstrate an empty sella, tortuous optic nerves, and flattening of the posterior aspect of the globes. CSF parameters are normal, except that the protein content may be slightly low. First-line medical treatment of IIH is acetazolamide, which presumably works by decreasing CSF secretion by the choroid plexus. Prompt therapy decreases the risk of vision loss. Weight loss is the only "disease-modifying therapy" for IIH.

FIGURE

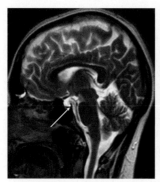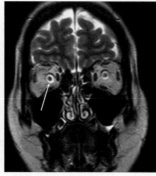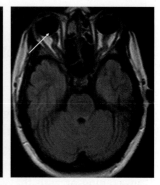

Characteristic MRI features of idiopathic intracranial hypertension. Left: Sagittal T2 MRI shows partially empty sella turcica (arrow). Middle: Coronal T2 images showing dilated perioptic CSF spaces (arrow). Right: Axial FLAIR images showing buckling of bilateral optic nerves and flattening of the posterior aspect of the optic globe (arrow). (Reprinted with permission from Hassan H, Das A, Baheti NN, et al. Teaching neuroimages: idiopathic intracranial hypertension: MRI features. *Neurology*. 2010;74(7):e24.)

QUESTIONS FOR SELF-STUDY

1. What is the anatomic reason for the physiologic blind spot? What is the reason for an enlarged blind spot in a patient with IIH? How would you evaluate a patient for an enlarged blind spot? What is the mechanism of papilledema in increased ICP?
2. Propose a mechanism to explain why transient visual obscurations often occur when patients with IIH go from a lying to a standing position.
3. A 40-year-old underweight woman presents with a new pattern of daily headache and bilateral papilledema. Her medical history is remarkable for migraines with aura. She is a smoker. Her only prescribed medication is an estrogen-containing contraceptive pill. Head CT without contrast is normal. LP shows on opening pressure of 35 cm H_2O_2. CSF analysis is unremarkable. What are the "red flags" for IIH in this patient? What additional testing is warranted to exclude important treatable cause of increased ICP in this patient?
4. What surgical options may be considered for patients with IIH who experience progressive visual loss despite optimal medical therapy?
5. LP is often easier to perform in a sitting rather than a lateral recumbent position. Invoking the principle of communicating vessels, explain why an LP performed in the sitting position yields falsely elevated measurement of ICP?

CHALLENGE

Patients with IIH may complain of diplopia. What extraocular movement is likely impaired? What is the probable cause of the diplopia? Why is it considered a "false localizing sign"?

REFERENCES

Markey KA, Mollan SP, Jensen RH, Sinclair AJ. Understanding idiopathic intracranial hypertension: mechanisms, management, and future directions. *Lancet Neurol*. 2016;15(1):78-91.

Mollan SP, Hornby C, Mitchell J, Sinclair AJ. Evaluation and management of adult idiopathic intracranial hypertension. *Pract Neurol*. 2018;18(6):485-488. pii: practneurol-2018-002009. [free online resource]

Movement Disorders

A Very Brief Introduction to Movement Disorders

... at meals the fork not being duly directed frequently fails to raise the morsel from the plate: which, when seized, is with much difficulty conveyed to the mouth. At this period, the patient seldom experiences a suspension of the agitation of his limbs.

James Parkinson[*]

The pathogenesis of most movement disorders is intimately linked to the deep gray matter nuclei known as the basal ganglia (BG). As an oversimplification, one can conceptualize the BG as gray matter relay stations that lie in between the external cortical gray matter and the internal thalamic gray matter. On midcoronal section, the main BG appear in approximately the following order from outside-to-inside: caudate, putamen, (two components of the striatum) globus pallidus externa (GPe), globus pallidus interna (GPi), subthalamic nucleus, and substantia nigra.

---

[*]James Parkinson (1755-1824) practiced general medicine in the small English town of Hoxton. He published the first detailed description of the eponymous disease in an essay "On Shaking Palsy." Parkinson was also an accomplished geologist. In awarding him a gold medal for his work on fossils, the Royal College of Surgeons commented: "The fruits of your exertions are distinguished by the stamp of simplicity and truth. They express the most laudable zeal in the pursuit and the promulgation of knowledge, for the benefit of mankind." (Cited in Lewis PA. James Parkinson: the man behind the shaking palsy. *J Parkinsons Dis.* 2012;2(3):181-187.)

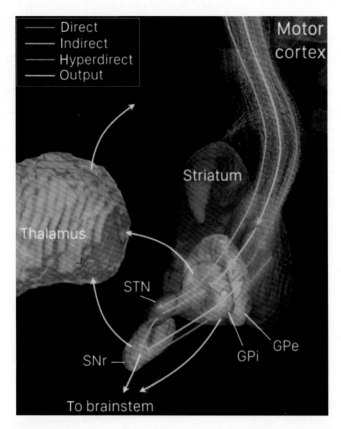

Basal ganglia and their major interconnections as shown by diffusion spectrum imaging of 30 subjects from the human connectome project. Direct, indirect, and hyperdirect pathways are visualized in different colors. GPe, external part of the pallidum; GPi, internal part of the pallidum; SNr, substantia nigra, pars reticulata; STN, subthalamic nucleus. (Credit: Andreashorn - Own work, CC BY-SA 4.0, https://commons.wikimedia.org/w/index.php?curid=46586775.)

In the classic model of Parkinson disease (PD; Chapter 39), degeneration of dopamine-producing neurons in the substantia nigra pars compacta results, via a series of suppression/facilitation steps, in inhibition of cortically mediated movements (hence: bradykinesia). This model does not explain many other salient features of PD, but yields a few important predictions, such as that stimulation of the STN will facilitate the output from the basal ganglia and improve bradykinesia. This prediction has been borne out, and deep brain stimulation of the STN is now an accepted strategy for managing PD. The model also predicts that decreased output from the striatum will result in excessive stimulation of the motor cortex and hyperkinesis. This is indeed the case in Huntington disease (HD; Chapter 41), a prototypical hyperkinetic disorder resulting from the loss of GABAergic neurons in the caudate nucleus.

Other hyperkinetic movement disorders discussed in this section include essential tremor (Chapter 40) and tardive dystonia (Chapter 43). Wilson disease, a very rare inherited movement disorder that can present with either hyperkinesia or bradykinesia, is included because it is not only treatable but potentially reversible (Chapter 42).

The section ends with a discussion of several conditions that lie in the borderland of movement disorders. Restless legs syndrome (RLS), one of the most common neurologic conditions, characterized by irresistible urge to move one's limbs is discussed in Chapter 44. Tourette syndrome (Chapter 45) is a common childhood-onset disorder characterized by motor and phonic tics. The final chapter is devoted to functional movement disorders, a common mimicker of organic movement disorders.

39 Parkinson Disease

Neurodegenerative bradykinetic movement disorder associated with loss of dopamine-producing cells in the substantia nigra

CORE FEATURES

1. Asymmetric resting tremor.
   A "pill-rolling" tremor involving index and thumb, and pronation/supination tremor in one hand are characteristic and often the first manifestation of PD. As the disease progresses, the tremor spread to both arms and may involve the legs and even the trunk.
2. Hypokinesia and bradykinesia.
   There is paucity (hypo) and slowness (brady) of movements (kinesia) that manifest in a slow and shuffling gait; "masked face" (hypomimia), with a decreased rate of eyelid blinking; soft voice (hypophonia); and small calligraphy (micrographia).
3. Rigidity.
   Increased muscle tone, with a ratchety quality (cogwheel rigidity), can be brought out with distraction maneuvers, such as asking the patients to draw imaginary circles in the air with one hand, while testing for rigidity in the other hand.
4. Postural instability.
   Postural reflexes are tested with the retropulsion test. The patient is asked to steady themselves quickly after a sudden backward pull on both shoulders. A positive test leads to patients taking more than two steps backward or falling. In the later stages of the disease, there is a festination on walking—as if the patient is trying to catch up to the center of gravity that lies in front of their base of support.
5. Response to L-dopa.
   PD is invariably responsive to L-dopa in the early stages, while in later stages, L-dopa is less effective and often complicated by dopa-induced dyskinesias.

SYNOPSIS

Parkinsonism is a hypokinetic syndrome whose cardinal features are depicted in the figure below. Parkinsonism can be a manifestation of an idiopathic neurodegenerative disorder (eg, PD) or rarer neurodegenerative disorders often referred to as "Parkinson plus" syndromes. Parkinsonism may also develop secondary to certain medications (dopamine-receptor blockers); vascular disorders; encephalitides; trauma; structural causes.

PD is usually a sporadic disease, but about 10% of patients carry a pathogenic mutation. Many of these mutations relate to α-synuclein protein, the principal constituent of Lewy bodies, which are the pathological hallmark of PD. Presumably, α-synuclein exerts a toxic effect on dopaminergic neurons, especially in the substantia nigra pars compacta, leading to apoptosis. Therapeutic strategies in PD focus on either increasing dopamine concentration or stimulating dopamine receptors in the brain. These strategies are highly effective in the early stages of the disease, but in later stages, treatment-resistant motor symptoms and nonmotor features become increasingly prominent and difficult to manage. Deep brain stimulation of the STN and globus pallidus may provide substantial relief for motor symptoms in treatment-recalcitrant cases.

PD is a prototypic movement disorder, but nonmotor symptoms are common and profoundly detrimental to patients' quality of life. Some symptoms— such as an impaired sense of smell, REM sleep disorder, depression, and constipation—can pre-date motor manifestations by years and even decades, while others, such as orthostatic hypotension and cognitive decline, emerge in later stages of PD. It has been hypothe-sized that nonmotor symptoms may be due to pathologic deposition of Lewy bodies outside of the basal ganglia—in the olfactory nerves (loss of smell), enteric nervous system (constipation), autonomic nervous system (orthostatic hypotension), thalamus, and cerebral cortex (cognitive decline).

FIGURE

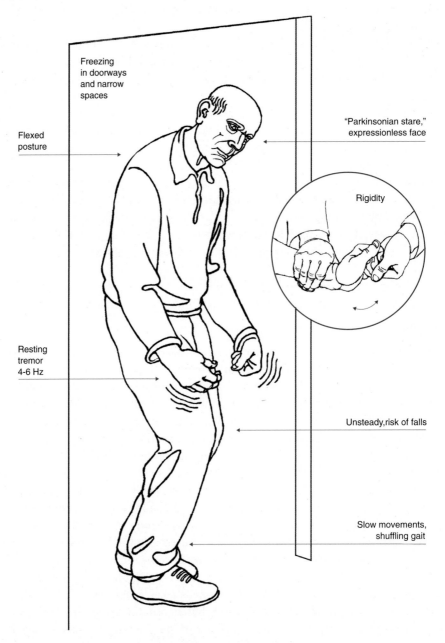

Cardinal features of Parkinsonism.

QUESTIONS FOR SELF-STUDY

1. Rigidity, an extrapyramidal symptom due to basal ganglia damage, and spasticity, which is due to corticospinal tract lesions, are both characterized by increased muscle tone. How would you differentiate spasticity from rigidity on examination? Define "cogwheeling," "lead-pipe," and "clasp-knife" phenomenon. Which of these terms apply to spasticity and which to rigidity?
2. Normal-pressure hydrocephalus (NPH) manifests with a short-stepped shuffling gait. What neurologic signs will assist you in differentiating a patient with a shuffling gait resulting from PD from a patient with NPH?
3. A 60-year-old man presents with rigidity, tremors, slow, and shuffling gait. PD is suspected, but nuclear medicine (NM) DaT scan is negative. What causes of parkinsonism are compatible with a normal NM-DaT scan?
4. A 90-year-old man with PD and mild dementia is admitted to the hospital with pneumonia. He becomes agitated in the evening ("sun-downing") and is given haloperidol to "calm him down." Within hours, he is unable to talk, walk, or feed himself. What is the underlying pathophysiologic explanation for his rapid decompensation?
5. An important question when evaluating a patient with a hypokinetic disorder is whether they have PD or one of the "Parkinson plus" syndromes. Match each set of "plus" clinical features in the Table below (middle column) with the syndrome that best exemplifies it (right column):

A	Myoclonus, dystonia, apraxia (inability to carry out a planned movement)	Progressive supranuclear palsy (PSP)
B	Visual hallucinations, episodic confusion, personality changes	Multiple system atrophy, cerebellar type (MSA-C)
C	Frequent falls, postural instability, apraxia of eyelid opening, and inability to look down on command	Multiple system atrophy, autonomic type (MSA-A)
D	Ataxia of limbs and trunk, lack of responsiveness to L-dopa	Corticobasal degeneration (CBD)
E	Prominent early autonomic symptoms including syncope, orthostatic hypotension, bladder, and sexual dysfunction	Dementia with Lewy bodies (DLB)

CHALLENGE

There are a number of ways in which dopamine concentration could be increased in the brain. One is to provide dopamine replacement therapy—carbidopa/levodopa. Suggest pharmacological strategies for activating dopamine receptors in the brain. Compare your responses with mechanisms of action of entacapone, ropinirole, and selegiline.

REFERENCES

Chaudhuri KR, Healy DG, Schapira AH; National Institute for Clinical Excellence. Non-motor symptoms of Parkinson's disease: diagnosis and management. *Lancet Neurol.* 2006;5(3):235-245.

Kalia LV, Lang AE. Parkinson's disease. *Lancet.* 2015;386(9996):896-912.

Perlmutter JS. Assessment of Parkinson disease manifestations. *Curr Protoc Neurosci.* 2009; Chapter 10:Unit10.1. [free online resource]

40 Essential Tremor

Progressive, usually familial, tremor disorder

CORE FEATURES

1. Insidious onset and slow progression of tremor of the upper extremities.
   Tremor may be present in adolescence but typically does not interfere with daily functioning till much later in life.
2. Action and postural tremor.
   Tremor is more evident when the patient is doing an action such as pouring water into a cup or while maintaining a posture with arms outstretched, rather than at rest.
3. Tremor is lessened with alcohol intake.
   This feature is observed in about half of patients with essential tremor (ET) but not in tremors of other etiologies.
4. Absence of other types of abnormal movements.
   No parkinsonian features or dystonia.
5. Family history of tremor.
   Family history is present in up to 70% of patients with ET.

SYNOPSIS

ET affects approximately 1% of the population worldwide. The designation "essential" implies that the underlying cause is unknown, and that tremor is the major, and usually the only, manifestation of the condition. Tremor is thought to originate by the oscillations in the cortico-ponto-cerebello-thalamo-cortical loop, but it is not known what drives these oscillations. The two best-established therapies for ET are beta-blockers and primidone. The more intractable cases may benefit from botulinum injections in selected muscles, or neurosurgical interventions—deep brain stimulation, thalamotomy, and thalamic thermoablation with ultrasound targeting the thalamic nucleus ventralis intermedius. Despite the clearly autosomal dominant nature of ET, its genetic basis remains unknown.

FIGURES

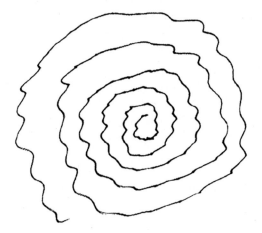

Drawing of Archimedes spiral by a patient with ET. (Reprinted with permission from Campbell WW. *Clinical Signs in Neurology: A Compendium.* Philadelphia, PA: Wolters Kluwer; 2015:Figure A.12.)

Handwriting of Samuel Adams, one of the Founding Fathers of the United States, shows evidence of ET. (Cited in Louis ED. Samuel Adams' tremor. *Neurology.* 2001;56(9):1201-1205.)

QUESTIONS FOR SELF-STUDY

1. A common clinical question is whether the patient's tremor is consistent with ET or PD. For each of the following tremor characteristics, please mark if it describes ET or PD tremor:

Frequency	3-5 Hz _____	4-8 Hz _____
Tremor maximal at	Rest _____	Action _____
Body parts affected	Jaw, tongue _____	Head, vocal cords _____
Improved with	L-dopa _____	Alcohol _____
Mostly symmetric	Yes _____	No _____

2. Physiologic tremor occurs in all healthy individuals. It is rarely visible to the naked eye but may be brought out by anxiety, stress, sleep deprivation, or excessive caffeine consumption. Enhanced physiologic tremor is an exaggerated version of the normal physiologic tremor and is not a sign of pathology. Describe how you would differentiate an enhanced physiologic tremor from ET by tremor frequency and unmasking maneuvers (action vs holding hands steady).

3. How would you differentiate tremor from other hyperkinetic movements such as myoclonus, chorea, or tics? What is the defining feature of a tremor?

4. The way a person speaks can yield important clues to the diagnosis. In PD, the speech may be hypophonic, while in ET, the speech may have a quavering quality when the vocal cords are involved. Another disorder that gives speech a stuttering quality is spasmodic dysphonia. Which vocal characteristics would help you distinguish between the two? How would vocal cord movements during phonation appear on laryngoscopy in ET and in spasmodic dysphonia?

5. You are evaluating a patient with an action tremor. What reversible causes of tremor must be excluded before making a diagnosis of ET?

CHALLENGE

Nearly all tremors and abnormal movements abate during sleep. Which tremor persists during sleep?

REFERENCES

Frucht S. Evaluation of patients with tremor. *Pract Neurol*. 2018:58-62. http://practicalneurology.com/2018/05/evaluation-of-patients-with-tremor/. [free online resource]
Haubenberger D, Hallett M. Essential tremor. *N Engl J Med*. 2018;378(19):1802-1810.
Louis ED. Samuel Adams' tremor. *Neurology*. 2001;56(9):1201-1205.

41 Huntington Disease

Autosomal dominant, progressive hyperkinetic disorder

CORE FEATURES

1. Progressive chorea.
   Chorea initially manifests in the hands and face and then progresses to involve all limbs and the trunk. Associated dystonia is common. The late stages may be marked by bradykinesia and rigidity.
2. Neuropsychiatric symptoms.
   Personality changes, mental inflexibility, obsessiveness, irritability, impulsivity, anxiety, depression, and apathy may precede or coincide with the onset of movement disorder. Cognitive symptoms are subtle early in the disease but become more prominent as disease progresses.
3. Caudate atrophy on magnetic resonance imaging (MRI).
   Loss of cells in caudate nucleus leads to caudate atrophy and enlargement of the frontal horns of the lateral ventricles ("boxcar ventricles").
4. Family history.
   De novo mutations are rare, and nearly all patients have an ancestor with Huntington disease (HD).
5. An abnormal number of CAG repeats in the Huntington gene (aka HTT or HD gene).
   Patients develop HD if they inherit more than 40 CAG repeats (full penetrance). Clinical manifestations may also be present with 36 to 40 CAG copies.

SYNOPSIS

"When either one or both parents show manifestations of the disease, one or more of the offspring invariably will suffer from the disease, if they live to adult life. But if by any chance, these children go through life without it, the thread is broken and the grandchildren and great-grandchildren of the original shakers will rest assured that are free from disease." These prescient observations by an American physician, James Huntington, which succinctly encapsulate the autosomal dominant mode of inheritance, were made decades before Gregor Johann Mendel's landmark discovery of the laws of inheritance became known, and more than 120 years before the discovery of the Huntington gene. A single copy of the Huntington gene that contains excessive CAG repeats is sufficient to cause the disease—this is the defining feature of an autosomal dominant disorder—because the mutant HTT protein contains an excess of glutamate and is toxic to GABAergic neurons within the caudate and putamen. The caudate atrophy is evident on brain MRI. At autopsy, the caudate volume is reduced by as much as 95%.

HD is presently an incurable, relentlessly progressive disorder that leads to death within 20 years of diagnosis. Tetrabenazine can improve the chorea, presumably via depletion of dopamine at the synaptic cleft, but may exacerbate depression. An in-depth understanding of the molecular mechanism of HD gives one hope that a successful genetic therapy will become available. A recent proof-of-concept study showed that intrathecal administration of the antisense oligonucleotide designed to inhibit HTT messenger RNA reduced concentrations of mutant huntingtin HTT in the spinal fluid (Tabrizi SJ, Leavitt BR, Landwehrmeyer GB, et al *N Engl J Med.* 2019;380:2307-2316.).

FIGURE

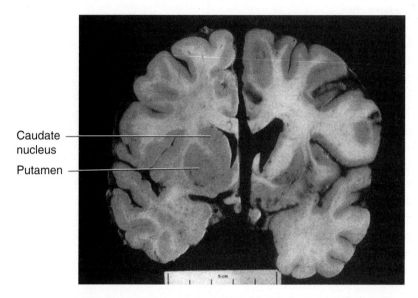

Caudate nucleus

Putamen

Normal cerebrum shown on the left is contrasted with cerebrum of a patient with Huntington disease (HD) shown on the right. Note the dilation of lateral ventricle and near-complete disappearance of the caudate head and putamen in HD. (From Strange PG. *Brain Biochemistry and Brain Disorders*. New York: Oxford University Press; 1992: Figure 11.2. Reproduced with permission of Oxford Publishing Limited through PLSclear.)

QUESTIONS FOR SELF-STUDY

1. How would you differentiate chorea from excessive fidgeting or tics?
2. Patients with HD often complain of poor sleep and weight loss. What potentially treatable symptom of HD should be considered that may be responsible for those complaints?
3. The 18-year-old son of a parent with HD develops bradykinesia and rigidity. What is the likely explanation?
4. A 35-year-old man complains of subtle involuntary movements of his fingers and toes. He suspects he is having early symptoms of HD, which affected his father and grandmother, but does not understand why he is developing symptoms so early in life: his father did not develop symptoms until age 40 years, and his grandmother not till her 50s. What is the genetic explanation for this observation? Explain why a healthy parent with 35 CAG copies on the Huntington gene may have a child, who is affected by HD.
5. An elderly man presents with new-onset chorea. Which reversible metabolic, iatrogenic, and endocrine etiology must be considered before attributing chorea to a neurodegenerative condition?

CHALLENGE

Genetic testing for HD is fraught with ethical dilemmas. Consider an asymptomatic adult whose grandfather had HD (proband). The man wants to find out whether he carries the gene for HD, while his mother, proband's daughter, does not wish to know her status. If the proband's grandson is allowed to proceed with testing and is found to carry the pathogenic mutation in HTT, the inevitable conclusion is that his mother, who wishes to remain agnostic to her risk, must also carry the pathogenic mutation. A similar situation arises when an asymptomatic progeny of HD proband wishes to undergo a preimplantation genetic test to ensure that the embryo does not carry the mutated gene but does not want to know their own status. Revealing the HD status of embryo unmasks the parent's status. Design a strategy for preimplantation testing for HD that would not reveal the parents' genetic status. (Hint: the strategy involves testing the parent's parents.)

REFERENCES

Caron NS, Wright GEB, Hayden MR. Huntington disease. In: Adam MP, Ardinger HH, Pagon RA, et al, eds. *GeneReviews®*. Seattle (WA): University of Washington; 1993-2019. https://www.ncbi.nlm.nih.gov/books/NBK1305/. [free online resource]

Ghosh R, Tabrizi SJ. Huntington disease. *Handb Clin Neurol.* 2018;147:255-278.

https://www.hda.org.uk/professionals/resources-for-professionals/best-practice-in-huntington-s-disease. [free online resource]

42 Wilson Disease

Autosomal recessive disorder of copper metabolism with neurologic, psychiatric, hepatic, and hematologic manifestations

CORE FEATURES

1. Abnormal movements.
   Tremor, including the classic, but uncommon "wing-beating tremor," dystonia, chorea, parkinsonism, and ataxia can be seen in WD.
2. Dysarthria.
3. Kayser-Fleischer ring (KFR).
   KFR is a brownish-yellow ring in the outer portion of the cornea composed of fine granular deposits of copper in the Descemet membrane. KFR is best appreciated on slit-lamp examination and is always present in patients with neurologic manifestations. KFR may disappear after chelation therapy.
4. Abnormal liver function test.
   WD may manifest as acute, recurrent, or chronic hepatitis, and even fulminant liver failure.
5. Elevated levels of copper in urine and decreased serum level of ceruloplasmin.
   Ceruloplasmin is the main transporter of copper in serum. Ceruloplasmin levels are low in WD because it is unstable unless loaded with copper.

SYNOPSIS

WD is an autosomal recessive disorder of copper metabolism. WD is due to a mutation in ATP7B gene which leads to a defective copper-transporting ATPase in the liver. This ATPase is responsible for detoxifying the body of excess copper by transporting copper from the hepatocytes into the bile. Mutations in the gene cause copper to accumulate in the liver (transaminitis, liver failure); brainstem and basal ganglia (bulbar and extrapyramidal symptoms); frontostriatal circuits (cognitive and psychiatric symptoms); and cornea (KFRs). More than 500 pathogenic mutations have been described to date. Thus, the sequencing of the entire ATP7B gene may sometimes be necessary to confirm the diagnosis.

WD typically presents in the second or third decade of life and is fatal if untreated. Progression may be halted with chelation therapy (D-penicillamine, trientine) and zinc, which blocks the absorption of copper in the gut. Treatment is lifelong with regular monitoring of copper levels in urine and serum. Patients with severe WD may be considered for liver transplantation.

FIGURE

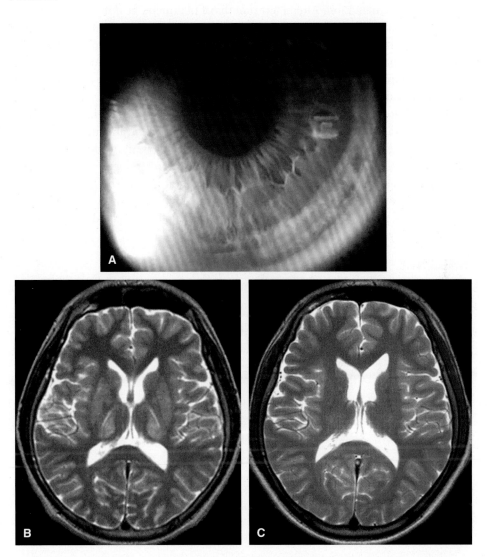

A, Slit-lamp examination of the cornea reveals Kayser-Fleischer rings, brown copper deposits in Descemet membrane. B and C, Brain MRIs of a patient with Wilson disease shows bilateral, symmetric T2-hyperintensities in putamen, thalami, posterior limbs of the internal capsules (A). After 4 years of treatment, the hyperintense lesions markedly improved (B). (A, Reprinted with permission from Vodopivecl, McGrath E, Vaitkevicius H. Teaching NeuroImages: Ocular findings in a patient with Wilson disease and venous sinus thrombosis. *Neurology*. 2017;88(7):e55-e56. B and C, Reprinted with permission from Park HK, Lee JH, Lee MC, et al. Teaching NeuroImages: MRI reversal in Wilson disease with trientine treatment. *Neurology*. 2010;74(17):e72.)

QUESTIONS FOR SELF-STUDY

1. Why is it important to test for WD asymptomatic relatives of patients with WD?
2. Liver transplantation is the definitive treatment of liver cirrhosis due to WD and may prevent neurologic deterioration as well. Based on your understanding of the copper metabolic defect in WD, suggest an explanation of why a patient can discontinue chelation therapy after liver transplantation.

3. A 40-year-old man with WD is unable to tolerate chelation therapy and is started on zinc supplementation. After a few months of treatment, he develops limb paresthesias and unsteady gait. Examination shows spastic-ataxic gait and stocking-glove distribution of sensory loss. Serum B12 level is normal. Which cause of reversible myeloneuropathy should be considered? Explain the likely biochemical mechanism of myeloneuropathy in this patient.

4. A 50-year-old woman develops cognitive difficulties, ataxia, dystonia, and tremor. Serum ceruloplasmin is low. WD is suspected, but KFRs are absent, and 24-hour urine shows a normal level of copper. She also has microcytic anemia with low iron levels and high levels of serum ferritin. What is the likely unifying diagnosis?

5. A previously healthy 7-year-old child is referred to a neurologist with new-onset difficulty walking and concerns for "possible cerebral palsy." The neurologist recognizes dystonia as the cause of gait impairment. Why is this history not consistent with cerebral palsy? A trial of which medication should be attempted that may effectively treat dystonia in this child?

CHALLENGE

Which inherited neurologic diseases may be successfully treated with organ transplantation?

REFERENCES

Bandmann O, Weiss KH, Kaler SG. Wilson's disease and other neurological copper disorders. *Lancet Neurol.* 2015;14(1):103-113. [free online resource]

Ferenci P, Caca K, Loudianos G, et al. Diagnosis and phenotypic classification of Wilson disease. *Liver Int.* 2003;23(3):139-142.

43 Tardive Dystonia

Dystonia due to treatment with dopamine-receptor blocking agents

CORE FEATURES

1. Dystonia.
   Dystonia is defined as co-contraction of agonist and antagonist muscles resulting in abnormal movements, postures, or tremulousness.
2. Dystonia is often triggered by a voluntary movement.
3. Dystonia may be relieved by a sensory trick or simple movement (*geste antagoniste*).
4. History of exposure to dopamine-receptor blocking drugs (DRBs).
   TD usually emerges following years of treatment with typical, or, less commonly, atypical antipsychotic agents. Rarely, TD may be seen after a short exposure to DRBs used to treat gastrointestinal ailments (metoclopramide and prochlorperazine).
5. TD does not resolve upon discontinuation of DRB agents.
   Unlike most drug-related side effects, TD rarely fully resolves upon drug withdrawal and may even emerge after DRB is discontinued.

SYNOPSIS

Dystonia is caused by *simultaneous* or near-simultaneous co-contraction of agonist/antagonist muscles. Dystonia manifests as abnormal postures, twisting movements, or tremulousness ("dystonic tremor"), which may be difficult to differentiate from true rhythmic tremors resulting from *sequential* contractions of agonist and antagonist muscles. Dystonia may result from inherited disorders. More than 15 genes have been implicated in diseases in which dystonia is a predominant feature, and dozens of other inherited diseases feature dystonia as part of a complex neurologic phenotype. Dystonia may also be a consequence of perinatal or acquired brain injury; encephalitis; stroke or other structural brain lesions; medication use—either acutely or after prolonged therapy (tardive).

Chronic use of DRBs is associated with tardive dyskinesia, a form of chorea, manifesting as lip pursing, lip-smacking, tongue protrusion, and, less commonly, tardive dystonia (TD). TD often involves the face and neck (retrocollis) and may be difficult to distinguish clinically from genetic dystonias. Outcomes are better when TD is recognized early, and DRB is successfully withdrawn.

FIGURE

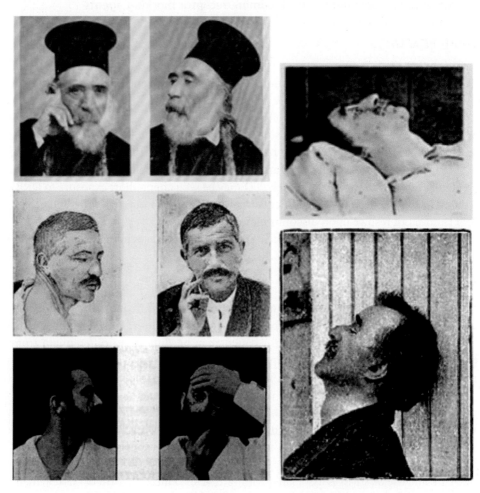

Illustrations of geste antagoniste in patients with inherited dystonia from cases presented by Brissaud in his 1894 Lesson. On the far right is a patient who tries to reduce torticollis by resting his head against a pillow or against the wall. (Reprinted with permission from Broussolle E, Laurencin C, Thobois S, et al. Early illustrations of geste antagoniste in cervical and generalized dystonia. *Tremor Other Hyperkinet Mov (N Y)*. 2015;5:332.)

QUESTIONS FOR SELF-STUDY

1. A 30-year-old woman presents to the emergency department (ED) with severe migraine and nausea. She receives a dose of intravenous metoclopramide and within a few minutes develops a bent-backward posture with rolling up of the eyes. She has difficulty speaking, but answers questions appropriately. What is the likely diagnosis and what medication(s) should be administered to abort these symptoms?
2. Describe the characteristic presentation of focal dystonia involving the eyelids; larynx; neck; arm; and hand.

3. A 60-year-old woman is started on olanzapine, an antipsychotic medication, "to help her sleep." She subsequently presents to the ED with fever, confusion, neck rigidity, and elevated serum CK levels. Assuming infectious causes have been excluded, what is the likely diagnosis? What is the optimal treatment of this condition?

4. A 50-year-old man who is on antipsychotics for bipolar disorder presents with new-onset facial and neck dystonia. What reversible cause of adult-onset dystonia in the adult must be excluded before making the diagnosis of TD?

5. A 25-year-old man with schizophrenia, on a stable regimen of risperidone, presents for evaluation of new-onset movement disorder. He appears restless, frequently getting up from the chair and continuously rocking back and forth. When asked to stay still, he is able to do so briefly, and then continues with the motions. What is the likely diagnosis? What can be done to lessen his urge to move without compromising the treatment of his schizophrenia?

CHALLENGE

Propose a plausible explanation as to the reasons blockade of dopamine receptors, which logically should lead to a hypokinetic disorder (parkinsonism), results in hyperkinetic tardive dystonia.

REFERENCES

Albanese A, Bhatia K, Bressman SB, et al. Phenomenology and classification of dystonia: a consensus update. *Mov Disord.* 2013;28(7):863-873.

Saifee TA, Edwards MJ. Tardive movement disorders: a practical approach. *Pract Neurol.* 2011;11(6):341-348. [free online resource]

44. Restless Legs Syndrome

A common condition characterized by episodic sensory tension relieved by movement

CORE FEATURES

1. Sensory discomfort or tension in the legs.
   Variably described as "crawling," "restless," "creeping," "pulling," and "itching," the sensation usually involves the legs but may spread to arms and trunk.
2. Irresistible urge to move ("akathisia").
   Akathisia arises in response to sensory tension but may occur without it.
3. Symptoms begin or worsen during a period of inactivity.
   Symptoms of restless legs syndrome (RLS) are worse in the evening hours, especially when trying to fall asleep and they may interfere with sleep. Symptoms usually resolve by early morning.
4. Moving or stretching the legs temporarily improves or relieves the symptoms.
5. Symptoms respond to dopamine agonist drugs.
   RLS may intensify after a period of successful treatment with dopaminergic drugs ("augmentation").

SYNOPSIS

RLS is among the most common neurologic disorders. About 10% of adults have symptoms of RLS. Prevalence increases with age and in patients with iron deficiency anemia, renal failure, pregnancy, and among those with a family history of RLS (heritability among twins is more than 50%). In severe RLS, which is uncommon, symptoms have a very detrimental effect on the quality of life because the movements disturb sleep and cause patients to avoid any activities requiring prolonged sitting. Other sleep problems frequently coexist: up to 90% of patients with RLS also exhibit periodic limb movements of sleep (PLMS). In PLMS, dorsiflexion of the big toes and ankles, and occasional flexion of the knees and hips occurs in trains of four or more during sleep. PLMS can be diagnosed with polysomnography that includes EMG of the anterior tibialis muscle.

The pathophysiology of RLS is unknown. Dysfunction of dopaminergic pathways and low levels of iron in basal ganglia and thalamus are likely contributing factors. All RLS patients should be screened for iron deficiency as patients with low ferritin respond well to iron supplementation and do not require long-term symptomatic therapy. Dopamine agonists, such as ropinirole, are highly effective in RLS, but the recognition that symptoms may intensify after a period of successful treatment ("augmentation") led some experts to recommend gabapentin and pregabalin as the first-line therapies.

FIGURE

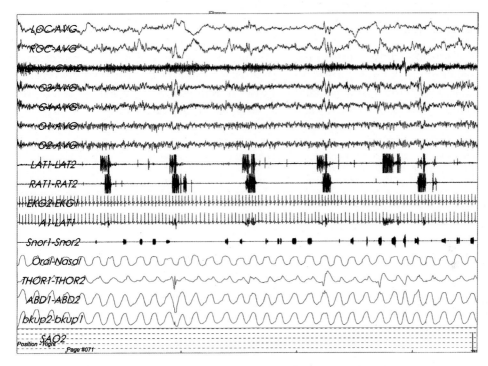

Polysomnogram shows a train of bilateral muscle contraction in the tibialis anterior muscles (LAT1 and RAT1 leads) consistent with periodic limb movements of sleep (PLMS). (Reprinted with permission from Geyer JD, Carney PR. *Atlas of Polysomnography*. 3rd ed. Philadelphia, PA: Wolters Kluwer; 2017:Figure 5.3.)

QUESTIONS FOR SELF-STUDY

1. A 90-year-old man with long-standing diabetes mellitus complains of unpleasant feelings in his legs. Which questions would you ask to determine whether his symptoms are likely due to RLS, diabetic neuropathy, arthritis, or cramps? (In practice, these common conditions often coexist.)

2. A 90-year-old woman with well-controlled RLS reports abrupt worsening of her symptoms. You review her medication history and note some changes compared to the last visit. Which prescription drug(s) or over-the-counter medications are known to exacerbate symptoms of RLS? If none of the medication changes can readily explain symptoms worsening, what laboratory testing should be ordered?

3. Which nonpharmacological therapies are beneficial in RLS?

4. A 70-year-old man is treated with ropinirole for RLS. He is requiring increasing doses to control his symptoms. During the doctor's visit, his wife reports changes in his personality: while normally frugal and taciturn, he lost thousands of dollars in a sports-betting website and made inappropriate comments to strangers. The patient's wife is concerned that he may be developing dementia as did his mother. What reversible cause of personality changes must be considered in this patient?

5. A 50-year-old man with a long-standing history of treated schizophrenia complaints that he cannot stop fidgeting. What is the most likely cause of these symptoms? What questions would you ask to try to distinguish this condition from RLS?

CHALLENGE

In hemochromatosis, serum and liver iron levels are elevated, but the iron concentration in the brain is normal. Suggest an explanation for this apparent discrepancy. Explain why iron supplementation in cases of RLS is effective when the serum iron concentration is low but not when the iron concentration is normal.

REFERENCES

Trenkwalder C, Allen R, Högl B, et al. Comorbidities, treatment, and pathophysiology in restless legs syndrome. *Lancet Neurol.* 2018;17(11):994-1005.

https://www.rls.org/. [free online resource]

Wijemanne S, Ondo W. Restless Legs Syndrome: clinical features, diagnosis and a practical approach to management. *Pract Neurol.* 2017;17(6):444-452. [free online resource]

45 Tourette Syndrome ▪️

Childhood-onset, hyperkinetic disorder characterized by motor and phonic tics

CORE FEATURES

1. Mean age of onset at 5 to 6 years of age.
   Symptoms tend to peak in prepubertal and early pubertal stages and subside by late adolescence. Most patients "grow out" of TS by the age of 18 years, but 30% will have persistence or reemergence of tics in adulthood.
2. Motor tics.
   Motor tics are "sudden, rapid, recurrent, nonrhythmic, stereotyped movements" (Diagnostic and Statistical Manual of Mental Disorders [DSM–5]). Earlier in the course of the disease, simple tics (blinking, squinting, pouting, etc) predominate, while more complex tics (touching, tapping, spinning, etc) tend to emerge later. Copying gestures of others (echopraxia) or obscene gestures (copropraxia) are examples of socially debilitating complex tics.
3. Phonic (or vocal) tics.
   Phonic tics are motor tics involving organs of phonation and articulation. They range from simple tics such as throat clearing or sniffing, to more complex ones—repeating one's own (palilalia) or others' (echolalia) words and phrases. Verbalizing obscenities, a form of vocal tics (coprolalia), occurs in up to 20% of patients with TS.
4. Premonitory urges prior to tics.
   A sensation of "discomfort," "tightness," "itchlike" sensation, often precedes the tics and is relieved by tics or movements. Tics can be briefly suppressed, but the urge to tic becomes difficult to control after a period of suppression. Tics tend to disappear during activities requiring sustained attention and motor control, such as playing a musical instrument.
5. Impaired attention and impulse control.
   Comorbid behavioral, psychiatric, and neurodevelopmental disorders occur in 90% of patients with TS. The most common comorbidity is attention deficit hyperactivity disorder (ADHD), followed by learning, obsessive-compulsive, and behavioral disorders. TS is also common in children with autistic spectrum disorder and global developmental delay.

SYNOPSIS

It is estimated that 20% to 30% of children exhibit tics at some point, but the persistence of motor and phonic tics for at least a year, as required for TS diagnosis, is seen in less than 1% of children, mostly in boys. Tics in TS may be difficult to distinguish from habits, stereotypies, or mannerisms, but there is evidence that TS is an organic movement disorder involving basal ganglia circuitry. Functional neuroimaging studies implicate dysfunction of basal ganglia-thalamocortical circuits in the genesis of TS. Disruptions in these circuits may impair the patient's ability to inhibit unwanted motor programs and may underlie the deficits in attention and impulse control that so frequently accompany TS. Tics respond to dopamine blocking or dopamine depleting agents (neuroleptics), which imply that TS is a hyperdopaminergic state. TS has a genetic component: first-degree siblings of a patient with TS have a 15-fold increased risk of tics.

FIGURE

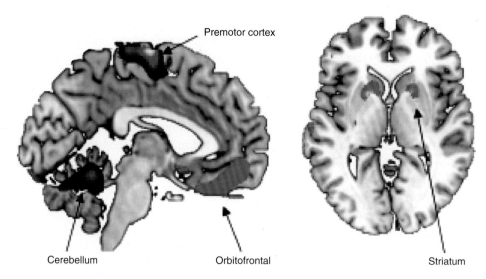

Metabolic pattern on FDG-PET scan in patients with Tourette syndrome (TS) shows increased premotor and cerebellar metabolism and decreased striatal and orbitofrontal metabolism compared to healthy controls. These findings suggest that symptoms of TS emerge through the abnormal activity of specific functional brain networks. (Reprinted with permission from Pourfar M, Feigin A, Tang CC, et al. Abnormal metabolic brain networks in Tourette syndrome. *Neurology.* 2011;76(11):944–952.)

QUESTIONS FOR SELF-STUDY

1. Which feature of muscle contraction is present in dystonia but absent in tics? Which sensory feature of tics is usually absent in dystonia? Do tics or dystonia persist during sleep?
2. Which subjective feature is present in complex tics (touching) but not compulsion (handwashing)?
3. What classes of medications have shown benefit in TS?
4. Given the frequent side effects of pharmacotherapy in children, medications are usually reserved for the more disabling cases of TS. As first line, various forms of cognitive behavioral therapy are recommended. Explain how premonitory urges can be harnessed to control tics with habit-reversal therapy.
5. TS is among the most heritable non-Mendelian disorders. Suggest a reason why efforts to identify a genetic basis of this disorder with whole-exome sequencing (WES) have largely failed. (Compare your answer with Marchuk DS, Crooks K, Strande N, et al. *PLoS One.* 2018;13(12):e0209185. [free online resource])

CHALLENGE

TS lies on the borderland between organic and functional movement disorders. How would you distinguish between the vocal and motor tics of TS from a functional tic disorder? (Compare your answer with Ganos C, Edwards MJ, Müller-Vahl K. "I swear it is Tourette's!": On functional coprolalia and other tic-like vocalizations. Psychiatry Res. 2016;246:821-826.)

REFERENCES

Cravedi E, Deniau E, Giannitelli M, Xavier J, Hartmann A, Cohen D. Tourette syndrome and other neurodevelopmental disorders: a comprehensive review. *Child Adolesc Psychiatry Ment Health*. 2017;11:59. [free online resource]

Jankovic J, Kurlan R. Tourette syndrome: evolving concepts. *Mov Disord*. 2011;26(6):1149-1156. [free online resource]

Robertson MM, Eapen V, Singer HS, et al. Gilles de la Tourette syndrome. *Nat Rev Dis Primers*. 2017;3:16097.

46 Functional Movement Disorders

Clinical syndromes defined by abnormal movements that are incongruent with any known neurologic cause

CORE FEATURES

1. Inconsistency of movements.
   Movements are often exaggerated during testing and abate when patients' attention is directed away from them or when patients are not observed.
2. Movements vary in type, amplitude, and frequency in a manner incongruent with organic movement disorders.
   For example, a tremor that varies in frequency and direction, or is "entrainable"—frequency changes to match the frequency of contralateral hand-tapping—is not seen with organic etiologies.
3. A pattern of gait that is incongruent with an organic neurologic disorder.
   "Acrobatic gait" with near falls and wild swaying requires a high degree of coordination, which is not compatible with the patient's complaint of loss of coordination. "Maladaptive gait" is when the patient drags the "weaker" leg behind him instead of circumducting it as would be expected in organic hemiparesis.
4. "Give-way weakness."
   The degree of weakness in confrontational testing is not commensurate with functional performance. For example, the patient is not able to lift their leg off the floor but is able to get up from a chair unassisted. Hoover sign takes advantage of the involuntary synergistic extension of the "paretic" leg when patients are asked to flex the unaffected contralateral leg against resistance, as shown on the figure below.
5. History of many medically unexplained symptoms.
   The patient undergoes multiple tests for a variety of nonspecific symptoms such as palpitations, nausea, abdominal pain, dyspepsia, menstrual and sexual dysfunction, and diffuse body aches. There may be a history of multiple surgeries without pathologic findings.

SYNOPSIS

Functional neurologic disorders (FNDs), of which roughly half are FMDs, account for as many as 15% of neurology outpatient visits. With a confusingly long list of symptoms and signs, and no laboratory or imaging findings to rely on, the diagnosis of FMD depends solely on the clinical acumen and experience of the evaluating physician. FMD is not a default diagnosis for any unusual condition that is not otherwise explained. As an example, genetically inherited dystonias were thought by many "too bizarre" to be an organic disorder until their genetic basis was discovered. Rather, the diagnosis of FMD depends on "positive" historical clues and examination findings that support such a diagnosis.

Because the abnormal movements in FMD appear very similar to voluntarily elicited movements, it has been postulated that patients produce symptoms via voluntarily motor pathways but are not fully aware that they are producing these movements. Consistent with this hypothesis is the finding of decreased functional connectivity between the right temporoparietal junction, which has been implicated in a sense of self-agency and sensorimotor regions (Maurer CW, La Faver, Ameli R, et al. *Neurology*. 2016;87(6):564-570).

The shift to neurologically grounded theories is a departure from historic conceptualization of conversion disorder as a reaction to psychological trauma. The current criteria of FND no longer require a history of psychologic trauma for diagnosis. Nevertheless, in a subset of patients with FND, psychological trauma likely is an important contributing factor and trauma therapy may sometimes be helpful or even curative. Other approaches includ specialized physiotherapy (using mirrors and video recording), cognitive behavioral therapy, and psychotherapy. The key prognostic factor is the patient's acceptance of the diagnosis of FND.

FIGURE

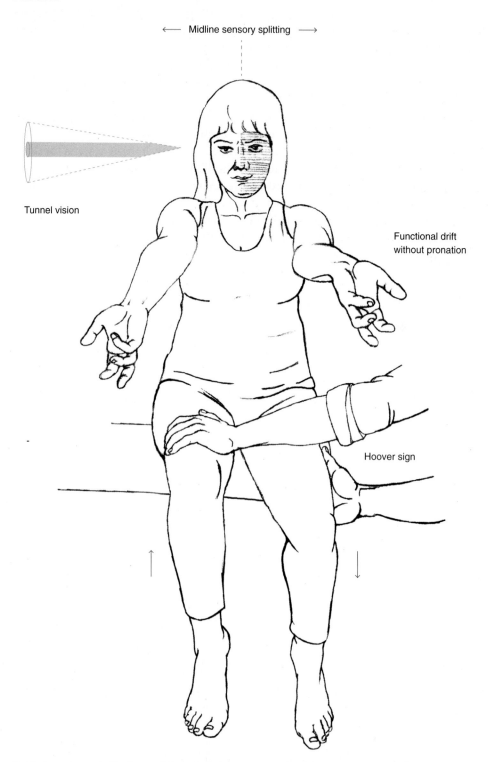

Typical nonorganic findings of functional neurologic disorder. In Hoover sign, there is forceful hip extension of the left "paretic" leg when patient is asked to flex the hip on the strong right side.

QUESTIONS FOR SELF-STUDY

1. It may sometimes be difficult to differentiate FND from fictitious disorders. What is the essential difference in the way the two conditions are defined?
2. Psychiatric comorbidities such as anxiety, depression, or psychoses are not more prevalent in FND than in organic neurologic conditions. However, patients with FND have more somatic dissociative symptoms. What questions would you ask to elicit a history of dissociative symptoms?
3. Bereitschaftspotential ("readiness potential"), detectable on electroencephalography (EEG), is generated by the supplementary motor area and precedes voluntary movement by 1 to 2 s. Explain how the presence or absence of Bereitschaftspotential can be used to differentiate functional from organic myoclonus of cortical origin.
4. Motor testing can be carried out under "make" or "break" conditions. In the "make" condition, the examiner keeps their arm steady and the patient is asked to push as hard as they can to overcome the examiner arm's resistance. In the break condition, the examiner pushes against the patient's limb until the examiner is able to overcome the patient's resistance. In neurologic paresis, the force generated in the two conditions is similar. Would you predict that a patient with FND performs better under "make" or "break" condition? (Compare van der Ploeg RJ, Oosterhuis HJ. *J Neurol Neurosurg Psychiatry*. 1991;54(3):248-251. [free online resource])
5. Approximately half of the patients with functional tremors report that their symptoms started abruptly, often following a putative trigger. Thus, the abrupt onset is an important clue to FMD. Which organic causes of tremors could also have abrupt onset?

CHALLENGE

Which functional neurological disorder can be diagnosed with a high degree of certainty using an objective test?

REFERENCES

Adams C, Anderson J, Madva EN, LaFrance WC Jr, Perez DL. You've made the diagnosis of functional neurological disorder: now what? *Pract Neurol*. 2018;18(4):323-330. [free online resource]

Edwards MJ, Bhatia KP. Functional (psychogenic) movement disorders: merging mind and brain. *Lancet Neurol*. 2012;11(3):250-260.

https://www.neurosymptoms.org/. [free online resource]

Disorders of Consciousness and Higher Cognitive Functions

A Very Brief Introduction to Disorders of Consciousness and Higher Cognitive Functions

The injury to the anterior part of the brain (frontal lobes) … does not damage a person's capacity to learn, perceive or remember… [yet] he is unable to form any lasting intentions, plan for the future, or determine the course of his behavior. He can only respond to signals he picks up from without… though his past remains intact, he is robbed of any possibility of the future…and loses precisely what makes a person human.

Alexander Luria*

The brain is composed of one hundred billion neurons and more than a hundred trillion synapses embedded in a matrix of over a hundred billion glial cells. It is supplied with a quarter gallon of oxygenated blood every minute via a network of 400 miles of capillaries. The brain is a delicate and high-maintenance organ that requires precisely adjusted homeostatic conditions for proper functioning. It is therefore unsurprising that a wide range of conditions—infections, electrolyte disturbances, dehydration, systemic illness, psychoactive substances, etc—can derail brain function and cause an acute confusional state (Chapter 47), otherwise known as delirium (Latin for "going off the furrow"). Even a relatively "minor" mechanical perturbation due to a head injury unaccompanied by any visible signs of brain damage belies a complex and long-ranging cascade of events—the release of excitatory neurotransmitters, the intracellular influx of calcium, hyperactivation of membrane pumps, glycolysis with increased lactate production, and impaired neuronal function. These changes manifest in a multiplicity of symptoms and a state of cerebral hypometabolism that can last for weeks and even longer (Concussion, Chapter 48). Brain dysfunction limited to a circumscribed, but strategically important area, can produce dramatic symptoms. A case in point is transient global amnesia (TGA, Chapter 49), which results from the disruption of hippocampal circuits that support the encoding of new memories ("anterograde amnesia"). Although TGA superficially resembles an acute confusional state, a careful mental status examination will show only memory deficits, while in delirium, there is marked inattention and multidomain cognitive deficits. Interestingly, anterograde amnesia may sometimes be seen after a concussion, suggesting hippocampal memory circuits are among the pathways that are disrupted in concussion.

Delirium, concussions, and TGA are acute and (usually) self-limited conditions. In contrast, dementias are chronic and progressive. Dementias cause a degree of cognitive decline that interferes with patients' social and occupational functions and, eventually, even the most overlearned daily activities. In the popular mind, dementia is synonymous with forgetfulness and memory loss. Indeed, Alzheimer disease (AD, Chapter 50), the best-known and most common form of dementia, is usually characterized by early and prominent amnesia. However, amnesia is not a presenting feature

---

*Alexander Romanovich Luria (1902-1977), a Russian-Jewish neuropsychologist and one of the fathers of modern neuropsychological assessment. His books include *The Frontal Lobes, Higher Cortical Function in Men,* and *The Neuropsychology of Memory.* The quotation in the epigraph is taken from a remarkable case history written by Luria, *The Man with a Shattered World. The history of a brain wound.*

of other dementias. Dementia with Lewy bodies (DLB, Chapter 51) typically presents with executive and visuospatial deficits, while memory is relatively spared early on. Frontotemporal dementia (FTD, Chapter 52) manifests with personality changes (behavioral variant) or language impairment (language variants). AD, DLB, and FTD are dementias associated with pathologic protein deposition (proteinopathies) that disrupt large-scale networks sustaining higher cognitive functions. Presenting symptoms depend on which of those circuits are affected first. However, not all dementias are "proteinopathies." Vascular dementia (Chapter 53) results from an array of cerebrovascular causes. The distinction between neurodegenerative and vascular etiologies is not as absolute as textbooks will suggest, and the majority of autopsied cases demonstrate pathologic protein deposition alongside vascular injury.

Dementias currently affect over 50 million people worldwide and cost more in healthcare expenditures than cancer and cardiovascular disease combined. The number of cases of dementia is expected to triple in the next decades due to an increase in life expectancy. Unfortunately, very few dementias are reversible. A potentially treatable etiology, normal pressure hydrocephalus (NPH), is discussed in Chapter 54. Other causes are listed in the table below. Though rare, these conditions must be considered before the diagnosis of an irreversible and incurable disease is made.

Potentially Treatable/Reversible Causes of Cognitive Decline

Endocrine	Organ Failure	Neoplastic	Vascular
Hypothyroidism and hyperthyroidism	Liver failure	Primary CNS lymphoma	Chronic subdural hematoma
Cushing disease	Heart failure	CNS neoplasms	Cerebral venous sinus thrombosis
Addison disease	Respiratory insufficiency	Metastatic brain disease	Dural arteriovenous fistula
Hyperparathyroidism		Neoplastic meningitis	Inflammatory cerebral amyloid angiopathy (CAA)
Infectious	**Toxic/metabolic**	**Autoimmune/ paraneoplastic**	**Miscellaneous**
HIV/AIDS	B12 deficiency	Autoimmune encephalitis	Seizures/TEA[a]
Neurosyphilis	Thiamine deficiency	Hashimoto encephalopathy	Wilson disease
Whipple disease	Alcohol abuse	Primary CNS angiitis	Head trauma
Lyme disease	Lead or other metal toxicity	Neurosarcoidosis	Normal pressure hydrocephalus
Brain abscess	Porphyria	Neuro-SLE[b]	Depression ("pseudodementia")
Chronic meningitis (tuberculous, cryptococcal, other fungal agents)	Psychoactive medications	Neuromorphea	

[a]TEA—transient epileptic amnesia.
[b]Systemic lupus erythematosus.

The section ends with Brain Death (Chapter 55). Brain death, the legal equivalent of death in Western countries, requires considerable neurologic skill for diagnosis.

REFERENCES

https://faculty.washington.edu/chudler/facts.html#brain. [free online resource]
https://www.who.int/en/news-room/fact-sheets/detail/dementia. [free online resource]

Delirium (Acute Confusional State)

An acute confusional state due to a variety of pathophysiologic stressors is especially prevalent among hospitalized and elderly patients

CORE FEATURES

1. Pathophysiologic stressor.
   Common stressors include infections, electrolyte imbalance, hypoxia, organ failure, myocardial infarction, pulmonary embolism, psychoactive medications, intoxications, withdrawal syndromes, surgery, burns, and dehydration.
2. Encephalopathy develops over hours to days.
   Symptoms may fluctuate throughout the day and are usually worse in the evening ("sundowning").
3. Altered level of arousal.
   Patients with *hyperactive* delirium are agitated and hypervigilant and may have visual hallucinations and delusions, while patients with *hypoactive* delirium are subdued, lethargic, uncooperative, and slow to respond.
4. Inattention.
   Patients are easily distractible, unable to follow a conversation, or carry out complex mental tasks.
5. Cognitive deficits across multiple domains.
   A mental status examination reveals deficits in language, memory, and visuospatial domains. These deficits represent a change from the patient's cognitive baseline.

SYNOPSIS

The "3A's" of delirium are **A**cute change in **A**rousal and **A**ttention. Because delirious patients may appear either hyper- or hypoaroused, and their ability to sustain attention fluctuates throughout the day, the diagnosis may be hidden on plain sight. Delirium is by far the most common acquired neuropsychiatric syndrome in hospital settings, yet it is estimated that two-thirds of delirium cases go unrecognized. Patients with preexisting dementia, the elderly and frail, and those who underwent a surgical procedure, are at the highest risk for experiencing delirium during hospitalization. The validated scales, such as the Confusion Assessment Method (CAM) Diagnostic Algorithm, facilitate accurate diagnosis and can be completed within minutes.

The cause of delirium is often evident from the medical context. Those without obvious cause must be screened for common infections, electrolyte imbalance, endocrine or vitamin deficiencies, and exposure to psychoactive medications and drugs of abuse. Select cases may require electroencephalography (EEG) (if subclinical seizures are suspected), magnetic resonance imaging (MRI) of the brain (to exclude a stroke or structural lesion), and lumbar puncture (to rule out central nervous system [CNS] infection or autoimmune encephalitis). The "3D's"—**D**ementia, **D**epression, and **D**elusional (psychotic) disorder—are well-known mimickers of delirium.

FIGURE

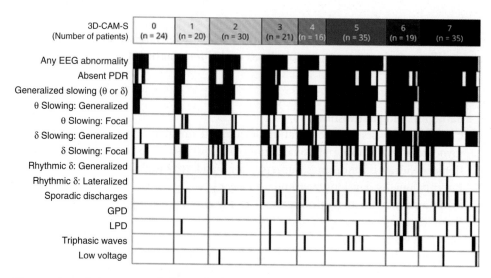

The number of electroencephalography (EEG) abnormalities (black cells) increases with higher delirium score. GPD, generalized periodic discharges; LPD, lateralized periodic discharges; PDR, posterior dominant rhythm. (Reprinted with permission from Kimchi EY, Neelagiri A, Whitt W, et al. Clinical EEG slowing correlates with delirium severity and predicts poor clinical outcomes. *Neurology.* 2019;93(13):e1260-e1271.)

QUESTIONS FOR SELF-STUDY

1. You are asked to evaluate a hospitalized 80-year-old man with altered mental status. On examination, he has occasional paraphasic errors and is unable to follow complex commands. Which questions on the mental status examination will help you differentiate delirium from aphasia in this patient?

2. Depressed patients may be inattentive and have psychomotor slowing. What historical clues—temporal profile, associated symptoms, or medical context—would favor the diagnosis of depression over hypoactive delirium?

3. Delirium may manifest with psychotic symptoms such as delusions and hallucinations. What is the main distinction between the type of hallucinations seen in psychotic disorders such as schizophrenia and those seen with delirium?

4. You are asked to evaluate a 90-year-old woman for "agitation." The patient is fidgeting, frequently getting up and down from a chair, and pacing the corridor. She denies being anxious or agitated. Her speech pattern is normal. She is oriented, is able to do serial 7's, spells "WORLD" backward, and scores a perfect score on Folstein Mini-Mental Examination. A review of medications shows that she was recently started on paroxetine for mild depression. Name the syndrome that can mimic agitation in this patient? What is the likely cause?

5. A 90-year-old confused woman is brought to the emergency department (ED) by her daughter. The patient was cognitively intact a day ago and complained of diarrhea. On examination, blood pressure is 100/60 mm Hg, the heart rate is 95 beats per minute. Temperature, pulse oximetry, and finger-stick glucose were within normal

limits. Mental status examination is consistent with hypoactive delirium. The BUN/creatinine ratio is 20:1. Otherwise, the electrolyte profile is normal. Infectious workup is negative. What is the probable cause of delirium? What test could help confirm your clinical suspicion? What is the treatment?

CHALLENGE

You are tasked with designing a program to decrease rates of delirium at your hospital. What interventions would you implement for at-risk patients? (Compare your answers with the NICE guidelines cited below.)

REFERENCES

Inouye SK. Westendorp RG, Saczynski JS. Delirium in elderly people. *Lancet.* 2014;383(9920):911-922. [free online resource]

https://www.nice.org.uk/guidance/cg103. [free online resource]

48 Concussion (Mild Traumatic Brain Injury)

A neurocognitive syndrome following a mild traumatic brain injury

CORE FEATURES

1. History of head injury.
   Head injury may be direct (blow to the head, blast injury) or indirect (whiplash).
2. Symptoms start on impact and evolve within minutes to hours.
   Upon impact, patients commonly experience "seeing stars," or, less commonly, brief loss of consciousness or a generalized seizure. More severe concussions may be associated with loss of memory for the period following injury—"anterograde amnesia," and sometimes even preceding injury—"retrograde amnesia."
3. Polysymptomatic presentation.
   Symptoms fall into several categories: somatic (headache is the most common, often with increased sensitivity to light and sounds); cognitive ("brain fog"); affective (irritability/lability); vestibular (dizziness, unsteadiness); visual (blurry vision); and sleep (sleep/wake cycle disturbance).
4. Symptoms resolve within days to weeks.
   In 10% to 15% of cases, symptoms may last for a year or longer.
5. No findings on noncontrast brain MRI or head CT.
   Abnormal findings such as skull fractures; epidural, subdural, subarachnoid or intraparenchymal bleeding; and brain swelling indicate a more severe form of traumatic brain injury (TBI). Neuroimaging is not required for the evaluation of concussion unless there are "red flags" (patient difficult to arouse; focal neurologic deficits; repeated vomiting; abnormal behavior).

SYNOPSIS

Concussion lies on the mild end of the spectrum of TBI but is perceived as quite disabling by the patient. By definition, the neurologic examination after a concussion is normal and the patient has a "perfect score" on the Glasgow Coma Scale (https://www.cdc.gov/masstrauma/resources/gcs.pdf. [free online resource]). Obtaining a head computed tomography (CT) on everyone with head trauma and neurologic symptoms will needlessly expose millions of patients to radiation and waste medical resources. The preferred approach is to stratify the need for neuroimaging studies based on the presence or absence of worrisome symptoms using validated assessment tools such as the Post-Concussion Symptom Scale. Guidelines on managing concussion for the medical professionals and laypeople—parents, coaches are available: https://www.cdc.gov/headsup/. [free online resource]

FIGURE

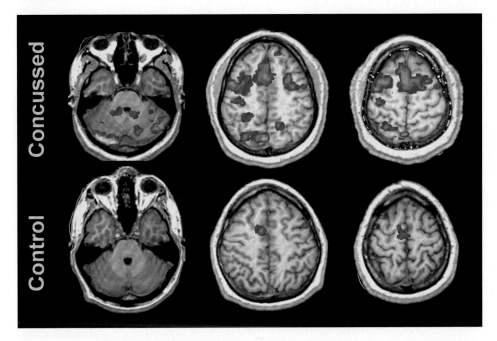

The concussed subject (upper panel) had significantly greater activation in cortical and subcortical regions a week after concussion compared to the control player (lower panel). (Courtesy of Kelly J. Jantzen, MD. In: Gean AD. *Brain Injury: Applications from War and Terrorism*. Philadelphia, PA: Wolters Kluwer Health/Lippincott Williams & Wilkins; 2014:Figure 5.25.)

QUESTIONS FOR SELF-STUDY

1. What are the critical elements of general and neurologic examination in a patient who sustained a head injury?
2. From this list of symptoms and clinical criteria, check off the ones that suggest a need for neuroimaging after concussion:

Age <2 y
Age 16-65 y
Amnesia for events shortly following a head injury
Difficulty sleeping in the days following the injury
Recurrent vomiting
Generalized seizure several hours after injury
Irritability
Mild headache
Receiving anticoagulants
Persistent drowsiness, difficulty waking up
Progressively worsening headache in the hours following the injury
Injury while intoxicated
Focal neurologic deficits (pupillary asymmetry, difficulty speaking or moving part of the body)
Evidence of basal skull fracture: bruising over mastoid (Battle sign), bruising under the eyes ("Raccoon eyes"), leakage of cerebrospinal fluid (CSF) from ears (otorrhea) or from the nose (rhinorrhea)

Compare your response with https://braininjuryguidelines.org/concussion/fileadmin/media/adult-concussion-guidelines-3rd-edition.pdf. [free online resource]

3. A 60-year-old man who sustained a fall on his face a few weeks previously reports new-onset positional headache that is worse on getting up. He has a persistent clear nasal discharge from the left nostril. The ED physician suspects a CSF leak. What imaging and laboratory testing should be carried out to test this hypothesis?

4. A 15-year-old boy fell off the bicycle and hit his head. He was not wearing a helmet. He has a large scalp hematoma, but no evidence of skull fracture. After 2 hours of observation in the ED, he reports a mild headache. Neurologic examination is normal. The decision is made to discharge him home with his parents. Which symptoms should his parents be instructed to monitor the child for which should prompt a return to the ED? (Compare your answers with CDC guidelines https://www.cdc.gov/headsup/providers/discharge-materials.html. [free online resource])

5. An 80-year-old woman is brought to the ED after a motor vehicle accident. Initially, she complains of severe neck and head pain but is lucid and has a normal neurologic examination. Within 2 hours, she becomes drowsy, dosing off in the middle of a conversation, and has less spontaneous movement on the right side. What is the most important diagnosis to consider that may explain the worsening mental status? Which testing must be urgently requested? If a noncontrast head CT is normal, what diagnosis may best explain the new onset of drowsiness and hemiparesis? What additional testing is required?

CHALLENGE

An interesting question is: what accounts for the loss of consciousness in mild TBI? The anatomical substrate of wakefulness is the ascending reticular activating system (ARAS), a loose network of nuclei within the pontomesencephalic tegmentum with projections to the thalami and cerebral cortex. Loss of consciousness typically occurs when there is insufficient oxygen or glucose to maintain cerebral function, as in syncope; when there is diffuse bihemispheric dysfunction, as in generalized seizures or drug effect; or if there is structural damage to the ARAS, as in pontine hemorrhages. Propose a mechanism that could explain the loss of consciousness in concussion. (Compare your answer with Chancellor SE, Franz ES, Minaeva OV, Goldstein LE. *Semin Pediatr Neurol.* 2019;30:14-25.)

REFERENCES

Dwyer B, Katz DI. Postconcussion syndrome. *Handb Clin Neurol.* 2018;158:163-178.
McCrory P, Meeuwisse W, Dvořák J, et al. Consensus statement on concussion in sport-the 5th international conference on concussion in sport held in Berlin, October 2016. *Br J Sports Med.* 2017;51(11):838-847. [free online resource]

49 Transient Global Amnesia

A syndrome of transient anterograde memory loss

CORE FEATURES

1. Acute onset of symptoms.
   Symptoms develop within minutes.
2. Dense anterograde amnesia.
   Anterograde (Latin for "going forward") amnesia—inability to encode new memories after symptom onset—is the defining feature of this condition. Some degree of retrograde (Latin for "going backward") amnesia—loss of memories acquired prior to symptom onset—may be present as well.
3. Only explicit memory is impaired, while implicit (procedural) memory and working (immediate term) memory remain intact.
   Nonmemory cognitive domains such as language, perception, general intelligence, and praxis are also intact.
4. The typical duration of amnesia is 4 to 6 hours.
   Patients may have no memory of the TGA episode. There are usually no long-term cognitive sequelae.
5. Punctate areas of diffusion restriction in one or both hippocampi.
   These characteristic MRI lesions typically appear 1 to 3 days after symptom onset and resolve within 2 weeks. The T2-weighted sequence may show a corresponding hyperintense signal within the hippocampus.

SYNOPSIS

TGA is a clinical diagnosis. A typical scenario involves a previously healthy, middle-age or older individual who suddenly appears to be "stuck in time" and unable to retain new information for more than a few minutes. Patients appear confused, repeatedly asking where they were and yet can speak, read, and write fluently; carry out arithmetic calculations; copy complex figures; and perform well on every cognitive task except for the tests of episodic memory. MRI of the brain is not required for diagnosis, but if obtained, it should be scrutinized for a lesion in the CA1 region of the hippocampus, which is highly characteristic of TGA. This MRI finding confirms the exquisitely localizing nature of this syndrome. Intriguingly, TGA is frequently triggered by physical stressors, such as immersion in cold water and strenuous exercise, or emotional stressors, blurring the boundary between psychology and neurology.

Rarely, a patient with a TGA-like presentation may have seizures involving memory circuits. This syndrome, termed transient epileptic amnesia (TEA), can generally be distinguished from TGA by its recurrent nature, shorter duration, associated epileptic features (olfactory or gustatory hallucinations, automatisms, staring spells), and response to antiseizure medications. TEA is very rare but important to recognize as it is one of the few causes of reversible memory loss.

FIGURE

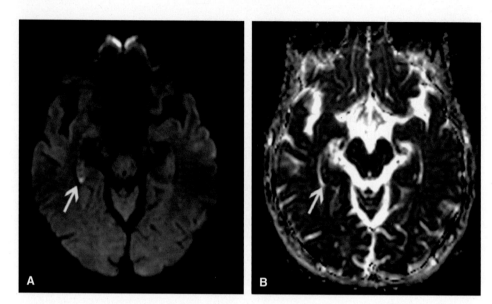

MRI of a 71-year-old man with TGA shows a small focus of restricted diffusion in the lateral portion of the right hippocampus (A, Diffusion-weighted imaging [DWI], arrow) and (B, Apparent diffusion coefficient [ADC] images, arrow). (Reprinted with permission from Cuello Oderiz C, Miñarro D, Dardik D, et al. Teaching NeuroImages: hippocampal foci of restricted diffusion in transient global amnesia. *Neurology*. 2015;85(20):e145.)

QUESTIONS FOR SELF-STUDY

1. A patient with TGA is able to remember and repeat seven digits of a phone number, but a minute later, he is unable to remember ever being asked to remember the digits. What does this observation teach us about the role of the hippocampus in immediate (working) memory and short-term (episodic) memory?

2. To a casual observer, a patient with TGA and a patient with delirium may appear similarly confused. What tests on mental status examination differentiate TGA from delirium?

3. An 18-year-old previously healthy woman was found by the police wandering in a park. She appears confused and is unable to state her name, her address, or current date but speaks in full sentences and follows simple commands. Immediate recall is 0/3 words. What features are highly atypical for TGA? What diagnosis does the inability to state one's name suggest? Which disorders should be considered on the differential diagnosis?

4. An 80-year-old man is brought to a neurologist for evaluation of memory loss. On testing, he has anterograde amnesia and a right homonymous quadrantanopsia. Assuming that a single lesion is responsible for both of these findings, which neighboring structures may be affected to yield this clinical picture? (For extra credit provide an alternative localization for this combination of symptoms.)

5. One of the most studied patients in the history of neurology—and possibly all of medicine—was H.M. As a young man, H.M. had undergone bilateral temporal lobectomies to control his seizures, which left him with life-long anterograde amnesia. Yet, he was able to learn complex new motor tasks. Explain in neuroanatomic terms, why the surgery led to the loss of declarative (conscious) memory while leaving intact nondeclarative (unconscious) memory.

CHALLENGE

A seemingly paradoxical feature of retrograde memory loss in TGA, head trauma, electroconvulsive therapy, and Alzheimer disease is that the more distant memories tend to be remembered better than the more recent memories. This phenomenon is known as the "Ribot gradient." Suggest an explanation for the Ribot gradient. (Compare your response with "the standard model of systems consolidation.")

REFERENCES

Arena J, Rabinstein A. Transient global amnesia. *Mayo Clin Proc.* 2015;90(2):264-272. [free online resource]
Bartsch T, Butler C. Transient amnesic syndromes. *Nat Rev Neurol.* 2013;9:86-97.

50 Alzheimer Disease

Dementia associated with deposition of β-amyloid plaques and neurofibrillary tau tangles

CORE FEATURES

1. Onset usually after 70 years of age; prevalence increases with age.
   Alzheimer disease (AD) affects 3% of people younger than 74 years, 17% of people aged 75 to 84 years, and 32% of people aged 85 years or older.
2. The ability to learn and retain new information is impaired early.
   AD is a predominantly amnestic syndrome, but several rare nonamnestic variants are also recognized: posterior cortical atrophy (visual-special deficits, apraxia), logopenic (primary progressive aphasia), and frontal (progressive apathy, behavioral disinhibition).
3. Symptoms evolve slowly over the course of years.
   Patients with AD live for 3 to 11 years after diagnosis, and some survive even longer.
4. Pathologic deposition of amyloid in the brain.
   Amyloid deposition can be measured *in vivo* with amyloid ligand–based positron emittion tomography (PET) scan and level of $A\beta_{1-42}$ in CSF. It is important not to overinterpret these findings as half of the people aged 85 years or older with no cognitive impairment have "abnormal" amyloid PET scan and $A\beta_{1-42}$ CSF level.
5. Pathologic deposition of phosphorylated tau in the brain.
   Phosphorylated tau (P-tau) is a marker of the intracellular neurofibrillary tangles, which, together with the extracellular amyloid plaques, constitute the "biologic signature of AD." P-tau deposition in the brain correlates with tau ligand–binding on PET and CSF P-tau levels.

SYNOPSIS

It may appear strange that a disease as prevalent as AD, the most common cause of dementia, was not named until the 20th century. This late recognition becomes more understandable if we bear in mind that extracellular β-amyloid plaques and intracellular neurofibrillary hyperphosphorylated tau tangles could only be appreciated with the advent of modern microscopy and specialized staining techniques. These neuropathologic findings were first described by Alois Alzheimer and still define the disease that bears his name. Recently, it became possible to quantitate amyloid and tau pathology in living persons using CSF assays and ligands-based positron emission tomography (PET) imaging.

AD starts insidiously and progresses slowly but inexorably. The sequential deposition of tau in the brain ("Braak staging") correlates with clinical and radiologic disease progression: tau deposition is first detected in the medial temporal and parietal lobes (early memory impairment; hippocampal and precuneus atrophy), then spreads to limbic regions and throughout the neocortex (global cognitive decline). Pathologic deposition of amyloid can be detected more than a decade before clinical symptoms develop. Acetylcholinesterase (AChE) inhibitors and memantine (NMDA receptor antagonist) modestly delay disease progression. Conversely, medications that have high "anticholinergic index"—anticholinergics, antipsychotics, antihistamines, and others—(https://www.health.harvard.edu/newsletter_article/anticholinergic-cognitive-burden-scale [free online resource]), worsen cognitive symptoms and should be avoided in AD whenever possible. Comprehensive guidelines on AD management are available in the NICE reference cited below.

FIGURES

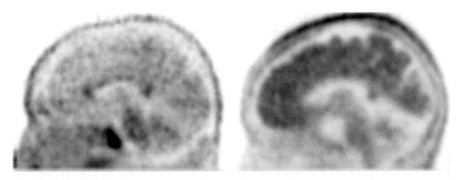

F-18 Flobetapil (Amyvid) scan of a healthy control (left) and patient with Alzheimer disease (right). There is a marked increase in amyloid plaques in the patient. (Courtesy of Robert Wagner, MD, Director of Nuclear Medicine, Loyola University Chicago, Stritch School of Medicine.)

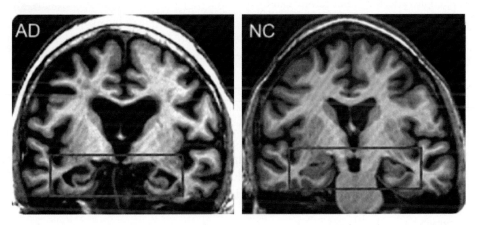

Medial temporal lobe atrophy is evident in Alzheimer diease (AD) (red rectangle) and is compared to normal medial temporal lobe volume in normal control (NC). (Reprinted with permission from Dr. Val Lowe, Mayo Clinic, Rochester, MN. In: McKeith IG, Boeve BF, Dickson DW, et al. Diagnosis and management of dementia with Lewy bodies: fourth consensus report of the DLB Consortium. *Neurology*. 2017;89(1):88-100.)

QUESTIONS FOR SELF-STUDY

1. Memory can be divided into encoding, storage, and retrieval functions. In free recall, patients are asked to memorize several words and repeat them after a few minute delay. Free recall is impaired if any of the memory functions are impaired. In cued

recall, patients are given a cue with each word and offered the cue to trigger their memories if they are unable to remember the word after a few minute delay. The cue facilitates the encoding of memory formation. In patients with AD and non-AD dementia who perform similarly poorly on free recall task, what would you predict their performance on cued recall to be—better or same as on free recall? Why?

2. In a small percentage of AD patients, AD is an autosomal-dominant disorder. What are some of the genes associated with early-onset autosomal dominant AD? Does the discovery of the genetic form of AD support the "amyloid theory" of AD pathogenesis or the "tau theory"?

3. A 75-year-old woman with mild AD develops confusion and visual hallucinations over the course of several days. Explain why these changes are not consistent with the evolution of AD. What questions would you ask and what testing would order to elucidate the etiology of her symptoms?

4. An 85-year-old man is brought by family members with concern for early dementia. The patient complains of poor memory. He has become more reclusive, rarely engages in conversation, and spends most of the day sleeping. He scores 28/30 on the Mini-Mental Status Examination (MMSE). Neurologic examination is otherwise unremarkable. The expanded dementia workup—brain MRI, screen for metabolic, endocrine, vitamin deficiencies, substance abuse testing and CSF studies for autoimmune encephalopathies, chronic infections, and amyloid and tau markers—is within normal limits. What potentially reversible cause of the patient's symptoms needs to be considered?

5. Even advanced AD pathology can be detected on a postmortem of individuals with no history of cognitive impairment. Explain the discrepancy between normal cognition and neuropathologic findings consistent with AD. Propose an explanation for why the risk of AD is higher among illiterate people.

CHALLENGE

There is a school of thought that AD should be defined not as a clinical syndrome of multidomain amnestic dementia but by the presence of the AD biomarkers. The advantage of this approach is that it focuses on AD-specific biologic mechanisms rather than the nonspecific clinical signs and symptoms. What are some of the drawbacks of defining disease in terms of biomarkers? (Compare your responses with McCleery J, et al. *Age Aging.* 2019;48(2):174-177. [free online resource])

REFERENCES

Dubois B, Feldman HH, Jacova C, et al. Advancing research diagnostic criteria for Alzheimer's disease: the IWG-2 criteria. *Lancet Neurol.* 2014;13(6):614-629.
https://www.alz.org/media/Documents/facts-and-figures-2018-r.pdf. [free online resource]
https://www.nice.org.uk/guidance/ng97/chapter/Recommendations. [free online resource]

51 | Dementia with Lewy Bodies

Dementia associated with parkinsonism and intraneuronal deposition of α-synuclein protein ("Lewy bodies")

CORE FEATURES

1. Executive dysfunction early on in the course.
   Attention and visuospatial domains are also affected early, while memory and language impairment are later manifestations.
2. Fluctuating levels of alertness.
   Abrupt onset of disorganized speech or behavior, inattention, altered consciousness ("zoning out," unresponsiveness) may be mistaken for delirium or syncope.
3. Visual hallucinations and illusions.
   Visual hallucinations, mostly of people and animals, occur in 80% of patients with early Dementia with Lewy Bodies (DLB). In contrast, visual hallucinations are uncommon in AD, though may be present in the advanced stage.
4. Parkinsonism.
   Parkinsonian features develop in approximately 85% of patients with DLB but are usually less severe than in Parkinson disease (PD).
5. Rapid eye movement sleep behavior disorder (RBD).
   RBD is a harbinger of synucleinopathies such as DLB or PD and may precede cognitive and motor manifestations by many years. In a patient with dementia, REM sleep without atonia on polysomnography, even without clinically overt RBD, supports the diagnosis of DLB.

SYNOPSIS

Clinical symptoms of DLB and AD overlap. Pathologically, most patients with DLB have amyloid plaques, while about half of patients with AD have synuclein deposition. However, for didactic purposes, it is helpful to highlight the contrasts between these two disorders. DLB presents with executive, visuospatial deficits and visual hallucinations. Correspondingly, there is occipital and posterior temporoparietal hypometabolism on fluorodeoxyglucose PET (FDG PET). Unlike AD, memory is relatively spared, and medial temporal lobes metabolism is relatively normal. DLB is a "synucleinopathy" characterized by α-synuclein inclusions, ("Lewy bodies"), within neurons of the cerebral cortex, brainstem, and substantia nigra. In contrast, AD is a "tauopathy." All synucleinopathies—PD, MSA, DLB—manifest parkinsonian features. When parkinsonian symptoms are subtle or absent, dopamine transporter imaging (DaT-SCAN) may be helpful diagnostically. DAT uptake in the basal ganglia is reduced in synucleinopathies but not in the other dementias. In DLB, as in AD, there is also loss of acetylcholine neurons, and patients with both dementias benefit from cholinesterase inhibitors.

FIGURE

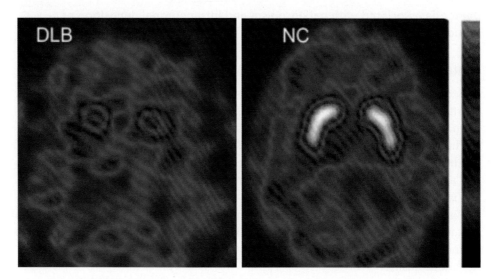

^{123}Iodine FP-CIT SPECT images in dementia with Lewy bodies (DLB) and normal controls (NC). There is minimal uptake in cases of DLB, which is restricted to the caudate ("period" or "full-stop" appearance) compared to the robust uptake in the caudate and putamen in NC ("comma" appearance). (Reprinted with permission from McKeith IG, Boeve BF, Dickson DW, et al. Diagnosis and management of dementia with Lewy bodies: fourth consensus report of the DLB consortium. *Neurology.* 2017;89(1):88-100.)

QUESTIONS FOR SELF-STUDY

1. What questions could you ask to elicit symptoms of executive and visuospatial deficits? Which tests best assess these cognitive domains?
2. Cognitive impairment is common in PD, and parkinsonism is common in DLB. What criteria are used to differentiate one synucleinopathy from the other?
3. A 70-year-old man diagnosed with AD has difficulty falling asleep. The treating physician prescribes a low dose of haloperidol. After a single dose, the patient becomes severely confused and has florid visual hallucinations. Which dementia is most consistent with this history? What is the pathophysiologic reason for the violent reaction to this antidopaminergic medication?
4. A 65-year-old cognitively intact woman with early parkinsonism is started on a dopamine agonist. Toward the end of the titration period, she becomes confused and has visual hallucinations. What is the most likely explanation?
5. A 40-year-old woman develops cognitive deficits, visual hallucinations, dystonia, and rigidity over a 2-month period. Which features argue against the diagnosis of DLB? What are the most likely etiologies? What ancillary testing should be carried out?

CHALLENGE

The perennial debate between "lumpers" and "splitters" plays itself out in connection to the two most common synucleinopathies—PD and DLB. Should these two clinically distinct disorders with similar underlying pathophysiology be considered as two ends of a spectrum or split into two separate categories? Present arguments for and against each position. (Compare your response with the dueling viewpoints presented by Berg D, et al. *Mov Disord*. 2014;29(4):454-462 and Boeve BF, et al. *Mov Disord*. 2016;31(11):1619-1622. [free online resource])

REFERENCES

Gomperts SN. Lewy body dementias: dementia with Lewy bodies and Parkinson disease dementia. *Continuum (Minneap Minn)*. 2016;22(2 Dementia):435-463. [free online resource]

McKeith IG, Boeve BF, Dickson DW, et al. Diagnosis and management of dementia with Lewy bodies: fourth consensus report of the DLB Consortium. *Neurology*. 2017;89(1):88-100. [free online resource]

52   Frontotemporal Dementia

Frontotemporal dementia, or frontotemporal lobar degeneration (FTLD), is a group of neurodegenerative diseases defined by deterioration in behavior, executive function, and language

CORE FEATURES

1. Peak age of onset, between ages 45 and 65 years.
2. Progressive deterioration in social behavior or language skills.
   Three main variants of FTD are recognized. The behavioral variant is the most common phenotype. It is characterized by early personality changes, behavioral disinhibition, socially inappropriate behavior, lack of empathy, selfishness, neglect of personal care, stereotypies, and compulsive behaviors. Primary progressive aphasia, a less common variant, is characterized by early deficits in language comprehension, production, and grammar. The semantic variant is characterized by impaired naming and comprehension but normal fluency and grammar.
3. No history of psychiatric disorder.
   This requirement may be difficult to ascertain as psychiatric disorders can mimic FTD. Compulsive behaviors of FTD may be misdiagnosed as an obsessive-compulsive disorder (OCD). Lack of sociability and personal hygiene may be mistaken for depression. Delusions and euphoria may be misdiagnosed as bipolar or psychotic disorder. Personality changes may be confused with narcissistic or schizoid personality disorder.
4. Family history of FTD.
   Family history is present in 40% of patients.
5. Frontotemporal atrophy on MRI.
   The frontal lobes, anterior temporal lobes, anterior cingulate cortex, and the insular cortex may be involved. The specific pattern of atrophy correlates with disease variants.

SYNOPSIS

Unlike AD and DLB, which are defined pathologically by abnormal accumulation of a specific protein, FTD is a group of clinical syndromes associated with several different proteins. The variants of FTD show considerable clinical overlap among each other and may overlap with atypical parkinsonian syndromes and motor neuron disease. The course of FTD is relentlessly progressive with an average life expectancy of 7 years. Information on symptomatic treatments and supportive advice are available through patient support organizations (https://ecdc.org.au/ftd-toolkit [free online resource]).

FTD is more likely than AD and DLB to run in families, but one needs to inquire not only about FTD diagnoses in relatives, but any dementia and psychiatric disorder. Certain pathological mutations—such as hexanucleotide expansion in C9orf72 gene, which causes a behavioral variant of FTD—predispose relatives of a proband to psychotic disorders. This example illustrates the artificiality of the distinction between psychiatric and neurologic diseases.

FIGURE

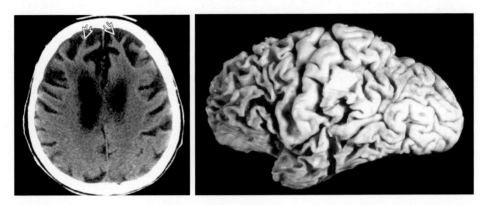

Frontal atrophy on CT head in a patient with FTD (arrowheads). The postmortem from a different patient shows "knife-edge" atrophy of the frontal and temporal lobes. (Courtesy of Dr. José Biller.)

QUESTIONS FOR SELF-STUDY

1. Brain MRI of a patient with FTD shows mainly right-sided temporal atrophy. Which of the three variants of FTD is more likely in this patient?

2. Age of onset younger than 65 years and early language deficits are atypical for AD but do not exclude this diagnosis. How can you differentiate AD from FTD in a patient with young-onset dementia and language deficits?

3. Psychologist Endel Tulving proposed a distinction between "episodic memory" that is linked to personal experience ("did you go biking this morning?") and semantic memory, which refers to impersonal knowledge of the world ("what is a bicycle?"). Episodic and semantic memory are forms of declarative (conscious) memory. There is also a nondeclarative (unconscious) form of memory (motor memory of riding a bicycle). Explain why the current classification of dementias, which differentiates AD from FTD, supports Tuvling's distinction between semantic and episodic memory.

4. A 60-year-old man with the behavioral variant of FTD develops muscle atrophy and weakness. Examination shows upper and lower motor neuron signs. What is the likely explanation? Where would you expect to see brain atrophy on his brain MRI?

5. A 65-year-old woman with FTD complains that her left hand is involuntarily grabbing objects. She needs to use the right hand to undo the unwanted actions of the left hand. What is the name of this phenomenon? What is its anatomic basis? In what other conditions can this phenomenon be seen?

CHALLENGE

Presence of the *C9orf72* mutation, the most common mutation associated with FTD, correlates with prominent somatic delusions. How would you "connect the dots" between a specific protein mutation and a specific clinical phenotype? (Compare your answer with Sivasathiaseelan et al, cited below.)

REFERENCES

Bang J, Spina S, Miller BL. Frontotemporal dementia. *Lancet.* 2015;386(10004):1672-1682. [free online resource]
Sivasathiaseelan H, Marshall CR, Agustus JL, et al. Frontotemporal dementia: a clinical review. *Semin Neurol.* 2019;39(2):251-263.

53 Vascular Dementia

■▬

Dementia due to an array of cerebrovascular disorders

CORE FEATURES

1. Early impairment in attention, information processing, and executive function.
   Symptoms are largely attributable to the disruption of frontostriatal circuits.
2. Personality changes.
   Lack of initiative, apathy, and depression are common.
3. Stepwise rather than insidious onset and stepwise rather than gradual progression are characteristic of vascular dementia (VaD).
   The onset of cognitive impairment may follow a stroke.
4. Corticospinal and corticobulbar signs.
   These include hemiparesis, dysarthria, pathologic hyperreflexia, Babinski sign, and gait impairment (hemiparetic gait or "frontal" gait—short-stepped and wide-based).
5. Stigmata of chronic cerebrovascular disease on brain MRI or head CT.
   Diagnosis of VaD requires a sufficient burden of cerebrovascular disease that can plausibly account for cognitive impairment—usually, one-third or more or subcortical white matter is affected.

SYNOPSIS

Broadly speaking, VaD can be described as "subcortical" dementia characterized by slowed processing speed, inattention and prominent early executive dysfunction, and personality changes, while AD is "cortical" dementia in which amnesia is followed by other A's of Aphasia, Apraxia, and Agnosia. Unlike the items on a supermarket shelf that are individually labeled, dementias are often difficult to assign a diagnostic label. Their symptoms are overlapping, and clinical-pathologic mismatch is common. In some series, more than 20% of patients diagnosed with AD had non-AD pathology on autopsy. Conversely, amyloid markers have been found in one-third of VaD cases. This observation may explain why cholinesterase inhibitors have been found beneficial in VaD. Despite the overlap, the distinction between vascular and neurodegenerative dementias is especially important for clinical research, since the experimental therapies are designed to target specific disease mechanisms. The mechanisms underlying VaD are vascular—large-artery atherosclerosis, small-vessel disease, arteriolosclerosis, cerebral microbleeds, superficial CNS siderosis, infarcts, and microinfarcts. The mainstay of management is the prevention of new strokes.

FIGURES

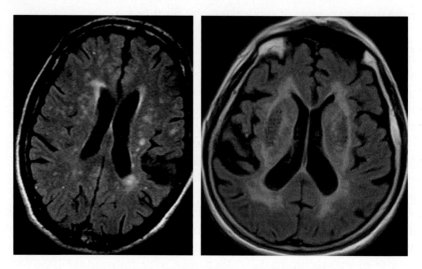

Brain MRI in patients with moderate (left) and severe (right) vascular dementia.

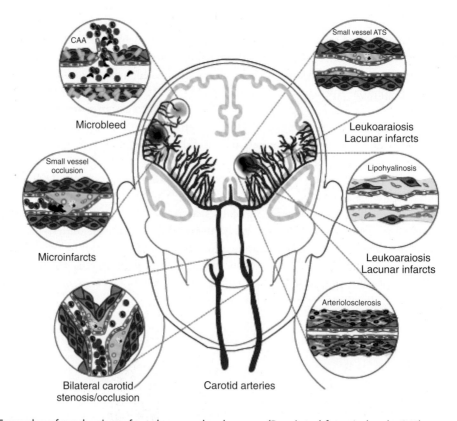

Examples of mechanism of cerebrovascular damage. (Reprinted from Iadecola C. The pathobiology of vascular dementia. *Neuron*. 2013;80(4):844-866. Copyright © 2013 Elsevier. With permission.)

QUESTIONS FOR SELF-STUDY

1. Explain why the Folstein Mini-Mental Status Examination (MMSE), a widely used screening tool for AD, is not sensitive for diagnosing VaD?
2. Because VaD involves frontal subcortical white matter, "frontal release signs" may be elicited on examination. Name some of the frontal release signs and describe how you would test for them.
3. A 50-year-old woman comes for an evaluation following a stroke. Her medical history is noteworthy for frequent migraines with aura. She has no vascular risk factors. Brain MRI shows a small subcortical infarction and an unexpectedly high burden of T2 lesions and lacunes. There is an involvement of white matter in the anterior temporal poles and external capsules. Her mother had "vascular dementia" and died from a stroke at age 60 years. What genetic condition should be considered? What is the underlying pathologic defect?
4. A 70-year-old woman had a brain MRI after a mild concussion. MRI did not show signs of traumatic brain injury but noted "several subcortical white matter T2 hyperintensities." The patient is concerned about possible vascular dementia. What is the prevalence of subcortical white matter lesions in this age group?
5. Multiple sclerosis (MS) and cerebrovascular disease both cause T2-hyperintense white matter lesions on MRI. There is a radiologic overlap in MRI appearance of these two conditions but also important differences. The inflammatory lesions of multiple sclerosis tend to form around small venules, while the microvascular lesions of the cerebrovascular disease result mainly from occlusion of small arteries. For each type of lesion, write down whether it is more typical of demyelinating or cerebrovascular disease:

Corpus Callosum Undersurface Lesions	
Wedgelike lesions in cerebellar surface	
Lesions in anterior temporal white matter	
Lesion that abuts the outer surface of the brainstem	
Lesions extending perpendicularly from the border of the lateral ventricles	

CHALLENGE

What conditions should be suspected if a patient with VaD has multiple small cortical hemorrhages? Explain why this disorder can be considered both vascular and amyloid.

REFERENCES

O'Brien JT, Thomas A. Vascular dementia. *Lancet*. 2015;386(10004):1698-1706.
Raz L, Knoefel J, Bhaskar K. The neuropathology and cerebrovascular mechanisms of dementia. *J Cereb Blood Flow Metab*. 2016;36(1):172-186. [free online resource]

54 Normal Pressure Hydrocephalus

A potentially reversible syndrome of cognitive and gait impairment associated with ventricular enlargement

CORE FEATURES

1. Gait apraxia.
   Gait is described as "marche a petit pas" (French for "gait with little steps") or "magnetic" because it is difficult to initiate, slow, wide-based, cautious, with reduced floor clearance.
2. "Frontal subcortical deficits."
   The early stages feature mostly executive dysfunction, inattention, and psychomotor slowing. Cognitive changes emerge after gait deficits become apparent, while the opposite is true for neurodegenerative dementias.
3. Urge incontinence.
   Initial urinary symptoms of frequency and urgency can progress to urinary incontinence.
4. Ventricular enlargement on CT or MRI without evidence of CSF obstruction ("communicating hydrocephalus").
   Enlargement of the ventricles in NPH is out of proportion to cortical atrophy, unlike neurodegenerative diseases in which there is both central and cortical atrophy.
5. Improvement in gait after "high-volume" lumbar puncture (LP).
   Typically, 30 to 50 mL of CSF needs to be removed to see a response (high-volume "tap test"). In cases with an equivocal response to LP, external lumbar drainage may be inserted for 2 to 3 days.

SYNOPSIS

The classic triad of gait disorder, cognitive decline, and urinary incontinence can plausibly be attributed to the disruption of frontal subcortical pathways. There is slowing in mentation and gait as may also be seen in subcortical dementia. Bladder symptoms are likely the result of interruption of the tonic inhibition from the frontal lobes to the pontine micturition center, a "master switch for micturition."

The diagnosis of NPH is not straightforward. The "classic triad" is present in less than half of patients at diagnosis, and individual components of this triad are common among patients with other cerebrovascular or neurodegenerative disorders, such as AD and PD. Enlargement of the ventricles invariably accompanies aging and what constitutes "pathologic enlargement" is not easy to define. The most important question when considering the diagnosis of NPH is whether the clinical and radiological features are best explained by the more common vascular or neurodegenerative conditions. The answer to this question will determine whether CSF "tap test" and, potentially, shunt placement should be pursued. Shunting improves gait in NPH and may have a positive effect on cognition, but patients with neurodegenerative dementias derive no benefit from the procedure and may experience worsening of the disease and serious complications such as shunt malfunction, infections, seizures, and subdural hematoma.

FIGURE

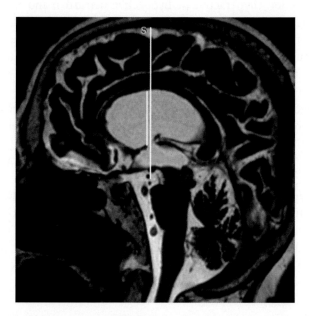

Midsagittal T2 MRI of a patient with NPH shows enlarged lateral ventricles and bowing of corpus callosum. The Z Evans index is the ratio of maximum axial length of the frontal horns (shorter line) to the maximum cranial axial length at the level of foramen monro (longer line); it is a measure of ventricular enlargement. (Reprinted with permission from Kantarci K, Irwin DJ, Jack Jr. CR, et al. Normal aging, dementia and neurodegenerative disease. In: Atlas SW, ed. *Magnetic Resonance Imaging of the Brain and Spine*. 5th ed. Philadelphia, PA: Wolters Kluwer; 2016:687:Figure 15.38.)

QUESTIONS FOR SELF-STUDY

1. What is the difference between gait ataxia and gait apraxia? How would patients with gait ataxia and gait apraxia perform when asked to draw an imaginary circle with their feet in the air or show how they pedal an imaginary bicycle while lying down?

2. Progressive supranuclear palsy (PSP), an extrapyramidal movement disorder with prominent gait abnormalities, early falls, and "subcortical" cognitive deficits, is a good mimicker of NPH. How would PSP and NPH patients perform on the "pull test," wherein a standing patient is asked to maintain their posture and avoid falling backward after a sudden pull on their shoulders from behind? What extrapyramidal features would be expected in PSP but not in NPH?

3. Hydrocephalus may be due to obstruction of CSF flow at any point from its origin in the choroid plexus to its entry into the venous sinuses. Name pathologic processes that could lead to hydrocephalus at the respective portion of the CSF pathway and the resulting size of the lateral and fourth ventricle:

Obstruction at the Level of ...	Pathology	Size of Lateral Ventricles	Size of the Fourth Ventricle
Foramen of Monro			
Cerebral aqueduct			
Foramina of Luschka/Magendie			
Subarachnoid space			

4. Urodynamic testing allows one to measure normal bladder filling pressure; bladder muscle contraction (hyperactive or hypoactive detrusor); and whether sphincter relaxes during bladder contraction or constricts (is in detrusor-sphincter dyssynergia or DSD). Predict filling volume, detrusor activity, and presence of DSD on urodynamic testing of patients with NPH; spinal cord injury; and diabetic autonomic neuropathy. (Compare your answers with Kavanagh A, et al. *Can Urol Assoc J.* 2019;13(6):E157-E176. [free online resource])

5. Walking speed has been called the "sixth vital sign." What are the major health outcomes that correlate with walking speed? (Compare your answer with Fritz and Lusardi's "white paper" cited below).

CHALLENGE

In NPH, the opening CSF pressure is normal, and there is no papilledema. Yet, clinical symptoms can be explained by invoking a "strain" on frontal subcortical fibers due to increased CSF pressure, and MRI shows "periventricular rimming" (high T2 signal) due to subependymal absorption of CSF. How could you reconcile the discrepancy between normal opening CSF pressure with the indirect evidence clinical and MRI evidence of elevated CSF pressure?

REFERENCES

Fritz S, Lusardi M. White paper. "walking speed: the sixth vital sign". *J Geriatr Phys Ther.* 2009;32(2):46-49. [free online resource]

Picascia M, Zangaglia R, Bernini S, Minafra B, Sinforiani E, Pacchetti C. A review of cognitive impairment and differential diagnosis in idiopathic normal pressure hydrocephalus. *Funct Neurol.* 30(4):217-228. [free online resource]

55 Brain death

Loss of brain function including brainstem reflexes; the legal equivalent to death in the United States

CORE FEATURES

1. History of a catastrophic brain injury.
   The most common causes are prolonged cardiac arrest; brain hemorrhage with herniation; and severe traumatic brain injury.
2. No responses to verbal or painful stimuli.
3. Absence of brainstem reflexes.
   In brain death, pupils are midsize and nonreactive to light. There are no extraocular movements on caloric testing, no corneal reflexes, no facial movements to noxious stimuli, no gag reflex, and no cough reflex on tracheal suctioning.
4. Absence of respiratory drive (apnea).
   After the patient is preoxygenated, the ventilator is disconnected. If there are no respiratory movements (no gasps), and CO_2 in arterial blood gas rises to >60 mm Hg, or 20 mm Hg over baseline, the test is consistent with apnea.
5. Exclusion of reversible causes of coma.
   Reversible causes of coma include hypotension; hypothermia; profound electrolyte or endocrine abnormalities; exposure to licit and illicit sedating substances (barbiturates); or neuromuscular agents (anesthetic agents, organophosphates). Other mimickers of brain death include severe Guillain-Barré syndrome and high cervical spine injury.

SYNOPSIS

Throughout human history, the boundary between life and death was fairly obvious. Breathing and heartbeat signified life and their absence, death. Anyone who could determine whether breathing and heartbeat have stopped could reliably pronounce a person dead. The invention of mechanical ventilators and other advances in critical care have introduced new complexities into the seemingly "black-and-white" issue. It became possible to maintain the patient's respiratory and circulatory functions in the absence of any clinically detectable brain activity. Is such a "brain dead" person dead or alive? The legal position in the United States and many other countries, and endorsed by the major medical societies, including the American Academy of Neurology, is that "complete loss of consciousness (coma), brainstem reflexes, and the independent capacity for ventilator drive (apnea), in the absence of any factors that imply possible reversibility," signifies "brain death," which is the equivalent of circulatory death. This definition allows for organ-sustaining support to be withdrawn from a brain dead patient and for their vital organs—heart, liver, kidney—to be harvested.

The concept of brain death, enshrined in law and accepted by the medical community at large, is not without detractors. It is difficult to be certain that there was indeed "complete cessation of brain activity" since clinical examination essentially only assesses motoric responses. Some small degree of cerebral activity is likely to be present after brain death and spreading neuronal depolarization can be reliably recorded after clinical diagnosis of brain death (Dreier JP, et al. Ann Neurol. 2018;83(2):295-310). In rare cases, even cortical and brainstem evoked potentials can be recorded from brain dead individuals (see references). On a practical level, the determination of brain death is prone to error. A recent survey found that only 25% of patients who were declared "brain dead" underwent the required neurologic testing necessary to establish brain death (Braksick SA, et al. Neurology. 2019;92:e888-e894). On an ethical level, the concept also raises a number of difficult issues, such as whether the brain death declaration serves the interest of the patient or the organ recipient (Clarke MJ, et al. Ann Thorac Surg. 2016;10:2053-2058).

FIGURE

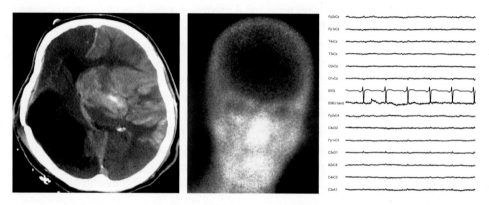

Left, Head CT scan of a patient with a catastrophic intracerebral hemorrhage, massive midline shift, and entrapment of the right lateral ventricle. Middle: "hot nose sign" on radionucleotide scan shows absent perfusion in the cerebrum but persistent perfusion of the face and nose via the extracranial carotid arteries consistent with the diagnosis of brain death. Right, "Flat EEG": there is no activity on cerebral leads, but ongoing cardiac activity on electrocardiography (ECG), consistent with, but not diagnostic of brain death. (Left, Courtesy of Dr. José Biller. Middle and Right, Reprinted with permission from Daffner RH, Hartman MS. *Clinical Radiology: The Essentials.* 4th ed. Philadelphia, PA: Wolters Kluwer Health/Lippincott Williams & Wilkins; 2013:Figure 12.52c and Reprinted with permission from Stern JM. *Atlas of EEG Patterns.* 2nd ed. Philadelphia, PA: Wolters Kluwer Health/Lippincott Williams & Wilkins; 2013:Figure 17.2.)

QUESTIONS FOR SELF-STUDY

1. Explain in simple terms the difference between "coma" and "brain death."
2. Why are certain complex motor movements, such as a "triple reflex" or the "Lazarus sign," compatible with the diagnosis of brain death, but the most feeble attempt at breathing is not?
3. Why is a "flat" (isoelectric) EEG a necessary but not a sufficient criterion of brain death?
4. Why do brain death determination criteria require that body temperature be higher than 36°C but not that it be lower than a certain threshold?

5. A patient receives high doses of neuromuscular blocking agents, which abolishes all motor responses and brainstem reflexes. This scenario is clinically indistinguishable from brain death. What ancillary test could help determine whether such a patient is indeed brain dead or completely paralyzed?

CHALLENGE

A patient has met all criteria for brain death, and the transplant team is summoned to extract vital organs. Should this procedure be performed with or without anesthesia? Find arguments for each position.

REFERENCES

Koenig MA, Kaplan PW. Brain death. *Handb Clin Neurol*. 2019;161:89-102.
Wijdicks EF, Varelas PN, Gronseth GS, Greer DM; American Academy of Neurology. Evidence-based guideline update. Determining brain death in adults: report of the Quality Standards Subcommittee of the American Academy of Neurology. *Neurology*. 2010;74(23):1911-1918. [free online resource]

Cerebrovascular Disorders

A Very Brief Introduction to Cerebrovascular Disorders

Falstaff: And I hear, moreover, his Highness is fall'n into same whoreson apoplexy.

Chief Justice: Well, God mend him! I pray you let me speak with you.

Falstaff: This apoplexy, as I take it, is a kind of lethargy, please your lordship, a kind of sleeping in the blood, a tingling.

Chief Justice: What tell you me of it? Be it as it is.

Falstaff: It hath it original from much grief, from study, and perturbation of the brain. I have read the cause of his effects in Galen, it is a kind of deafness.

William Shakespeare, 2 Henry IV*

As pointed out by Falstaff, stroke—the older term is "apoplexy" (Greek: "stricken down")— is a highly morbid condition with diverse clinical manifestations. Our understanding of stroke mechanisms has been refined since Galen. Ischemic strokes, which comprise approximately 85% of all strokes, are the result of a blockage in one or more of the precerebral or cerebral arteries, usually due to atherosclerosis or embolism. A thorough understanding of neurovascular syndromes presupposes knowledge of cerebrovascular anatomy, which will be briefly reviewed here.

The arterial supply of the brain derives from paired carotid arteries and paired vertebral arteries (VAs). The carotid arteries give rise to the "anterior circulation" of the brain, which supplies the anterior two-thirds of the cerebral hemispheres and some of the basal ganglia. The vertebral arteries give rise to the "posterior circulation" that supplies the posterior aspect of the cerebral hemispheres, some of the basal ganglia, the thalami, the brainstem, and the cerebellum. The anterior and posterior circulations are connected via the circle of Willis and other collateral connections.

This section describes some of the more common vascular syndromes associated with steno-occlusive disease of the larger arteries of the anterior circulation—internal carotid artery (ICA) and middle cerebral artery (MCA) (Chapters 56 and 57)—and the posterior circulation—vertebral arteries (VAs), basilar artery (BA), and posterior cerebral artery (PCA) (Chapters 58-60). We also discuss classic lacunar stroke syndromes in the brainstem and elsewhere that are the result of small-vessel disease (Chapters 61 and 62) and the devastating syndrome of intracerebral hemorrhage that usually results from rupture of intracranial arterial perforators (Chapter 63). Another kind of hemorrhagic stroke—nontraumatic subarachnoid hemorrhage (SAH)—is a dreaded complication of a ruptured brain aneurysm (Chapter 64).

On the venous side, cerebral drainage is accomplished via the deep and superficial venous systems, which empty out into the venous sinuses within the dural meninges via

---

*William Shakespeare (1564-1616), plausibly the greatest dramatist of all time, may also have been the most medically erudite. Shakespeare's understanding of medicine is all the more remarkable as his formal education was limited to high school. References to neurologic diseases in Shakespeare's plays have been collated in Paciaroni and Bogousslavsky. 'William Shakespeare's neurology'. *Prog Brain Res.* 2013;206:3-18).

"bridging veins." Rupture of "bridging veins" into the space between the dura and the cerebrum results in subdural hematomas, not an uncommon condition in the elderly (Chapter 65). Strokes due to thrombosis of cerebral venous sinuses accounts for only about 1% of all strokes, but is important to keep in mind in the differential diagnosis as it requires a different type of intervention than arterial ischemic stroke (Chapter 66).

Stroke is the second most common cause of death and of lost disability-adjusted life years in Western countries. Because strokes evolve rapidly and carry high morbidity, any new maximal at onset focal neurologic syndrome of unknown etiology should be presumed to be vascular until proven otherwise and evaluated and managed emergently. The intravenous clot buster, tPA (alteplase), improves long-term functional outcomes in ischemic stroke when given within 4.5 hours of symptom onset. Large artery occlusive (LAO) ischemic stroke may be amenable to modern neurointerventional techniques of clot retrieval up to 24 hours of stroke onset. All stroke patients benefit from comprehensive care afforded by specialized stroke units and control of vascular risk factors to prevent stroke recurrence.

REFERENCES

Benjamin EJ, Blaha MJ, Chiuve SC, et al. Heart disease and stroke statistics-2017 update: a report from the American Heart Association. *Circulation*. 2017;135(10):e146-e603. [free online resource]

Southerland AM. Clinical evaluation of the patient with acute stroke. *Continuum (Minneap Minn)*. 2017;23(1, Cerebrovascular Disease):40-61.

van der Worp HB. Clinical practice. Acute ischemic stroke. *N Engl J Med*. 2007;357(6):572-579.

56 Cervical Internal Carotid Artery Dissection

Tear and hematoma in the inner layer of the walls of the internal carotid artery may lead to brain or retinal ischemia

CORE FEATURES

1. Ipsilateral head, face, and neck pain.
   Pain is the most common presenting symptom and may precede other symptoms by hours to days. Head pain is often gradual in onset, but some patients may present with a thunderclap headache.
2. Horner syndrome.
   Miosis and ptosis—without anhidrosis—can be observed in half of the patients with internal carotid artery dissection (ICAD). Acute onset of a postganglionic Horner syndrome should be presumed to be due to ICAD until proven otherwise.
3. Ipsilateral visual symptoms.
   Ipsilateral retinal ischemia causes amaurosis fugax (Greek: "fleeting obscuration") or, uncommonly, permanent monocular visual loss.
4. Contralateral motor-sensory deficits.
   Cerebral ischemia causes focal hemispheric syndromes and aphasia if the dominant hemisphere is involved.
5. Pulsatile tinnitus.
   Tinnitus is due to flow turbulence through a narrowed ICA segment. A carotid bruit may be present on auscultation.

SYNOPSIS

Dissection of the extracranial ICA may be a result of major neck trauma (motor vehicle accident, attempted strangulation), a trivial trigger (painting a ceiling, riding a roller coaster), or even occur spontaneously. Cervical ICAD is more common than intracranial ICAD because the cervical segment of the ICA is more mobile and may come into contact with the transverse processes of the upper cervical vertebrae when the neck is stretched. Headache and neck pain are presumably the result of irritation of pain-sensitive fibers along the wall of the carotid artery. Horner syndrome is a result of the interruption of the oculosympathetic fibers to the eyelid and pupil as they ascend into the cranium along the extracranial ICA. A combination of ipsilateral amaurosis fugax due to retinal artery ischemia and contralateral hemispheric symptoms localizes the vascular lesion to the ICA. Magnetic resonance angiography (MRA) and computed tomography angiography (CTA) are noninvasive imaging alternatives to conventional catheter cerebral angiography, the previous gold standard for the diagnosis of ICAD. Color duplex ultrasound of the carotid arteries may be used to detect the mural hematoma and the thrombus.

ICAD is an important cause of stroke especially in younger patients with no traditional risk factors for stroke. Among the older population with vascular risk factors, the high-grade atherosclerotic carotid disease is by far the more common cause of carotid ischemia. High-grade symptomatic cervical atherosclerotic carotid artery disease requires carotid revascularization with either carotid endarterectomy (CEA) or carotid artery stenting (CAS) and optimal medical management (antiplatelet therapy, high-dose statin therapy, and optimal control of risk factors such as hypertension and diabetes). Symptomatic cervicocephalic arterial dissections tend to recanalize spontaneously and generally require no intervention beyond antiplatelet therapy.

FIGURE

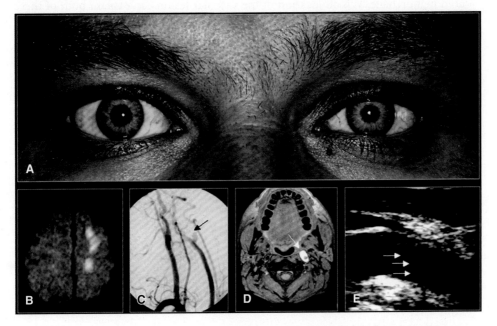

Findings in ICA dissection. A, Partial Horner syndrome (left-sided miosis and ptosis). B, Multiple left frontoparietal acute ischemic lesions on DWI. C, Carotid angiography with evidence of left extracranial ICA occlusion. D, ICA mural hematoma (arrow) due to dissection evident on MRI scan. E, Intimal flap (arrows) appearance on Duplex scan, a pathognomonic sign of dissection. (Reprinted with permission from Mazzucco S, Rìzzuto N. Teaching neuroimage: Horner syndrome due to internal carotid artery dissection. *Neurology.* 2006;66(5):E19.)

QUESTIONS FOR SELF-STUDY

1. Is pupillary asymmetry due to Horner syndrome more apparent in a fully lighted or in a dimmed room? Explain your answer.
2. Which of the features of extracranial ICAD would be absent in symptomatic extracranial ICA atherosclerotic disease?
3. A 70-year-old healthy woman presents after few-minute episodes of blurry vision in her right eye. Carotid Doppler ultrasound reveals atherosclerotic plaque of the right ICA with >70% diameter stenosis. What is the recommended course of management of the symptomatic right ICA steno-occlusive disease in this patient? If the patient also has 60% left ICA diameter stenosis, what would be the recommended management for that artery? Is there a difference in recommendation based on whether carotid stenosis is symptomatic or not?

4. A 70-year-old man with history of hyperlipidemia and cigarette smoking presents with horizontal binocular diplopia and left hemiparesis. Brain MRI confirms a right pontine stroke. Do you need to obtain a color duplex carotid ultrasound as part of his stroke workup? Make an argument for and against imaging of the carotid arteries in this clinical setting.

5. A 55-year-old young man presents with acute-onset headache and right hemiparesis. Brain MRI shows ischemic changes in the left MCA distribution and subarachnoid hemorrhage. Which location of the vascular lesion can explain both of these findings? Explain why these MRI findings are not compatible with an extracranial ICAD.

CHALLENGE

Internal carotid artery does not supply the brainstem. How would you explain "brainstem signs" (ipsilateral CN III or CN XII palsies) that are seen in about 10% of patients with ICAD?

REFERENCES

Brott TG, Halperin JL, Abbara S, et al. 2011 ASA/ACCF/AHA/AANN/AANS/ACR/ASNR/CNS/SAIP/SCAI/SIR/SNIS/SVM/SVS guideline on the management of patients with extracranial carotid and vertebral artery disease: executive summary. *Stroke.* 2011;42(8):e420-e463. [free online resource]

Gaba K, Ringleb PA, Halliday A. Asymptomatic carotid stenosis: intervention or best medical therapy? *Curr Neurol Neurosci Rep.* 2018;18(11):80. [free online resource]

Schievink WI. Spontaneous dissection of the carotid and vertebral arteries. *N Engl J Med.* 2001;344(12):898-906.

57 Middle Cerebral Artery Territory Infarction

A cerebrovascular syndrome due to internal carotid artery (ICA) or middle cerebral artery (MCA) steno-occlusive disease

CORE FEATURES

The table lists features of complete left and right MCA territory infarctions.

	Left MCA Syndrome (Dominant Hemisphere)	Right MCA Syndrome (Nondominant Hemisphere)
1. Higher cortical functions	Global aphasia	Left hemispatial neglect; cortical sensory deficits (agraphesthesia, astereognosis)
2. Visual field loss	Right homonymous hemianopia	Left homonymous hemianopia
3. Motor deficits	Right face/arm > leg weakness Dysarthria	Left face/arm > leg weakness Dysarthria
4. Sensory deficits	Right face/arm > leg hemisensory deficits	Left face/arm > leg hemisensory deficits
5. Early imaging findings	CT: "dense MCA" sign and "insular ribbon" sign MRI brain: restricted diffusion in MCA territory	

SYNOPSIS

The table highlights clinical features of a "complete MCA" syndrome, which may occur with a stem MCA occlusion. More limited aphasia syndromes and visual field defects (eg, inferior homonymous quadrantanopia) arise from the more distal MCA branch occlusions. Because the cerebral territory supplied by the MCA includes the frontal eye fields, gaze deviation to the side of the lesion is present in the acute phase, along with the expected contralateral motor-sensory deficits (involvement of lateral and central aspects of the motor and sensory cortices); aphasia (left perisylvian region involvement in the dominant hemisphere); contralateral neglect (higher level sensory integration areas in the nondominant hemisphere); and homonymous hemianopia (optic radiations). Strokes in the anterior cerebral artery (ACA) distribution are much less frequent. They often present with neuropsychiatric symptoms, such as abulia, agitation, perseveration, memory impairments, and crural predominant hemiparesis of the contralateral limbs. The etiology of most large-vessel strokes is cardioembolism or atheroembolism.

FIGURES

Right-side visual
field cut

Aphasia

Right face and arm >
leg weakness

Right face and arm >
leg numbness

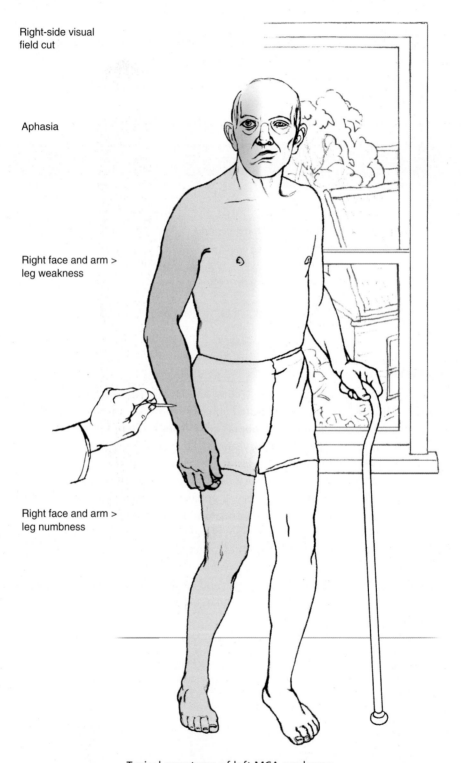

Typical symptoms of left MCA syndrome.

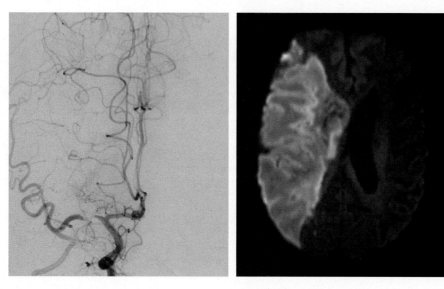

Occlusion of M1 segment of right MCA on cerebral angiogram (left). DWI restrictive diffusion lesion in complete right MCA territory infarction (right).

QUESTIONS FOR SELF-STUDY

1. Patients with aphasia may be mistaken for patients with acute confusional states. What mental status tests help differentiate aphasia from an acute confusional state?
2. Which language deficits would be expected with occlusion of the superior division of the left MCA and which language deficits with occlusion of the inferior division of the left MCA?
3. How does the neuroanatomy of the primary motor cortex (motor homunculus) explain why MCA territory infarctions produce a greater degree of weakness in the face and arm, while ACA territory infarctions produce greater weakness in the leg than in the arm?
4. Explain why a large acute MCA territory infarction is not associated with depressed consciousness, while a much smaller infarction involving the thalami or upper brainstem may result in coma? If a patient with an MCA territory infarction becomes drowsy and obtunded 2 to 3 days after symptom onset—what is the likely explanation? What is the definition of "malignant MCA infarction"? What surgical intervention may be considered for malignant MCA infarction?
5. A 65-year-old woman with a right MCA syndrome has an irregularly irregular pulse. ECG confirms atrial fibrillation. What is the likely stroke mechanism? What is the recommended secondary stroke prevention strategy in such a patient?

CHALLENGE

The vestibulo-ocular reflex (VOR) elicits eye deviation to the contralateral side when the head is rotated. Explain how the VOR helps differentiate gaze deviation due to a supratentorial vascular lesion from gaze deviation due to an infratentorial vascular lesion. Explain "Doll's eye reflex" in terms of the VOR. Why is Doll's eye reflex not compatible with the diagnosis of brain death?

REFERENCES

Huttner HB, Schwab S. Malignant middle cerebral artery infarction: clinical characteristics, treatment strategies, and future perspectives. *Lancet Neurol.* 2009;8(10):949-958.

Navarro-Orozco D, Sánchez-Manso JC. *Neuroanatomy, middle cerebral artery.* In: *StatPearls.* Treasure Island, FL: StatPearls Publishing; 2019. Available from https://www.ncbi.nlm.nih.gov/books/NBK526002/. [free online resource]

58 Posterior Cerebral Artery Territory Infarction

A cerebrovascular syndrome due to steno-occlusive disease of posterior cerebral arteries (PCAs)

CORE FEATURES

	Right Occipital (Nondominant PCA) Infarction	Left Occipital (Dominant PCA) Infarction	Bilateral Occipital (Bilateral PCA) Infarction
1. Visual field loss	Left homonymous hemianopia with macular sparing	Right homonymous hemianopia with macular sparing	"Cortical blindness"
2. Visual inattention	Neglect of the left visual field		Denial of blindness and confabulation (Anton syndrome)
3. Visual hallucinations and illusions	More common than with left-sided lesions		Visual hallucinations common
4. Visual processing deficits	Loss of topographic orientation	Anomia (especially for colors) Alexia without agraphia (if splenium of corpus callosum is involved)	
5. Early imaging findings	CT head: dense PCA sign MRI: restriction diffusion in PCA territory		

SYNOPSIS

Homonymous hemianopia in PCA infarction is the result of damage to the retrochiasmatic visual pathways at the level of the optic radiations, which connect the lateral geniculate nucleus of the thalamus to the primary visual cortex, or to the primary visual cortex itself in the occipital lobe. Patients may also experience deficits in higher order visual information processing—hemivisual neglect or inability to visually piece together a picture into a coherent whole (simultanagnosia). Patients with bilateral watershed infarctions in the boundary zones between the PCA and MCA territories—usually from global hypoperfusion—present with simultanagnosia and propasognosia (inability to recognize familiar faces) but have a different pattern of visual field defect than in PCA territory strokes. An interesting "disconnection syndrome" occurs if there is damage to the left visual field and the splenium of the corpus callosum. Patients are unable to read letters on the right side of their visual field (right homonymous hemianopia) nor transfer visual information from the intact left visual field to the language areas of the dominant hemisphere (due to callosal damage). As a result, language is effectively disconnected from the visual input. Patients are unable to read but are able to write ("alexia without agraphia"). In addition to visual symptoms, patients with PCA occlusion proximal to branches to the midbrain and thalamus may experience hemibody motor deficits (midbrain cerebral peduncle), hemisensory, cognitive, and behavioral symptoms (thalamic involvement).

FIGURE

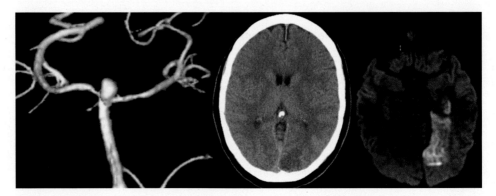

Right: Tip of the basilar aneurysm, which was treated endovascularly. Middle: Endovascular procedure was complicated by left PCA territory stroke—hypodense signal on noncontrast head computed tomography (CT). Left: Brain DWI sequence shows the extent of left PCA territory infarction.

QUESTIONS FOR SELF-STUDY

1. How would you test for visual neglect in a patient with a visual field defect?
2. Explain why the commonly used stroke screen, F-A-S-T (face, arm, speech, time), is likely to miss a PCA territory stroke.
3. Why are pupillary light reflexes not impaired in patients with cortical blindness?
4. An 80-year-old woman presents with a right-side eye deviation, left hemiparesis, and a dense left homonymous visual field loss. Brain MRI shows infarction in both the right MCA and PCA territories. Which common variant in the posterior circulation can explain a stroke that ostensibly involves both the anterior and posterior circulation? How would the visual field defect in a patient with MCA/PCA territory stroke differ from that in a patient with a PCA territory infarction?
5. A 30-year-old woman presents within 3 days postpartum with headaches and bilateral visual blurring. Her blood pressure is 190/90 mm Hg. MRI shows nonenhancing bilateral, symmetrical occipital lobe T2-hyperintense lesions. There is no diffusion restriction. MRA and MRV of the brain are normal. What is the likely diagnosis? What is the next step in management?

CHALLENGE

"Blindsight" may occur among cortically blind persons who are able to navigate their way in space and reach for objects without being able to consciously perceive them. Suggest the neuroanatomic basis for this unusual phenomenon. What visual pathways must be intact to allow blindsight?

REFERENCES

Arboix A, Arbe G, García-Eroles L, Oliveres M, Parra O, Massons J. Infarctions in the vascular territory of the posterior cerebral artery: clinical features in 232 patients. *BMC Res Notes*. 2011;4:329. [free online resource]

Nouh A, Remke J, Ruland S. Ischemic posterior circulation stroke: a review of anatomy, clinical presentations, diagnosis, and current management. *Front Neurol*. 2014;5:30. [free online resource]

59 Basilar Artery Occlusion

Basal artery territory stroke due to basilar artery atherothrombosis or embolism from the heart or proximal arteries

CORE FEATURES

1. Alteration in consciousness.
   Symptoms range from confusion to coma if the ascending reticular activating system (ARAS) within the upper brainstem tegmentum is involved.
2. Bilateral motor deficits.
   Disruption of the corticospinal tracts results in quadriparesis or quadriplegia. Hemiparesis may occur if the stroke involves half of the brainstem.
3. Dysphagia and dysarthria.
   Disruption of the corticobulbar tracts may cause impairment or inability to articulate and swallow (anarthria and aphagia).
4. Extraocular movement abnormalities.
   Distal basilar artery occlusion (BAO) can mimic a CN III palsy, while middle BAO is more likely to cause gaze palsies. A variety of peculiar oculomotor deficits such as ocular bobbing (abrupt downward jerks of both eyes with a slow return to midposition), rotational-torsional nystagmus, etc, have been described in BAO.
5. Stuttering course.
   Unlike other ischemic strokes which typically present in acute-at-onset, "stroke-like" fashion, BAO tends to follow a stuttering or subacute course due to progressive intracranial arterial stenosis and occlusion.

SYNOPSIS

BAO presents with a bewildering variety of manifestations. In addition to headache, which is most common and least specific, symptoms include vertigo (ischemia of the vestibular nuclei and pathways); visual disturbances (occipital lobes); unilateral or bilateral hypesthesia or anesthesia (medial lemnisci, spinothalamic tracts, or thalamic nuclei); tinnitus and hearing loss (cochlear nuclei or lateral lemnisci); drop attacks (transient ischemia of the corticospinal tracts); ataxia (cerebellum or cerebellar pathways); Horner syndrome (oculosympathetic pathways in the brainstem); and confusion, amnesia, dreamlike behavior (thalamic nuclei and medial temporal lobes). Other rare and more difficult-to-localize symptoms that may herald a BAO include pathological fits of laughter ("fou rire prodromique") and visual hallucinations ("peduncular hallucinosis"). The nature and severity of symptoms are determined by the site of arterial occlusion—proximal, middle, or distal basilar artery—and the extent of the collateral circulation.

The "locked-in syndrome," the dreaded complication of BAO, is a result of a large medial pontine stroke which leaves only blinking and vertical eye movements under voluntary control. Alexandre Dumas described this condition as a "soul trapped in a body that no longer obeys its commands" ("Count of Monte Cristo"). Counterintuitively, patients with locked-in syndrome rate their quality of life similar to healthy subjects (Lulé D, Zickler C, Häcker S, et al. Life can be worth living in locked-in syndrome. *Prog Brain Res*. 2009;177:339-51.).

FIGURES

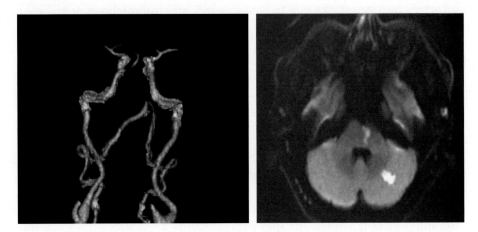

Basilar artery occlusion (BAO) with patchy ischemia in brainstem and cerebellum. Patient made a full recovery.

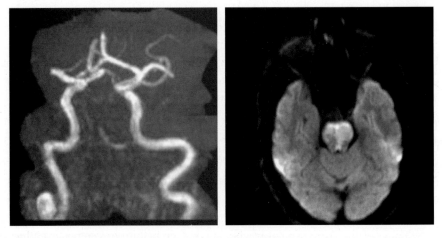

MRA (left) shows BAO. MRI shows no rim around the brainstem and apex toward ventricular surface; these features predict poor recovery.

QUESTIONS FOR SELF-STUDY

1. The locked-in syndrome does not affect higher cognitive functions as attested by the autobiographical account by J-D. Bauby, who wrote *The Diving Bell and the Butterfly* with 200,000 blinks after being locked-in by a stroke. Explain how to differentiate locked-in syndrome from coma at a bedside.

2. A 40-year-old man presents to the ED with acute-onset headache, drowsiness, and vertigo. Brainstem ischemia is suspected, but brain MRI and extracranial and intracranial MRA are normal. The patient reports several similar attacks since his 20s. His symptoms typically recover within an hour, except for headaches, which may last for several hours. What is the likely diagnosis?

3. A 50-year-old woman presents to the ED with diplopia, ataxia, and bilateral facial weakness of 3-day duration. Muscle stretch reflexes are absent in both upper and lower limbs. Brain MRI and MRA are normal. What is the likely diagnosis? Which blood test could confirm your diagnostic suspicion?

4. Syncope, a very common symptom, is usually due to a transient drop in blood pressure. Exceptionally, syncope can be due to a BAO, in which case, other brainstem symptoms usually suggest this diagnosis. Explain why BAO can cause syncope, while a carotid artery occlusion can not. Based on this insight, explain why a carotid duplex ultrasound study is not recommended for syncope workup. (For other unnecessary but commonly performed tests after syncope, see Mendu et al., referenced below).

5. What is an early sign of BAO that may be seen on the noncontrast head CT?

CHALLENGE

Most cases of syncope are due to impaired control of baroreceptor reflex (vasovagal syncope) or orthostatic hypotension. Cardiac causes, such as congestive heart failure, valvular heart disease, cardiac arrhythmias, are less common but important not to miss. Neurologic causes of syncope are rare. Neurologic and neurovascular testing—head CT, electroencephalography (EEG), and carotid ultrasound—have very low yield and are not indicated in cases of uncomplicated syncope (no focal neurologic symptoms or postictal confusion). In addition to BAO, what other unusual causes of syncope are due to intracranial pathology?

REFERENCES

Mattle HP. Basilar artery occlusion. *Lancet Neurol.* 2011;10(11):1002-1014.
Mendu ML, McAvay G, Lampert R, Stoehr J, Tinetti ME. Yield of diagnostic tests in evaluating syncopal episodes in older patients. *Arch Intern Med.* 2009;169(14):1299-1305. [free online resource]

60 Cervical Vertebral Artery Dissection

An ischemic syndrome due to dissection of the extracranial vertebral artery

CORE FEATURES

1. Neck pain.
   Half of the patients report posterior neck pain ipsilateral to the vertebral artery dissection. The pain is often described as similar to musculoskeletal pain.
2. Headache.
   Two-thirds of patients report headaches, which are usually occipital and unilateral. Neck and head pain may precede ischemic symptoms by hours to days.
3. Dizziness and vertigo.
   These symptoms are reported by most patients. Vomiting without any other gastrointestinal symptoms should raise suspicion of a neurologic or neurotologic etiology.
4. History of a "triggering event."
   Only half of the patients with vertebral artery dissection (VAD) can identify a potential trigger, which can range from the obvious (motor vehicle crash) to the trivial (sneezing, heavy lifting, swinging a racket, yoga, cervical chiropractic manipulation).
5. Clinical symptoms and signs suggestive of vertebrobasilar ischemia.
   Vertigo, diplopia, dysarthria, and ataxia are common symptoms due to ischemia of the brainstem and cerebellum. A lateral medullary infarction (Wallenberg syndrome) and medial medullary infarction (Déjerine syndrome) are classic syndromes of vertebral artery dissection.
6. Brain and neck MRA or CTA show narrowing or occlusion of the vertebral artery.
   MRI may show restriction diffusion in vestibulobasilar territory distribution.

SYNOPSIS

VAD is a very rare cause of stroke overall but is not very rare among stroke patients younger than 45 years without vascular risk factors. Unilateral neck and head pain and dizziness are nonspecific symptoms but raise the question of VAD. When VAD is suspected, a dedicated CTA or MRA of the head and neck should be pursued without delay. Ischemic stroke due to either embolization or hypoperfusion develops in 90% of patients with VAD. Although many clinicians favor short-term anticoagulation in the acute phase, the Cervical Artery Dissection in Stroke Study (CADISS; Lancet Neurology. 2015;14(4):361-367) study could not confirm the superiority of oral anticoagulation over antiplatelet therapy. Patients with cervical arterial dissection tend to have a good recovery. Unlike steno-occlusive atherothrombotic strokes, dissected arteries usually recanalize spontaneously within a few months of the dissection.

FIGURE

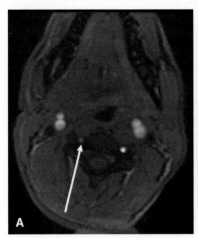
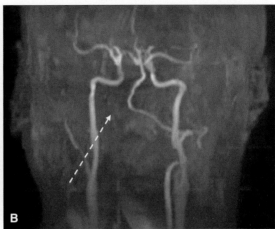

A, Time-of-flight MRA shows decreased caliber of the right vertebral artery with irregularity of flow signal at the C2 level (solid arrow). B, No flow signal in the right vertebral artery intradurally (dashed arrow). These findings are consistent with right extracranial vertebral artery dissection. (Reprinted with permission from Kornbluh A, Twanow JD. Teaching neuroimages: Adolescent Wallenberg syndrome with overlooked signs: ipsipulsion and ipsilateral facial palsy. *Neurology.* 2018;91(20):e1949-e1950.)

QUESTIONS FOR SELF-STUDY

1. Dizziness and vertigo are common concerns among patients evaluated in the ED. In only a small minority of cases, the cause of vertigo is posterior fossa ischemia or hemorrhage. However, it is essential not to miss these vascular causes, as misdiagnosis can lead to catastrophic sequelae. Which findings on neurologic examination are incompatible with the diagnosis of peripheral vertigo?

2. Lateral medullary syndrome of Wallenberg is a classic crossed brainstem syndrome that can follow VAD, or from atherothrombotic occlusion of vertebral artery or posterior inferior cerebellar artery (PICA). Name the neuroanatomic tracts/structure(s) which are responsible for the following findings in a patient with Wallenberg syndrome:

   - The patient veers to one side when asked to walk straight despite normal strength on confrontational testing.
   - The patient has pain on the left side of the face and right side of the body.
   - Horner syndrome.
   - The patient has normal strength throughout due to sparing of which tracts?
   - Several months after a lateral medullary infarction, a patient complains of increased sweating on the left side of his body and absent sweating on his right side.

3. A 50-year-old woman with difficult-to-control arterial hypertension and a history of cervical carotid artery dissection presents with left-sided headache, neck pain, and dizziness. MRA of the head and neck vessels shows a left VAD and a 5-mm

unruptured right posterior communicating artery aneurysm. Which underlying diagnosis could account for these findings and her medical history? What is the likely mechanism of uncontrolled hypertension? What other rare conditions predispose a patient to arterial dissections?

CHALLENGE

Horner syndrome could result from cervical dissection of either the cervical ICA or the vertebral arteries in the neck. Explain the mechanism of Horner syndrome in these two types of cervical arterial dissection. Explain how pharmacologic testing can differentiate Horner syndrome due to cervical ICA dissection from Horner syndrome due to a vertebral artery dissection. Why would you expect loss of sweating with Horner syndrome from VAD but not from ICAD?

REFERENCES

Caplan LR. Dissections of brain-supplying arteries. *Nat Clin Pract Neurol.* 2008;4(1):34-42. [free online resource]
Gottesman RF, Sharma P, Robinson KA, et al. Clinical characteristics of symptomatic vertebral artery dissection: a systematic review. *Neurologist.* 2012;18(5):245-254. [free online resource]

61 "Crossed" Brainstem Vascular Syndromes

Ischemic stroke due to occlusion of one of the arterial perforator branches supplying the brainstem

CORE FEATURES

The table summarizes clinical findings in several named crossed brainstem syndromes. Letters in superscript reference syndrome name.

	Ventral Midbrain Syndromes	Ventral Pontine Syndromes	Dorsal Pontine Syndromes[f]	Dorsal Pontine Syndromes [M-F]	Ventral Medullary Syndrome
1. Ipsilateral cranial nerve deficits	CN III[W,B,C]	CN VI [R M-G] CN VII [M-G]	CN VI + PPRF (horizontal gaze palsy); CN VII		CN XII[D]
2. Contralateral hemiparesis (arm and leg)	Yes [W,B]	Yes [R, M-G]	Yes	Yes	Yes
3. Contralateral sensory deficits				Yes (spinothalamic tract; sparing face)	Yes (medial lemniscus; sparing face)
4. Ipsilateral cerebellar signs	Yes [C] (superior cerebellar peduncle)			Yes, hemiataxia (pontocerebellar tract)	
5. Ipsilateral extrapyramidal signs	Yes [B] (red nucleus)				

Millard-Gubler (M-G), Raymond (R), Foville (F), and Marie-Foix (M-F) are pontine syndromes; Weber (W), Benedikt (B), and Claude (C) are midbrain syndromes.

SYNOPSIS

Brainstem ischemic strokes are usually due to occlusion of perforating arteries that arise from the vertebral or basilar artery or their respective branches: posterior inferior cerebellar artery (PICA), anterior inferior cerebellar artery (AICA), superior cerebellar artery (SCA), and PCA. Brainstem stroke syndromes typically involve only one side of the brainstem, but their clinical manifestations are often "crossed", with cranial nerve deficits ipsilateral to the lesion and hemibody motor-sensory deficits contralateral to the lesion. The ventral-dorsal coordinate of the lesion can be deduced based on which of the cranial nerves are involved. CN III palsy implies midbrain level; CN VI palsy—pontine level, CN XII palsy—medullary level. The lateral-medial coordinate can be deduced based on which of the long tracts are involved: motor tracts in more medial lesions and spinothalamic tracts in more lateral lesions. The table lists classic named brainstem syndromes, with the exception of the laterally medullary syndrome of Wallenberg, which is discussed in the chapter on vertebral artery dissection (Chapter 60).

Noncontrast head CT is useful to rule out a brainstem hemorrhage but is not sensitive to ischemia in the posterior fossa. MRI with diffusion-weighted imaging (DWI-MRI) is recommended when a brainstem infarction is suspected, with the caveat that some infarctions, particularly involving the midbrain and caudal tegmentum pontis, should not be excluded by early DWI-negative MRI.

FIGURE

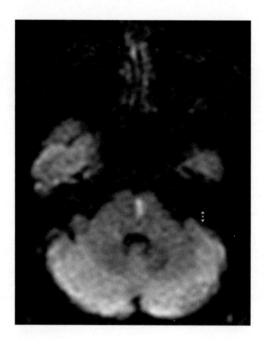

Brain DWI sequence shows a left paramedian pontine infarction.

QUESTIONS FOR SELF-STUDY

1. Vertigo—an illusion of motion when the person is stationary—is a common symptom. A rare but important cause of new-onset vertigo is a brainstem stroke. Describe how to perform HiNTS a battery of tests, which can help "rule out" brainstem lesion as a cause of vertigo with a sensitivity that exceeds that of brain MRI. HiNTS consists of Head Impulse test (unilateral "positive" test is reassuring for peripheral cause); spontaneous or gaze-evoked Nystagmus (absence is reassuring for a peripheral cause of vertigo); ocular Skew deviation (absence is reassuring for a peripheral cause of vertigo); and abnormalities in smooth pursuit and saccadic eye movements (absence is reassuring for a peripheral cause). (Compare your response with LaPlant et al. Vertigo: A hint on the HiNTS examination at http://www.nuemblog.com/blog/hints. [free online resource])

2. Explain the anatomical basis for horizontal gaze paresis—the inability to move both eyes passed the midline on one direction—in dorsal pontine syndromes.

3. Explain the anatomical basis for the "one and a half syndrome" (patient only able to move one eye out).

4. Suggest localization for a lesion that causes tongue paralysis and flaccid quadriplegia sparing the face.

5. Millard-Gubler syndrome features facial paresis ipsilateral to the lesion and paresis of arm and leg contralateral to the lesion. The pattern of facial weakness is "peripheral" (both upper and lower facial muscles are involved). Explain how a central nervous system (CNS) lesion can account for a "peripheral" pattern of facial palsy.

CHALLENGE

A pontine stroke can cause an ipsilateral facial palsy and a contralateral hemiparesis (Millard-Gubler syndrome) as well as a contralateral facial palsy and a contralateral hemiparesis (Raymond syndrome). What is the neuroanatomic basis for the facial weakness in these two brainstem syndromes? Explain the laterality of facial symptoms in the two syndromes.

REFERENCES

Brandt T, Dieterich M. The dizzy patient: don't forget disorders of the central vestibular system. *Nat Rev Neurol.* 2017;13(6):352-362. [free online resource]

Oppenheim C, Stanescu R, Dormont D, et al. False-negative diffusion-weighted MR findings in acute ischemic stroke. *AJNR Am J Neuroradiol.* 2000;21(8):1434-1440.

Querol-Pascual MR. Clinical approach to brainstem lesions. *Semin Ultrasound CT MR.* 2010;31(3):220-229.

62 Lacunar (Small-Vessel) Syndromes

Ischemic stroke due to occlusion of small penetrating end- arteries and arterioles

CORE FEATURES

Note that this table describes five common lacunar syndromes, not five features of one syndrome.

Symptoms	Localization
1. Pure motor hemiparesis	Contralateral corticospinal tract at the level of the internal capsule, corona radiata, pons
2. Pure sensory stroke (hemisensory deficits)	Contralateral posterolateral thalamus, often in the territory of the thalamogeniculate artery
3. Sensorimotor stroke (hemisensory deficits and hemiparesis)	Contralateral thalamus and adjacent posterior limb of the internal capsule
4. Ataxic hemiparesis	Basal pons
5. Dysarthria-clumsy hand syndrome	Basal pons, contralateral internal capsule

SYNOPSIS

Lacunar infarctions are small lesions less than 15 mm in diameter, round or ovoid in shape. They result from occlusion of small penetrating end-arteries and arterioles in the deep, subcortical regions of the cerebrum and brainstem. Lacunar infarctions in clinically eloquent areas account for 30% of all ischemic strokes but represent a small fraction of all lacunar infarctions (most are "silent infarctions"). Lacunes are found alongside other stigmata of vascular aging and disease: subcortical infarcts, white matter hyperintensities, enlarged perivascular (Virchow-Robin) spaces, and microbleeds. Population-based studies have shown that a higher burden of white matter vascular lesions correlate with worse long-term cognitive and gait outcomes. Hence, the importance of controlling vascular risk factors—arterial hypertension, diabetes mellitus, hyperlipidemia, obesity, and cigarette smoking—even in patients without a stroke history.

FIGURE

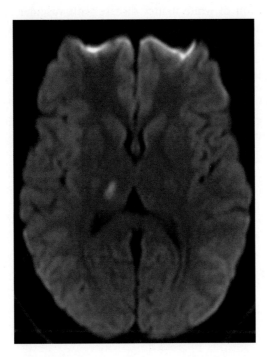

Brain DWI shows a left thalamic lacunar infarction.

QUESTIONS FOR SELF-STUDY

1. A 65-year-old former smoker with a history of arterial hypertension presented to the ED following a 15-minute episode of numbness around the right side of his mouth and right hand. Neurologic examination and noncontrast head CT were normal. What is the name of this syndrome? What is the probable etiology? What is the appropriate workup?

2. A 60-year-old woman presents with a 20-minute episode of blurry vision on the right. She describes a progressive loss of vision coming in from the right side toward the center. This is the third time she had similar symptoms in the last 4 years. The examination is normal. Stroke workup, including brain MRI and MRA, is unremarkable. What is the likely diagnosis?

3. An 80-year-old previously healthy man presented with acute-onset uncontrollable, nonrhythmic flinging movements of the left arm. Assuming the cause of symptoms is a lacunar infarction, what is the most likely localization? What is the name of this syndrome?

4. A 90-year-old woman develops severe pain on the left half of her body, which was previously affected by a stroke. Where is the likely localization of the stroke? What is the likely etiology of this pain syndrome?

5. Which sleep disorder is a risk factor for stroke?

CHALLENGE

How is the progression of white matter disease with vascular aging graded on the Fazekas scale? (Compare your answer with Forbes reference below.)

REFERENCES

Forbes K. MRI brain white matter change: spectrum of change – how can we grade? *J R Coll Physicians Edinb.* 2017;47:271-271. [free online resource]

Regenhardt RW, Das AS, Lo EH, Caplan LR. Advances in understanding the pathophysiology of lacunar stroke: a review. *JAMA Neurol.* 2018;75(10):1273-1281.

Southerland AM. Clinical evaluation of the patient with acute stroke. *Continuum (Minneap Minn).* 2017;23(1, Cerebrovascular Disease):40-61.

63 Hypertensive Intracerebral Hemorrhage

Hemorrhage in brain parenchyma associated with long-standing arterial hypertension

CORE FEATURES

1. Rapid neurologic deterioration.
   Progression of symptoms from normal to obtunded and comatose within minutes to hours is highly characteristic of large intracerebral hemorrhages.
2. Severe headache.
3. Vomiting at symptom onset.
4. Dramatic elevation in blood pressure.
   Systolic blood pressure is much higher than at baseline and may exceed 220 mm Hg.
5. Noncontrast head CT shows bright (hyperdense) signal within the brain parenchyma. Brain MRI was considered inferior to noncontrast head CT for imaging of parenchymal bleeding because acute blood appears isointense on T1- and T2-weighted MR sequences. However, with the addition of gradient echo and T2* susceptibility–weighted sequences, which are exquisitely sensitive to acute blood products, the sensitivity of brain MRI is comparable to that of head CT.

SYNOPSIS

Hypertensive ICH results from the rupture of small penetrating arterioles. The most common locations for spontaneous hypertensive ICH are the putamen, thalamus, cerebellum, and pons. Lobar hemorrhages require evaluation for nonhypertensive causes. Rapid evolution and severity of symptoms is a result of rapid hematoma expansion and mass effect. Increasing intracranial pressure may explain such common manifestations of ICH as extreme blood pressure elevation, headaches, and vomiting. Other neurologic manifestations will depend on the location of ICH and whether there is intraventricular bleeding, hydrocephalus, and compartmental shifts with brain herniation. Arterial hypertension remains the most common cause of spontaneous ICH. Other important causes include cerebral amyloid angiopathy (CAA); ruptured CNS vascular malformations; oral anticoagulant therapy (vitamin K antagonists, direct oral anticoagulants), antiplatelet therapy, heparins or thrombolytic agents; sympathomimetic drugs (cocaine, amphetamines); bleeding diatheses (leukemia, hemophilia, thrombocytopenia, disseminated intravascular coagulation [DIC], coagulopathy); primary or secondary neoplasms; systemic or primary CNS vasculitis; CNS infections, cerebral hyperperfusion syndrome after carotid artery stenting (CAS) and carotid artery endarterectomy (CEA); and cerebral venous sinus thrombosis (CVST).

FIGURES

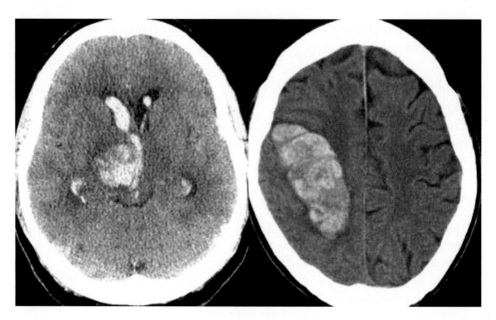

Left: Thalamic hypertensive hemorrhage with rupture into the ventricles. Right: Lobar hematoma due to coagulopathy of liver disease in a patient with alcohol use disorder.

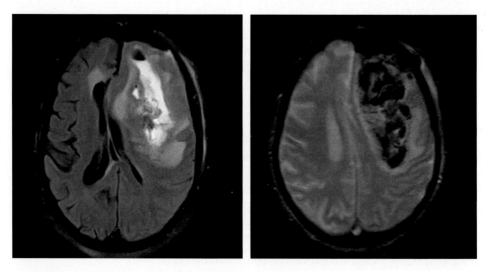

Fluid-attenuated inversion recovery (FLAIR) MRI of a lobar hemorrhage with subfalcine herniation and midline shift (left). GRE sequence on a subsequent MRI highlights the area of hemorrhage (dark signal, right). The second MRI was done after the patient had a frontal craniotomy.

QUESTIONS FOR SELF-STUDY

1. A "found down" patient is brought to the ED. Noncontrast head CT shows a large ICH. What are the most important laboratory tests to obtain at this time?
2. A 75-year-old man with long-standing arterial hypertension presents with new-onset headache, vomiting, and falling. He is alert and oriented. Cranial nerves are intact. Motor and sensory examinations are normal. However, he is unable to sit or stand unassisted. Assuming ICH is the diagnosis, what is the likely location of the hematoma?
3. Indications for surgical intervention are not well established for spontaneous ICH, except in one clinical scenario where there is broad consensus that emergent surgical hematoma removal is indicated. What is this scenario?
4. A 75-year-old normotensive man is brought to the ED with new-onset headache and left hemiparesis. Noncontrast head CT shows an acute hematoma in the right frontal subcortical white matter and evidence of smaller foci of old hemorrhages in the left occipital and parietal lobes. What is the likely cause of ICH in this patient?
5. What are common funduscopic findings of long-standing, poorly controlled arterial hypertension? (Compare your responses with https://eyewiki.aao.org/Hypertensive_retinopathy#Physical_examination. [free online resource])

CHALLENGE

The dramatic medical case history presented below illustrates many of the cardinal features of a hemorrhagic stroke. Suggest a pathologic mechanism that may explain the sequence of changes in the pupillary size described by the attending physician.

> "He was in a very good mood in the morning and his guests commented … how well he looked. He was sitting in a chair—as the subject of some sketches …—when he suddenly complained of a terrific occipital headache. He became unconscious within a minute or two. When seen 15 minutes later, he was pale and sweating profusely and totally unconscious. Pupils were at first equal, but in a few minutes, the left pupil became widely dilated… Systolic blood pressure was well over 300 mm Hg, diastolic was 190 mm Hg… [15 minute later] breathing a little irregular. BP fallen to 240/120… [30 minute later] right pupil still widely dilated, left pupil from moderate constriction become moderately dilated… [15 minute later] Pupils approximately equal. Breathing irregular. [1 minute later] Breathing stopped …."

The patient was Franklin Delano Roosevelt, 32nd US President. For more detail on FDR's medical history, see http://www.fdrlibraryvirtualtour.org/graphics/07-38/7.5_FDRs_Health.pdf. [free online resource]

REFERENCES

Hemphill JC III, Greenberg SM, Anderson CS, et al. Guidelines for the management of spontaneous intracerebral hemorrhage: a guideline for healthcare professionals from the American Heart Association/American Stroke Association. *Stroke*. 2015;46:2032-2060. [free online resource]

Hobson EV, Craven I, Blank SC. Posterior reversible encephalopathy syndrome: a truly treatable neurologic illness. *Perit Dial Int*. 2012;32(6):590-594. [free online resource]

64 Nontraumatic Subarachnoid Hemorrhage

Most commonly, SAH is the result of rupture of an intracranial aneurysm into subarachnoid space

CORE FEATURES

1. Thunderclap headache.
   "Worst headache of my life." Sudden headache that is maximal in intensity at onset is highly suspicious for SAH, but more gradual headaches are also compatible with this diagnosis. Some patients may have a history of thunderclap headache prior to SAH ("sentinel bleed").
2. Altered level of consciousness.
   The level of arousal at presentation correlates with prognosis. A clear sensorium predicts better outcomes; coma portends the worst prognosis.
3. Noncontrast head CT shows blood in the subarachnoid space.
   The sensitivity of noncontrast head CT for SAH within hours of bleeding is very high when read by an experienced neuroradiologist. As blood resolves, sensitivity decreases and only 50% of patients will have subarachnoid blood on noncontrast head CT one week following the bleed.
4. Blood and blood products (bilirubin) in the cerebrospinal fluid (CSF).
   The absence of red blood cells (RBCs) in the CSF at the time of presentation excludes the diagnosis of SAH. Xanthochromia, a yellow tinge of the CSF due to the presence of bilirubin, may not be observable at onset as it develops within 12 hours of bleeding and dissipates within 3 weeks.
5. Cerebral aneurysm visualized on CT or MR angiogram.
   Conventional catheter cerebral angiography is traditionally considered the gold standard for diagnosis of cerebral aneurysms, but the noninvasive CTA can detect aneurysms as small as 2 mm in diameter and is usually adequate for ruling out aneurysms.

SYNOPSIS

Intracranial aneurysms are present in approximately 3% of the general population, but very few of them will rupture. Risk factors for aneurysmal rupture include arterial hypertension, cigarette smoking, heavy alcohol consumption, and drug abuse, particularly of cocaine. Brain aneurysmal rupture is a catastrophic event. Thunderclap headache and syncope (in half of the patients), rapidly followed by meningismus, depressed consciousness, focal deficits, and seizures, is a characteristic sequence following SAH. Ten percent of patients with aneurysmal SAH die before reaching a hospital. One-third of the survivors remain neurologically devastated.

Patients with SAH should promptly undergo cerebrovascular imaging to determine the source of bleeding. In 80% of cases, nontraumatic SAH is caused by a ruptured cerebral aneurysm. Because the risk of aneurysmal rerupture within 1 month is as high as 40%, it is recommended that treatment—either surgical (clipping) or endovascular (coiling)—should not be unduly delayed. Nonaneurysmal causes of SAH include intracranial arterial dissections, ruptured arteriovenous malformation, dural arteriovenous fistulae, bleeding diatheses, cocaine abuse, primary or systemic CNS vasculitis, cerebral amyloid angiopathy, reversible cerebral vasoconstriction syndrome, and perimesencephalic SAH.

FIGURES

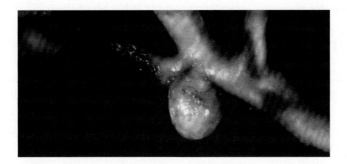

Brain aneurysm near vessel bifurcation on a postmortem.

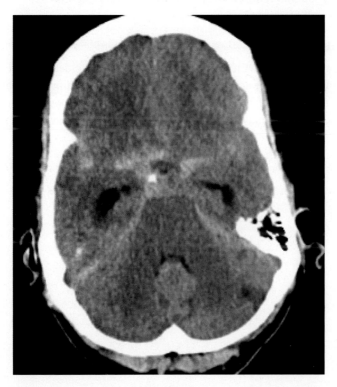

"Star sign" of SAH in a noncontrast head CT. Note also the radiographic evidence of early hydrocephalus with enlargement of the temporal horns.

QUESTIONS FOR SELF-STUDY

1. What is a "three-tube test"? Explain how the "three-tube" test could help differentiate SAH from a traumatic LP. (Note that this test is only reliable if no RBCs are found in the third tube.)

2. A 40-year-old man admitted for aneurysmal SAH underwent a successful aneurysmal clipping. Five days following the procedure, he became obtunded and hemiparetic. Noncontrast head CT does not show acute bleeding. What is the likely explanation for the neurologic deterioration? What pharmacologic strategy should be used to prevent this complication?

3. Five weeks following an aneurysmal SAH and successful endovascular clipping of the brain aneurysm, the patient's condition begins to decline: he is mentally slow and has difficulty walking. Head CT shows newly enlarged ventricles. What is the likely explanation for the neurologic deterioration in the context of his medical history?

4. A patient who presents with thunderclap headache requires stat head CT and, if negative, an LP to rule out SAH. If these studies are normal, urgent brain MRI, MRA of the brain and neck, and MRV are recommended. Explain the necessity of each of these tests.

5. A 25-year-old woman presents to the ED with a thunderclap headache 2 weeks following an uneventful delivery. She is obtunded and hemiparetic. MRA shows multiple segmental areas of intracranial arterial constriction. What is the likely diagnosis? How would you differentiate this entity from primary angiitis of the central nervous system (PACNS)?

CHALLENGE

A CSF sample of a patient with suspected SAH has been accidentally left in the refrigerator for a few days. Laboratory staff is reluctant to test the sample for xanthochromia because they are concerned that the results would be a false positive due to cell lysis. Explain why xanthochromia only occurs if there is RBC lysis in vivo but not ex vivo.

REFERENCES

Al-Shahi R, White PM, Davenport RJ, Lindsay KW. Subarachnoid haemorrhage. *BMJ*. 2006;333(7561):235-240. [free online resource]

Lawton MT, Vates GE. Subarachnoid hemorrhage. *N Engl J Med*. 2017;377(3):257-266.

65 Acute and Chronic Subdural Hematoma

Bleeding into subdural space due to tearing of "bridging veins"

CORE FEATURES

	Acute SDH (<3 d)	Chronic SDH (>3 wk)
1. Symptoms evolve over…	Hours to days	Weeks to months
2. Head trauma precedes symptom onset	Yes, usually	Often no history of head trauma or trivial head trauma weeks prior to symptom onset
3. Headache	Common, often severe	In half of the patients, often mild
4. Altered mental status	Symptoms range from acute encephalopathy to stupor and coma	Cognitive decline and behavioral changes in half of the patients
5. Non-contrast head CT	Crescent of bright signal in subdural space, often with mass effect on the brain	Crescent of dark signal in subdural space; neomembrane around the hematoma

SYNOPSIS

Subdural hematoma most often results from tears of "bridging veins" in the subdural space as they course from the cortex to the dural sinuses. Prominent cerebral atrophy, which occurs with advanced age and chronic alcohol use disorder, leads to stretching of the bridging veins in the subdural space and predisposes to SDH. The use of oral anticoagulant therapy is another major risk factor. Acute subdural hematoma (aSDH) is usually diagnosed promptly if there is a history of head trauma and rapid evolution of neurologic symptoms. A "stat" noncontrast head CT will then demonstrate the characteristic crescent of acute blood over one or both cerebral hemispheres, sometimes with mass effect. Chronic subdural hematoma (cSDH), on the other hand, presents a diagnostic challenge. Symptoms of cSDH evolve slowly, over weeks or months, and are usually nonlocalizing—headaches, subtle behavioral and cognitive changes. When patients with known cSDH experience acute neurologic worsening, rebleeding into the old hematoma should be suspected—so-called "acute-on-chronic SDH." As cSDH is one of a few reversible causes of cognitive decline, it should always be considered in the differential diagnosis of rapidly progressive dementia.

There are no specific medical interventions for SDH, other than promptly reversing a coagulopathy or low platelet count if present. Surgical options include twist drill or burr hole opening, with or without drainage, and, in the more severe cases, craniotomy.

FIGURE

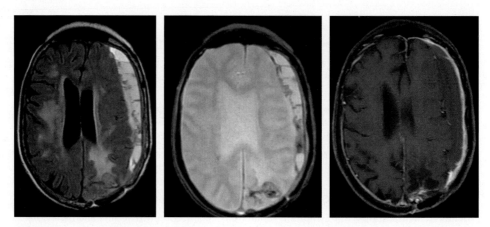

Acute on chronic subdural hematoma with mass effect in adjacent frontoparietal temporal lobes and rightward midline shift in a patient with lung and ovarian cancer with brain metastases and numerous falls. T2 FLAIR sequence shows the subdural hematoma as well as metastatic parenchymal lesions (left). Susceptibility-weighted imaging (SWI) sequence shows small areas of acute bleeding within the subdural hematoma and the intraparenchymal metastatic lesion (middle). T1-weighted image with contrast shows pseudomembrane over the subdural hematoma, indicating chronicity (right).

QUESTIONS FOR SELF-STUDY

1. A 6-month-old infant is brought to the ED by her mother with failure to thrive and vomiting. On examination, the infant is drowsy but arousable. Multiple bruises are noted on both arms. Retinal hemorrhages are present on funduscopy. Nonenhanced head CT shows both acute and cSDHs. Which diagnosis best explains all of these findings?

2. A 60-year-old man presents with a new-onset seizure. Head CT shows a small SDH. What are the nontraumatic etiologies of SDH to be considered in this context? Which additional testing is necessary?

3. Explain why the appearance of blood on noncontrast head CT changes from hyperdense (bright) in the acute phase, to isodense relative to the cortex in the subacute phase, to hypodense (dark) after 2 weeks.

4. The following case history is taken from "*That to study philosophy is to learn to die,*" an essay by Michel de Montaigne published in 1580:

   "...A brother of mine, Captain St Martin, a young man, three-and-twenty years old, who had already given sufficient testimony of his valour, playing a match at tennis, received a blow of a ball a little above his right ear, which, as it gave no manner of sign of wound or contusion, he took no notice of it, nor so much as sat down to repose himself, but, nevertheless, died within five or 6 hours..."

What is the likely diagnosis? How do you explain the "lucid period" between initial trauma and subsequent demise? What would you expect a head CT to show?

5. Epidural hematoma is most often the result of the traumatic rupture of the middle meningeal artery. Blood accumulates rapidly in the epidural space between the skull and the dura. The pace of progression is typically much faster than in SDH due to the higher pressure in the arteries compared to the veins. An epidural hematoma usually requires urgent surgical intervention. One way to differentiate epidural from a subdural hematoma on CT is that epidural hematomas generally do not cross suture lines. Provide an anatomical explanation for why epidural hematomas "respect" suture lines, while subdural hematomas do not.

CHALLENGE

A patient is brought to the ED with depressed mental status, worsening right-sided hemiparesis and a dilated right pupil. Head CT head shows a large, right frontoparietal convexity subdural hematoma with early transtentorial herniation. How can you explain a right-sided hemiparesis in a patient whose intracranial lesion is on the right side? What is the name of this syndrome?

REFERENCES

Adhiyaman, Asghar M, Ganeshram KN, Bhowmick BK. Chronic subdural haematoma in the elderly. *Postgrad Med J*. 2002;78(916):71-75. [free online resource]
Vega RA, Valadka AB. Natural history of acute subdural hematoma. *Neurosurg Clin N Am*. 2017;28(2):247-255.

66 Cerebral Venous Sinus Thrombosis

Thrombosis of the deep and superficial cerebral veins and dural sinuses can lead to venous infarctions and increased intracranial pressure

CORE FEATURES

1. Headache.
   Headache is the most common and may be the only manifestation of cerebral venous sinus thrombosis (CVST). Onset is gradual, rarely "thunderclap."
2. Papilledema.
   Observed in 40% of patients with CVST, it is a sign of increased intracranial pressure.
3. Stroke.
   Acute onset of focal neurological deficits with imaging evidence of one or more strokes not fitting an arterial distribution pattern.
4. Seizures.
   Reported in 40% of patients with CVST, seizures are much more common in venous than in arterial ischemic strokes.
5. Signs of CVST on neuroimaging.
   In the proper clinical context, the abnormal signal within the venous sinuses and absence of flow on MRV make the diagnosis of CVST highly likely. An "empty delta sign" on contrast-enhanced CT or MRI is a sign of superior sagittal sinus thrombosis.

SYNOPSIS

CVST is a challenging diagnosis. Presentations are highly variable and include new-onset headaches, raised intracranial pressure syndrome, strokes, new-onset seizures, cavernous sinus syndrome, and depressed consciousness due to thalamic involvement. Time course is also highly variable, ranging from hyperacute—onset to nadir within a few hours—to subacute-to-chronic, unfolding over many weeks or longer. CVST should be considered in the differential diagnosis of an array of syndromes, including stroke, especially in young patients and in patients with predisposition to venous thrombosis (pregnancy or peripartum period, malignancy, hypercoagulable disorder) Features favoring venous over arterial strokes on imaging include the presence of multiple infarctions, often with hemorrhagic transformation; infarctions not confined to a single arterial territory; large infarctions with cortical sparing; diffuse brain or bilateral thalamic edema; and intraparenchymal and SAHs.

FIGURE

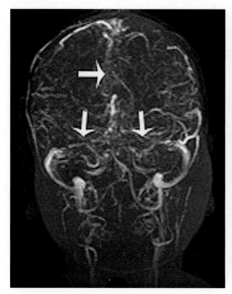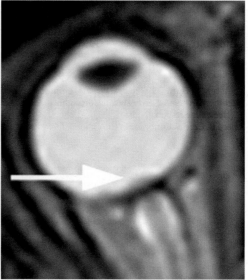

MR venography demonstrated partial thrombosis of the superior sagittal sinus, torcula, and proximal transverse sinuses (arrows). Close-up of the right eye shows protrusion of optic nerve papilla into the globe (arrow) consistent with increased intracranial pressure from sinus thrombosis. (Reprinted with permission from Zimmer JA, Garg BP, O'Neill DP, et al. Teaching neuroimage: MRI visualization of papilledema associated with cerebral sinovenous thrombosis in a child. *Neurology*. 2008;71(7):e12-e13.)

QUESTIONS FOR SELF-STUDY

1. A 5-year-old girl presents with signs of raised intracranial pressure. She has had several days of fevers and progressive ear pain. Examination shows a bulging right tympanic membrane and effusion. Can you provide a unifying explanation of this child's clinical course?

2. What is the first-line treatment for CVST? What interventions should be considered in a patient with CVST whose neurologic status is deteriorating despite first-line therapy?

3. A 25-year-old healthy woman on estrogen-containing contraceptives develops CVST. What laboratory tests are indicated to elucidate the possible etiology?

4. Although venous infarctions may appear to be quite extensive of MRI, they are often not as debilitating as arterial ischemic strokes, likely because the signal abnormalities are due to vasogenic rather than cytotoxic edema. How would you differentiate vasogenic from cytotoxic edema with diffusion-weighted imaging (DWI) and apparent diffusion coefficient (ADC) MRI sequences?

5. Explain why the loss of signal in one or more of the intracranial venous sinuses is not an absolute diagnostic criteria of CVST. What anatomical venous variant could be mistaken for venous thrombosis on MRV or computed tomography venography (CTV)?

CHALLENGE

Bilateral edematous thalamic strokes raise the possibility of thrombosis of the deep intracranial venous system draining venous flow from both thalami. However, bilateral thalamic strokes can also be due to arterial etiologies. Explain how an occlusion of a single intracranial artery could result in bilateral thalamic infarctions.

REFERENCES

Bousser MG, Ferro JM. Cerebral venous thrombosis: an update. *Lancet Neurol.* 2007;6(2):162-170.
Guenther G, Arauz A. Cerebral venous thrombosis: a diagnostic and treatment update. *Neurologia.* 2011;26(8):488-498. [free online resource]
Ichord R. Cerebral sinovenous thrombosis. *Front Pediatr.* 2017;5:163. [free online resource]

Epilepsy

A Very Brief Introduction to Epilepsy

...in the midst of his conversation he stopped and became silent... from his behavior, now staring at the ground with fixed gaze and eyes wide open without moving an eyelid, again closing them, compressing his lips and raising his eyebrows, we could perceive plainly that a fit of madness of some kind had come upon him.

Miguel de Cervantes Saavedra[*]

Epilepsy, from the Greek "to seize," affects 3% of the population in advanced economy countries and an even higher proportion in emerging economies. The first known description of a generalized seizure, with attribution to the moon god, comes from a 4000-year-old Assyrian tablet: "his neck turns left, his hands and feet are tense and his eyes wide open, and from his mouth froth is flowing without his having any consciousness." Otherworldly origins of epilepsy, widely accepted in antiquity and even to this day among some societies, were denied by the rationalistically inclined physicians since the time of Hippocrates, the "Father of Medicine," who declared epilepsy to be "no more divine than any other disease" and attributed its cause—"as of the more serious diseases generally"—to the brain.

The groundwork for the modern understanding of epilepsy was laid in the 19th century. John Hughlings Jackson, the pioneering English neurologist, defined epilepsy as "occasional, sudden, excessive, rapid, and local discharge of gray matter." Jackson further hypothesized that a type of seizure in which twitching starts in one part of the body and progresses to involve the neighboring muscle groups is a result of the propagation of the discharge through somatotopically organized cortical matter. This insight provided crucial support for the foundational principle of neurology that focal neurologic deficits localize to specific focal lesions within the nervous system and led to the development of modern neurologic examination.

A seizure must be differentiated from paroxysmal events of nonepileptic etiology. A comprehensive listing of seizure mimickers can be found at https://www.epilepsydiagnosis.org/epilepsy-imitators.html. A thorough history obtained from the patient and bystanders who witnessed the event is indispensable for diagnosis. Physical examination may also offer important clues: lateral tongue biting is highly suggestive of a generalized tonic-clonic seizure (GTCS), while temporary focal paralysis following a seizure (Todd's paralysis) may point to an underlying structural lesion that precipitated a seizure. Once a seizure diagnosis is confirmed, the clinician will need to try to identify its proximate cause. Common seizure triggers include intracerebral lesions (strokes, neoplasms), head trauma, drug exposure or drug withdrawal, metabolic disturbances, and, in children, any febrile illness ("Febrile Seizures," Chapter 69). The search for cause of seizure will depend on the clinical context and may include testing of serum electrolyte

---

[*]Miguel de Cervantes Saavedra (1547-1616), a contemporary of William Shakespeare, was a singular influence on Spanish language and literature. A son of a physician, Cervantes was well versed in medicine, and his works include clinically precise descriptions of many medical conditions. For a review of neurologic diseases mentioned in Cervantes' magnum opus, *Don Quixote*, see Palma JA and Palma F. Neurology and Don Quixote. Eur Neurol. 2012;68(4):247-57.

levels, with special attention to glucose, sodium, and renal function; brain magnetic resonance imaging (MRI) using "epilepsy protocol" that allows for detection of subtle structural abnormalities, such as focal cortical dysplasia and mesial temporal sclerosis; toxicology screen; cerebrospinal fluid (CSF) analysis if there is a suspicion for central nervous system (CNS) infection or subarachnoid hemorrhage (SAH); autoimmune antibody panel if autoimmune epilepsy is suspected; and genetic testing where there is a possibility of an inherited epilepsy syndrome. A seizure with no identifiable cause— an "unprovoked" seizure—carries a substantial risk of seizure recurrence and raises the question of whether the patient needs to be started on an antiseizure medication to lower the risk of subsequent seizures. The risk of epilepsy is especially high in patients with an abnormal neurological examination, brain lesions on MRI, abnormal electro-encephalography (EEG), and those who experienced a seizure during sleep. Although traditionally the diagnosis of epilepsy required two unprovoked seizures, presently even a single unprovoked seizure in a patient whose risk of recurrence is more than 60% will satisfy criteria for the epilepsy diagnosis and warrant antiseizure therapy. Patients with unprovoked seizures should receive standard "seizure precautions"—to avoid working at heights, near heavy machinery, scuba diving, ladder climbing, unobserved swim-ming, and tub baths. The legal requirement with regard to driving limitations follow-ing a seizure varies by state and country (https://www.epilepsy.com/driving-laws [free online resource]).

EEG helps to stratify the risk of recurrence after a first event and to determine sei-zure type—focal onset versus generalized. Focal-onset seizures arise within one hemi-sphere and are associated with focal EEG abnormalities (Chapter 67). If a focal-onset seizure spreads to the other hemisphere, conscious awareness will be lost, manifesting either in complex automatisms ("fit of madness" described by Cervantes in the epi-graph), motor behavioral arrest, or tonic-clonic seizures (Chapter 68). Generalized-onset seizures originate as synchronous abnormal discharges in both hemispheres and, as a rule, present with loss of consciousness (LOC) at the onset. It may be difficult to distinguish generalized-onset seizures from focal-onset seizures that quickly become "generalized," but it is important to clarify the seizure type whenever possible as etiol-ogies and treatments will differ depending on whether seizures are generalized or focal onset. Once the seizure type is known, the clinician will have to determine whether the seizure pattern fits in with one of the epilepsy syndromes, and this determination will guide optimal treatment. Several classic epilepsy syndromes are discussed in this sec-tion: Childhood Absence Epilepsy (Chapter 70), Juvenile Myoclonic Epilepsy (Chapter 71), Lennox-Gastaut (Chapter 73), and West Syndrome (Chapter 72).

REFERENCES

Magiorkinis E, Sidiropoulou K, Diamantis A. Hallmarks in the history of epilepsy: epilepsy in antiquity. *Epilepsy Behav.* 2010;17(1):103-108.

Pohlmann-Eden B, Beghi E, Camfield C, Camfield P. The first seizure and its management in adults and children. *BMJ.* 2006;332(7537):339-342. [free online resource]

Scheffer IE, Berkovic S, Capovilla G, et al. ILAE classification of the epilepsies: position paper of the ILAE Commission for Classification and Terminology. *Epilepsia.* 2017;58(4):512-521. [free online resource]

Focal Seizures ▪

Focal-onset seizures originate within a neural network located in one hemisphere

CORE FEATURES

Focal seizures are classified according to whether they are accompanied by loss of awareness (focal impaired-awareness seizures, FIAS, vs focal aware seizures, FAS) and according to their presumed sites of origin. This section contains a listing of common sites of origin of focal seizures and the typical symptoms with each locus of origin.

1. Temporal lobe seizures.
   The temporal lobe seizures, the most common focal seizures, begin with sensory (olfactory, gustatory, auditory, vertiginous), emotional (fear), cognitive (déjà vu, jamais vu), or autonomic (epigastric rising sensation, tachycardia, pallor) symptoms and may evolve into complex oral and manual automatisms, behavioral arrest, or bilateral tonic-clonic seizures. Temporal lobe seizures are usually due to hippocampal sclerosis.
2. Frontal lobe seizures.
   Symptoms include Jacksonian march (unilateral tonic-clonic movements starting in one muscle group spreading to adjacent muscle groups); bilateral asymmetric tonic posturing with vocalization or speech arrest; aphasia or dysphasia (if Broca area is involved); hyperkinetic automatisms; olfactory hallucinations; autonomic symptoms (palpitations, altered respiration, epigastric sensation, flushing, piloerection, lacrimation); and forced thoughts.
3. Frontoparietal operculum seizures (rolandic seizures).
   This subtype of frontal seizures is the hallmark of a common epilepsy syndrome—childhood epilepsy with centrotemporal spikes (CECTS). Children with CECTS have twitching and tingling of one side of the face or tongue, sometimes accompanied by drooling and impaired articulation. If seizures occur during sleep, they can progress to GTCS. CECTS is typically self-limited and may not require antiseizure medications.
4. Parietal lobe seizures.
   Unilateral paresthesias and dysesthesias are the most common symptoms and may spread along the body in a Jacksonian march. Visual, vertiginous, and gustatory hallucinations, as well as disturbances of body image (somatic illusion), can occur as well. Receptive language impairment points to the involvement of the dominant parietal hemisphere.
5. Occipital lobe seizures.
   Elementary visual hallucinations or transient loss of vision (ictal amaurosis) are the most frequent manifestations. Blinking, forced eye closure, eyelid fluttering, head and eye deviations, and nystagmus may occur as well.

SYNOPSIS

Classifying focal seizures by lobe of origin is convenient, but several caveats must be kept in mind. First, a seizure may originate "silently" in one area of the brain but cause clinical manifestations when it reaches a different brain area. Thus, a parietal lobe seizure that spreads to the temporal lobe and manifests as déjà vu will perfectly mimic a mesial temporal lobe–onset seizure. Secondly, focal seizure symptoms are rarely pathognomonic for a specific brain lobe and often overlap with symptoms of neighboring lobes due to rapid seizure spread. Third, focal seizures can originate in multiple areas, rather than a single region, as is often observed during intraoperative epilepsy monitoring. Finally, the brain lobes are large structures, and each can give rise to a variety of characteristic seizure syndromes depending on which specific area of the lobe is involved. For example, there are seven distinct types of frontal lobe seizures currently recognized. Despite these caveats, by carefully analyzing the ictal semiology, EEG, and brain MRI findings, one can be reasonably assured of the locus of origin of the seizures in most cases. Identifying the site of origin of the ictal focus is no mere academic exercise: the success of surgical resection, an increasingly utilized approach for drug-resistant focal epilepsy, is critically dependent on the correct localization of the site of seizure origin (ictogenic focus).

FIGURES

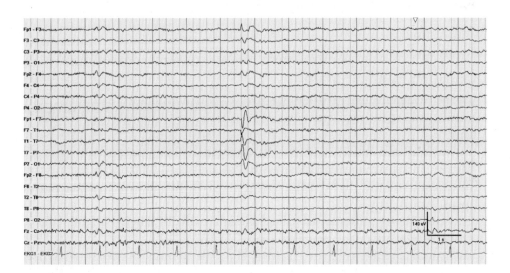

EEG shows a left anterior temporal sharp wave in a 35-year-old woman with mesial temporal lobe epilepsy and left hippocampal atrophy (mesial temporal sclerosis) on MRI. (Courtesy of Dr Jorge Asconapé, Loyola University Chicago, Stritch School of Medicine.)

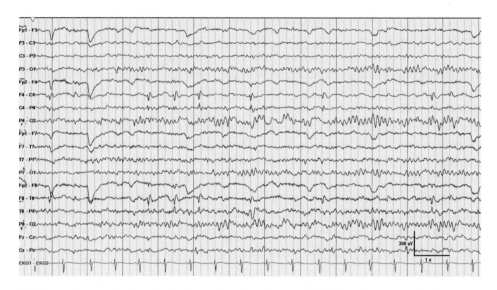

EEG in an 8-year-old girl with benign rolandic epilepsy of childhood. Note the right centrotemporal spikes with phase reversal at C4 and T8. (Courtesy of Dr Jorge Asconapé, Loyola University Chicago, Stritch School of Medicine.)

QUESTIONS FOR SELF-STUDY

1. Define "epileptic aura." Provide examples of common sensory, emotional, autonomic, and cognitive epileptic auras. What is the pathophysiologic basis of epileptic aura?

2. Lateral head and eye deviation may be observed in both hemispheric strokes and seizures. In a stroke, the head and eye turn "toward" the site of the brain lesion, while in epileptic seizures, the head and eyes are typically turned away from the seizure focus. Explain why.

3. In occipital lobe seizures, visual hallucinations are visually simple—brightly colored flashes of light, spots, and geometric shapes. In parietal lobe seizures, the visual hallucinations are more complex—pictures of people, animals, or scenes. What does this observation teach us about the role of the occipital and parietal lobes in the processing of visual information?

4. As a rule, a seizure which manifests with bilateral motor activity involves both hemispheres and is associated with an impaired level of awareness and EEG evidence of bihemispheric ictal activity. In a patient with bilateral tonic-clonic activity, who is awake and responsive and has normal ictal EEG, psychogenic nonepileptic seizure disorder (PNES) should be strongly suspected. Yes, there is one focal epileptic seizure that is an exception to the rule that bilateral motor activity does not occur without impaired awareness or EEG correlate. Which focal seizure should be considered on the differential of PNES?

5. How would you distinguish visual migraine aura from epileptic visual auras based on the pace of symptom evolution and the duration of aura?

CHALLENGE

What are the indications for seizure surgery in patients with focal epilepsy? What modalities—other than EEG and brain MRI—can be utilized to identify the ictogenic focus?

REFERENCES

https://www.epilepsydiagnosis.org/epilepsy/focal-epilepsy-groupoverview.html. [free online resource]

Kumar A, Sharma S. *Complex partial seizure.* In: *StatPearls [Internet].* Treasure Island, FL: StatPearls Publishing; 2019. Available at https://www.ncbi.nlm.nih.gov/books/NBK519030/. [free online resource]

68 Generalized Tonic-Clonic Seizures ∎

Seizures due to synchronous discharges in both hemispheres manifesting as loss of consciousness and bilateral motor activity

CORE FEATURES

1. Abrupt loss of consciousness.
   GTCS begin abruptly and cause patients to fall. Any premonitory signs—aura, lateralized jerking, confusion—imply a focal onset and suggest the diagnosis of "focal to bilateral tonic-clonic seizures" rather than GTCS.
2. Tonic phase is characterized by bilaterally increased tone.
   As the torso goes into flexion and extension, respiratory muscles contract, and the air is expelled against the closed glottis, giving rise to "the epileptic cry." The eyes are wide open and rolled back; the forearms are flexed and the legs extended. Flushing or cyanosis, sweating, and drooling often accompany the tonic phase which usually lasts less than a couple of minutes before giving way to the clonic phase.
3. Clonic phase is characterized by sustained, rhythmic, symmetrical, decelerating contractions of limb and facial muscles.
   The clonic phase usually lasts about a minute and gives way to the postictal phase.
4. Postictal phase is characterized by unresponsiveness followed by confusion.
   At the conclusion of GTCS, patients are first unresponsive, immobile, hypotonic, and then lethargic and confused. Confusion usually resolves in less than an hour, but patients often report cognitive and affective symptoms that linger for hours and days. Headaches (commonly) and psychosis (rarely) may occur in the postictal phase.
5. EEG shows generalized fast rhythmic spikes in the tonic stage and decelerating bursts of spikes and slow waves in the clonic phase.
   Ictal EEG is often uninterpretable due to motion artifact. During the postictal period, the EEG background is slow and irregular.

SYNOPSIS

In the popular imagination, GTCS—formerly referred to as "grand mal," or "big sickness"—ranks among the most feared diseases. Despite the dramatic presentation, most GTCS self-terminate within minutes and do not result in long-term harm. The only intervention required from bystanders is to ensure that patients do not harm themselves during the seizure by removing sharp objects in the vicinity, placing a cloth under the patient's head, and turning patients to the lateral decubitus position after the seizure is over. Seizures that do not resolve spontaneously within a few minutes are referred to as status epilepticus (SE), a neurologic emergency that requires prompt and aggressive seizure medications in a monitored setting. SE is associated with irreversible brain injury and significant mortality, especially in elderly individuals.

Eliminating or reducing the frequency of GTCS is of the utmost importance. Fewer seizures means less motor vehicle accidents, drownings, falls and burns, and a lower risk of sudden unexpected death in epilepsy (SUDEP), a major contributor to excess mortality among patients with epileptic seizures. Moreover, seizures have a very detrimental effect on patients' quality of life and are associated with significant "invisible disability" (social isolation, anxiety, depression, cognitive dysfunction).

FIGURE

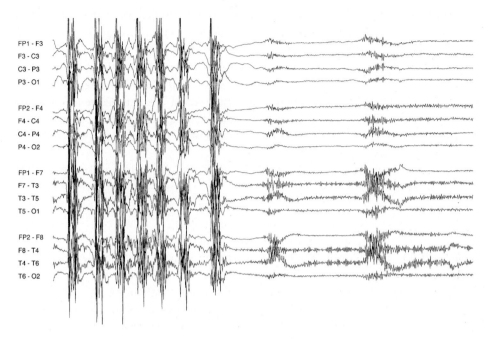

Termination of a clonic-tonic-clonic seizure (grand mal). Postictal EEG attenuation was associated with bursts of decerebrate or decorticate posturing. (Reprinted with permission from Blume WT, Holloway GM, Kaibara M, et al. *Atlas of Pediatric and Adult Electroencephalography*. Philadelphia, PA: Wolters Kluwer Health/Lippincott Williams & Wilkins; 2010:Figure 4-3.64.)

QUESTIONS FOR SELF-STUDY

1. It is sometimes challenging to determine an episode of loss of consciousness results from a seizure or syncope, especially when syncope is accompanied by myoclonic jerks. Which of the clinical features listed in the table below favor the diagnosis of seizure and which favor the diagnosis of syncope?

Tongue laceration
Déjà vu or jamais vu before loss of consciousness
Emotional stress
Head-turning during spell
Unusual movements or abnormal behavior
Confusion after a spell
Amnesia for the event
Sweating before spell
Spell associated with prolonged sitting or standing

Compare your responses with Sheldon R, Rose S, Ritchie D, et al. Historical criteria that distinguish syncope from seizures. *J Am Coll Cardiol*. 2002;40(1):142-148. [free online resource].

2. What is the most common cause of breakthrough seizures among patients with well-controlled epilepsy?

3. A 25-year-old recently married woman with well-controlled generalized epilepsy is considering starting a family. What advice would you give her regarding the choices of antiseizure medications and vitamin supplementation?

4. Seizures that do not spontaneously stop within 5 min or recur without full recovery in between episodes are considered to be status epilepticus (SE). What are the first steps in managing SE? What are the first- and second-line antiseizure medications used in SE? What testing should be considered in a patient with no prior seizure history who presents with SE? (Compare your response with American Epilepsy Society guidelines cited below.)

5. What are nonpharmacologic approaches to the treatment of drug-resistant generalized epilepsy?

CHALLENGE

To determine whether seizure onset is focal or generalized may be challenging. What features during and following a seizure suggest a focal onset? Did the patient described on the 4000-old Assyrian tablet—"his neck turns left, his hands and feet are tense and his eyes wide open, and from his mouth froth is flowing without his having any consciousness"—more likely have GTCS or focal to tonic-clonic seizure? Which antiseizure medications are effective for focal to tonic-clonic seizures, but not for GTCS?

REFERENCES

Glauser T, Shinnar S, Gloss D, et al. Evidence-based guideline: treatment of convulsive status epilepticus in children and adults. Report of the guideline Committee of the American Epilepsy Society. *Epilepsy Curr.* 2016;16(1):48-61. [free online resource]

Mahler B, Carlsson S, Andersson T, Tomson T. Risk for injuries and accidents in epilepsy: a prospective population-based cohort study. *Neurology.* 2018;90(9):e779-e789.

Tomson T, Sveinsson O, Carlsson S, Andersson T. Evolution over time of SUDEP incidence: a nationwide population-based cohort study. *Epilepsia.* 2018;59(8):e120-e124. [free online resource]

69   Febrile Seizures ▬

A generalized seizure during a febrile illness in a child who does not have epilepsy

CORE FEATURES

1. Onset between 6 months and 5 years of age.
   The peak of FS is between 2 and 3 years. Seizures in a febrile child who is younger than 6 months raise suspicion of CNS infection.
2. Febrile illness.
   FS usually occurs when body temperature is ≥39°C (102°F) but may manifest prior to fever onset or during defervescence.
3. Tonic-clonic seizure in most cases.
   FS do not manifest as myoclonic seizures, infantile spasms, or nonconvulsive attacks.
4. Most FS will self-terminate within minutes.
   "Simple FS," which comprises 75% of FS, typically lasts less than a few minutes and have a postictal period of less than a few minutes. "Complex FS" lasts longer than 15 min; have ictal or postictal focal deficits; and may recur during the same febrile illness. FS lasting more than 30 min is "febrile status epilepticus"; it accounts for 5% of all FS. Febrile SE is a neurologic emergency, which requires aggressive therapy, often with multiple antiseizure medications, in a closely monitored setting.
5. Absence of any "seizure triggers" other than fever.
   FS cannot be diagnosed if the child has CNS infection, septic embolization, significant metabolic disturbance, toxic exposure, hemolytic-uremic syndrome, or head trauma.

SYNOPSIS

FS occurs in up to 5% of children and is by far the most common childhood seizure. Though frightening to parents and onlookers, the brief clonic-tonic seizure during a febrile illness is usually benign and requires neither a workup nor hospital admission. Parents should be reassured that the child will suffer no long-term consequences and warned about the risk of recurrence during febrile illness. The risk of recurrence is higher if the child presents at a younger age; has a lower temperature at seizure onset or a shorter lag from fever to seizure; has neurodevelopmental delay; or a family history of FS.

The risk of developing epilepsy in a child who had one simple FS is about 1%, which is not much higher than the baseline population risk of epilepsy. In contrast, complex FS carry an increased risk of epilepsy and require additional testing, especially when there are ictal or postictal focal neurological deficits. Febrile status epilepticus may be associated with language and motor delay and subsequent hippocampal atrophy on brain MRI. Children with prolonged or recurrent FS, or febrile status epilepticus, should be prescribed midazolam nasal spray or rectal diazepam to be deployed by caretaker in case of seizure recurrence.

QUESTIONS FOR SELF-STUDY

1. How would you differentiate FS from shivering?
2. What are the indications for an LP to rule out an intracranial infection in a child with fever and a seizure? (Compare your answer with the American Academy of Pediatrics recommendations referenced below.)
3. A parent of a child with simple FS is requesting that the child be prescribed a daily antiseizure medication to prevent a recurrence. Explain why prophylactic therapy with antiseizure medication is not recommended despite the risk of febrile seizure recurrence.
4. A mother refuses a flu vaccine for her child because "flu vaccines cause seizures" (https://www.cdc.gov/vaccinesafety/concerns/febrile-seizures.html). Explain why her decision may increase the child's risk of FS.
5. An otherwise healthy 1-year-old girl experienced a prolonged seizure during each febrile illness and once following routine vaccination. She is diagnosed with complex FS. During a follow-up, parents report that she has developed occasional jerky movements of the arms, had a single episode of unprovoked hemiclonic seizures, and is losing her language skills. Which features of this history are not consistent with the diagnosis of FS? Which rare genetic condition should be considered in this context?

CHALLENGE

Explain why the medical consensus is not to consider recurrent FS as an epilepsy syndrome.

REFERENCES

Leung AK, Hon KL, Leung TN. Febrile seizures: an overview. *Drugs Context*. 2018;7:212536. [free online resource]
Subcommittee on Febrile SeizuresAmerican Academy of Pediatrics. Neurodiagnostic evaluation of the child with a simple febrile seizure. *Pediatrics*. 2011;127(2):389-394. [free online resource]
Whelan H, Harmelink M, Chou E, et al. Complex febrile seizures-a systematic review. *Dis Mon*. 2017;63(1):5-23.

Childhood Absence Epilepsy

Idiopathic generalized epilepsy syndrome in children

CORE FEATURES

1. The typical age of onset is 5 to 7 years.
   Onset after 12 years of age suggests an alternative epilepsy syndrome.
2. Episodes of abrupt unresponsiveness lasting about 10 s.
   A child will typically stop in their tracks and stare absently during the seizure. Behavioral automatisms such as lip-smacking can occur but never loss of motor tone. Episodes end as abruptly as they begin, and the child resumes the interrupted activity. Absence seizures may recur dozens of times a day.
3. Absence seizures are provoked by hyperventilation.
   Asking the child to blow rapidly on a pinwheel or a strip of paper for 3 to 5 min provokes an absence seizure in >80% of patients with childhood absence epilepsy (CAE).
4. Absence seizure correlates with a run of generalized, synchronous, and symmetrical spike and slow-wave 3 Hz discharges on EEG.
   These discharges arise suddenly from normal EEG background.
5. Normal neurologic examination.
   Children with CAE have normal development but may have attention deficit hyperactivity disorder, anxiety disorder, and learning disorders; screening for these comorbid conditions is recommended.

SYNOPSIS

Absence seizures resemble daydreaming or absent-mindedness, and so are easy to overlook. But once the diagnosis is suspected, it is usually easy to confirm with the hyperventilation maneuver, which brings out the seizure and the characteristic EEG changes. Most patients with CAE respond to therapy, either with an older drug, ethosuximide, or one of the other antiseizure medications (valproic acid, lamotrigine). Up to 90% of children with CAE "grow out" of seizures by early adolescence, at which point antiseizure medications can usually be tapered off. Atypical features—a continuation of absence seizures into adolescence, development of generalized tonic-clonic seizures or myoclonic seizures, complex automatisms—suggest an alternative epilepsy diagnosis, such as juvenile absence, juvenile myoclonic epilepsy (JME), or focal-onset seizures.

FIGURE

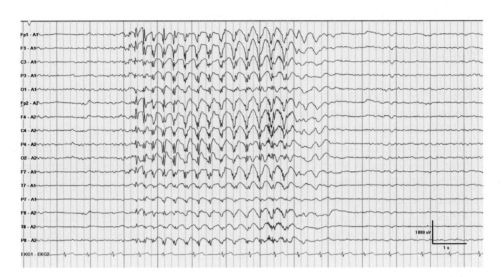

EEG shows a generalized spike-wave discharge in a 6-year-old girl with childhood absence epilepsy. The generalized spike-wave discharge was associated with a blank stare and behavioral arrest. (Courtesy of Dr Jorge Asconapé, Loyola University Chicago, Stritch School of Medicine.)

QUESTIONS FOR SELF-STUDY

1. Daydreaming is a far more common cause of a child's transient "unresponsiveness" than CAE. Which of the following features are characteristic of daydreaming and which of CAE:

   a. Duration of 1 min or longer

   b. Occurrence when the child is tired or bored

   c. Can interrupt an activity, such as playing a musical instrument, eating

   d. 3-Hz eyelid flickering during an episode of unresponsiveness

   e. Able to "snap out" of the episode with distraction or touch

2. A less benign alternative diagnosis to CAE is focal-onset seizure with impaired awareness. Which of the following features are characteristic of focal-onset seizure with impaired awareness rather than CAE.

   a. Onset with an aura such as rising epigastric sensation, a sudden unexplained feeling of fear or joy, experience of déjà vu or jamais vu

   b. Lasts minutes, not seconds

   c. Complex automatisms—wandering around, stereotypic behavior

   d. Evolves into tonic-clonic convulsions

   e. All of the above

3. Explain why brain imaging is not necessary for children diagnosed with CAE but is necessary for children diagnosed with focal seizures.

4. A 5-year-old child presents with brief "staring spells," which may be accompanied by chewing and lip-smacking. The physician diagnoses "seizures" and prescribes carbamazepine. The child's mother reports that the medication is not effective and the physician increases the dose. Within 3 days, the child becomes confused and unresponsive and is brought to the ED. Routine blood tests, urine toxicology, carbamazepine blood levels, CSF analysis, and brain imaging are all normal. Assuming the child's diagnosis is CAE, what would you expect the EEG to show? Explain how EEG done prior to starting antiseizure medication may guide the correct choice of therapy. Which antiseizure drugs may be pro-epileptic in generalized onset seizures?

5. The absence seizures are typically brief, abate on their own, and do not lead to injuries. Make an argument for treating CAE with antiseizure medications.

CHALLENGE

A 2-year-old child presents with atypically long-lasting absence seizures. Her father suffers from epilepsy and has involuntary contraction of the limbs triggered by exercise. Her older brother was diagnosed with alternating hemiplegia. Could you suggest a unifying genetic diagnosis for this family? What tests could confirm your suspicion? Which dietary intervention can prevent neurologic symptoms in all family members?

REFERENCES

Matricardi S, Verrotti A, Chiarelli F, Cerminara C, Curatolo P. Current advances in childhood absence epilepsy. *Pediatr Neurol.* 2014;50(3):205-212.

Kessler SK, McGinnis E. A practical guide to treatment of childhood absence epilepsy. *Paediatr Drugs.* 2019;21(1):15-24. [free online resource]

Idiopathic generalized epilepsy typically presenting in adolescence

CORE FEATURES

1. Typical age of onset is 12 to 18 years.
   When JME is diagnosed in adulthood, pointed questioning usually discloses a history of myoclonic jerks in adolescence.
2. Myoclonic jerks are brief, sudden, single, or irregularly repetitive jerks involving arms and shoulders.
   Myoclonic jerks are more frequent upon awakening, when tired, stressed, or sleep-deprived.
3. Generalized tonic-clonic seizures.
   GTCS occur in over 90% of patients at some point in the disease course. GTCS may be preceded by a train of myoclonic jerks of increasing frequency and intensity.
4. Absence seizures.
   Absence seizures occur in about half of patients.
5. Bilaterally symmetric 4 to 6 Hz polyspike and wave complexes on interictal EEG.
   EEG background is normal, without generalized slowing. Interictal polyspike and wave complexes are more likely to be present when patients are sleep-deprived or with intermittent photic stimulation ("photoparoxysmal response"). Myoclonic jerks correspond to short runs of 10 to 20 Hz polyspike discharges.

SYNOPSIS

Occasional brief jerking of the arms may seem like a detail too insignificant to mention to a healthcare professional but is a critical clue to the diagnosis of JME. This symptom must be explicitly queried about in any patient with generalized tonic-clonic or absence seizures, even those who present outside of a typical age window for JME. Diagnosis of JME is confirmed if interictal EEG shows the characteristic 4 to 6 Hz polyspike and wave complexes, which can usually be brought out with sleep deprivation or photic stimulation. Like CAE, JME usually responds well to treatment. Unlike CAE, JME patients usually do not "grow out" of their seizures and may require life-long antiseizure therapy.

A minority of children with JME have mood, anxiety, and personality disorders and may have mild executive dysfunction on cognitive testing, but overall neurologic development in JME is normal. Cognitive decline, progressive ataxia, or abnormal EEG background is not compatible with JME and suggests the much more ominous diagnosis of progressive myoclonic epilepsy.

FIGURE

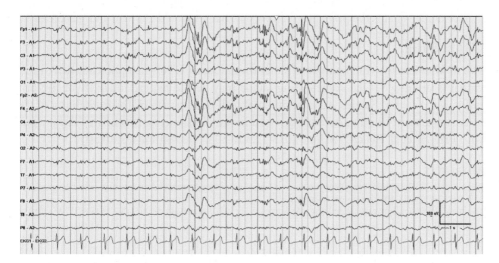

EEG during drowsiness in a 35-year-old man with juvenile myoclonic epilepsy shows brief bursts of generalized spike-wave and polyspike-wave activity with a frontocentral predominance. (Courtesy of Dr Jorge Asconapé, Loyola University Chicago, Stritch School of Medicine.)

QUESTIONS FOR SELF-STUDY

1. "Hypnic jerks" are myoclonic movements that occur as an individual is falling asleep. They are common and nonpathologic. How can you differentiate hypnic jerks from myoclonic jerks by history?
2. GTCS may be a manifestation of a generalized epilepsy syndrome or a "focal to bilateral tonic-clonic" seizure. What questions would you ask patients and bystanders who have witnessed a seizure that may help you decide whether the affected individual is more likely to have had generalized or a "focal to bilateral tonic-clonic" seizure?
3. What is the first-line antiseizure therapy for patients with JME? What would be the antiseizure medication of choice for a woman with JME who is planning a pregnancy?
4. Among photosensitive individuals, as are patients with JME, visual flicker may induce seizures. Visual flicker may be induced when driving with the sun setting behind the trees, looking at shimmering lights reflected on snow or water, checkered tablecloths, computer monitors, or video games. What precautions should photosensitive individuals take to decrease the risk of seizures? (Compare your answer with https://www.epilepsy.com/learn/triggers-seizures/photosensitivity-and-seizures. [free online resource])
5. A 17-year-old woman with newly diagnosed JME is started on valproic acid. The dose is slowly titrated to the point where she no longer experiences myoclonic jerks, but she develops short-term memory, confusion, disorientation, hypersomnia, and blurred vision. On examination, she has psychomotor slowing, slurred speech, and ataxia.

Urine toxicology screen is negative, and the valproic acid blood level is in the high-normal range. Routine laboratory testing, neuroimaging, and LP results are unremarkable. What is the probable diagnosis? What test could confirm your suspicion?

CHALLENGE

The mechanism by which photic stimulation induces a GTCS in a photosensitive individual is unknown. One contributing factor may be the hyperexcitability of the primary visual cortex. Suggest an experimental technique by which the excitability of the visual cortex can be quantitatively assessed in human subjects. (Compare your answer with Brigo F, et al. *Epilepsy Behav.* 2013;27:301-306. [free online resource])

REFERENCES

Renganathan R, Delanty N. Juvenile myoclonic epilepsy: under-appreciated and under-diagnosed. *Postgrad Med J.* 2003;79(928):78-80. [free online resource]

Yacubian EM. Juvenile myoclonic epilepsy: challenges on its 60th anniversary. *Seizure.* 2017;44:48-52. [free online resource]

72 | West Syndrome and Infantile Spasms

Severe epileptic encephalopathy of early infancy associated with hypsarrhythmia

CORE FEATURES

1. Age of onset is usually between 4 and 6 months.
   Onset is within the first year in 90% of cases.
2. Epileptic spasms (infantile spasms).
   Epileptic spasms are sudden, few-seconds long contractions of the neck, trunk, and limb muscles. There may be a brief loss of alertness during the spasms. Spasms may occur in clusters, especially upon awakening.
3. Hypsarrhythmia on interictal EEG.
   This random, chaotic, high-voltage, nonsynchronous spikes, and slow-wave pattern is more likely to be present during non-REM sleep. It is absent in about one-third of cases.
4. Developmental regression following onset of spasms.
   At long-term follow-up, up to 90% of patients have a moderate-to-severe learning disability and approximately one-third of children have autism spectrum disorders.
5. Resolution of spasms and hypsarrhythmia within days of starting adrenocorticotropic hormone (ACTH) therapy in about half of patients.
   Other treatment options include high-dose oral prednisone and vigabatrin. In West syndrome associated with tuberous sclerosis complex, VGB controls spasms in up to 95% of patients and is the drug of choice.

SYNOPSIS

The triad of West syndrome is epileptic spasms, intellectual disability, and hypsarrhythmia on EEG, but only epileptic spasms and one of other two features are required for diagnosis. The epileptic spasms can be flexor, extensor, or mixed flexor-extensor. They may be subtle—like a head nod (neck flexor) or a shrug (shoulder flexion), or more dramatic—full-body flexion resembling salaam greeting (hence the older term "salaam seizures"). Epileptic spasms recur up to many hundreds of times per day in some patients, and may occur during sleep. Epileptic spasms have a number of EEG correlates, but EEG features do not predict the semiology, except that longer ictal duration tends to be associated with behavioral arrest and spasm clusters. Several other seizure types—tonic, clonic, or focal seizures—can occur as well in addition to epileptic spasms.

West syndrome is unique among epileptic encephalopathies in being steroid responsive. Shorter time to diagnosis and therapeutic response are associated with better developmental outcomes. Unfortunately, most patients still suffer from global intellectual disability despite treatment, and about one-third will go on to develop other seizure disorders, such as Lennox-Gastaut syndrome (LGS), which is discussed in the next chapter.

FIGURE

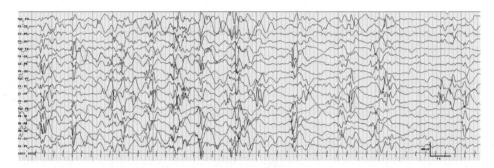

EEG in a 7-month-old baby with West syndrome. Note the marked disorganization of the background with multifocal epileptiform discharges characteristic of hypsarrhythmia. (Courtesy of Dr Jorge Asconapé, Loyola University Chicago, Stritch School of Medicine.)

QUESTIONS FOR SELF STUDY

1. A number of epileptic encephalopathies of infancy present with myoclonus rather than epileptic spasms. How does the duration of epileptic spasms compare to myoclonic seizure? How does the duration of an epileptic spasm compare with tonic seizures?

2. A 2-month-old infant boy is diagnosed with WS. Noncontrast head CT and MRI show calcified subependymal nodules, cortical tubers, and frontal lobe cortical dysplasia. What is the underlying diagnosis? What findings would you expect on a dermatologic examination? Which test can confirm your diagnostic suspicion?

3. Provide an example of a rare, but potentially reversible cause of WS. What is the recommended treatment?

4. A 12-month-old girl presents with myoclonic jerks of the head and arms. Her development is normal. Awake and asleep interictal EEG is normal. What is the likely diagnosis?

5. A 6-month-old infant boy presents with brief episodes of arching of the back, dystonic posturing of the limbs, and failure to gain weight for the past 2 months. He is suspected of having infantile spasms, but prolonged video EEG, which captures multiple episodes, is normal, and his neurologic development is unremarkable. What nonneurologic treatable disorder must be considered? Which tests may confirm your diagnostic suspicion?

CHALLENGE

Underlying causes in epileptic encephalopathies include congenital or acquired structural brain abnormalities, chromosomal and genetic disorders such as Down syndrome, tuberous sclerosis complex, Miller-Dieker lissencephaly syndrome, and others. Identifying the etiology often does not affect the management of epilepsy with the important exception of metabolic causes. In metabolic epilepsy, identifying the specific metabolic defect can lead to targeted treatment that may lead to amelioration or even reversal of symptoms. What are some of the metabolic causes of epilepsy that are potentially amenable to replacement therapy or dietary intervention? What ancillary tests may be required to identify the metabolic defect? (Compare your response with Salar S, Moshé SL, Galanopoulou AS. Metabolic etiologies in West syndrome. *Epilepsia Open*. 2018;3(2):134-166 [free online resource] and https://www.epilepsydiagnosis. org/aetiology/metabolic-groupoverview.html. [free online resource])

REFERENCES

Go CY, Mackay MT, Weiss SK, et al. Evidence-based guideline update: medical treatment of infantile spasms. Report of the guideline development subcommittee of the American Academy of Neurology and the Practice Committee of the Child Neurology Society. *Neurology*. 2012;78(24):1974-1980. [free online resource]

Osborne J, Lux AL, Edwards SW, et al. The underlying etiology of infantile spasms (West syndrome): information from the United Kingdom Infantile Spasm Study (UKISS) on contemporary causes and their classifications. *Epilepsia*. 2010;51(10):2168-2174.

Widjaja E, Go C, McCoy B, Snead OC. Neurodevelopmental outcome of infantile spasms: a systematic review and meta-analysis. *Epilepsy Res*. 2015;109:155-162.

73 Lennox-Gastaut Syndrome

Severe, childhood-onset epileptic encephalopathy characterized by multiple seizure types

CORE FEATURES

1. Age of onset is between 3 and 5 years.
   The range of age of onset is from 1 to 7 years.
2. Tonic seizures during sleep are the most characteristic seizure type-recorded in 90% of patients.
   Tonic seizures during slow-wave (non-REM) sleep or on awakening last less than 10 s and may go unnoticed.
3. A multiplicity of seizure types.
   Atypical absence seizures occur in two-thirds of patients and atonic seizures (drop attacks) in about half of patients. GTCS, focal seizures, epileptic spasms, myoclonic, and myoclonic-atonic seizures are less frequent.
4. Progressive cognitive and behavioral regression.
   Language regression, intellectual disability, labile mood, aggressiveness, loss of relationships, social isolation, and autistic behaviors are the common accompaniments of LGS.
5. Slow, <2.5 Hz spike-and-wave and fast, >10 Hz activity on EEG during slow sleep is required for diagnosis.
   In the awake state, there may be focal or multifocal spike-and-wave or sharp-slow-wave complexes. Ictal EEG depends on seizure type.

SYNOPSIS

LGS usually develops in patients with prenatal or postnatal brain insults such as anoxic-ischemic injury, stroke, brain trauma, CNS infection, brain malformations, and congenital disorders, but in a minority of patients, there is no identifiable cause ("cryptogenic LGS"). Traditionally, LGS has been characterized by a triad of frequent seizures of multiple types, intellectual disability, and diffuse, slow spike-and-waves on interictal EEG. Yet, no one feature is specific for LGS. Differential diagnosis of epileptic encephalopathies with multiple seizure types includes epilepsy with myoclonic-atonic seizures and Dravet syndrome.

Seizures in LGS are notoriously difficult to control. They may recur many times a day despite multiple antiseizure medications. To complicate matters, an antiseizure medication effective for one kind of seizure may exacerbate another type of seizure. The majority of patients experience status epilepticus (SE) that can last for hours, days, and even weeks. SE may manifest as any seizure type—absence, tonic, and myoclonic seizures, or there may be ongoing electroencephalographic epileptic activity without overt clinical manifestations—"subclinical SE," which is a major contributor to poor cognitive outcomes in LGS. Long-term prognosis is poor with moderate-to-profound intellectual disability in 90% of patients.

FIGURE

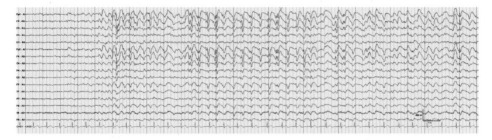

EEG shows a burst of slow generalized spike-wave in an 8-year-old boy with Lennox-Gastaut syndrome. (Courtesy of Dr Jorge Asconapé, Loyola University Chicago, Stritch School of Medicine.)

QUESTIONS FOR SELF-STUDY

1. What is "epileptic encephalopathy"? How does it differ from "developmental encephalopathy"? Does every child with intellectual disability and seizures have "epileptic encephalopathy"?
2. Background EEG is abnormal in LGS, but normal in the generalized idiopathic epilepsies such as childhood absence seizures and JME. What is a normal EEG background in an awake adult whose eyes are closed? How is it different from the normal EEG background of a healthy child?
3. A 7-year-old boy with LGS has adjusted doses of three antiseizure medications with a resultant decrease in seizure frequency and improvement of EEG. However, his parents report that his cognitive performance has declined during this period. In addition, to the natural progression of LGS, what potentially reversible cause of cognitive worsening should be considered?
4. A previously healthy, normally developing 5-year-old girl has language regression. She has difficulty understanding her parents and peers and expressing herself. Her hearing test is normal. She plays well with other children and does not engage in repetitive or ritualistic behaviors. Which treatable epileptic encephalopathy should be considered? How would you differentiate this syndrome from LGS?
5. A drop attack is a sudden, unprovoked, momentary loss of muscle tone without the associated loss of consciousness. Drop attacks are a very common cause of falls and injuries in patients with LGS. What are the nonepileptic causes of drop attacks?

CHALLENGE

A sometimes effective surgical intervention in LGS is corpus callosotomy, which interrupts the interhemispheric spread of the epileptic activity. Describe symptoms of disconnection syndromes that result from this procedure. (Compare your answer with Asadi-Pooya AA, Sharan A, Nei M, Sperling MR. Corpus callosotomy. *Epilepsy Behav.* 2008;13(2):271-278. [free online resource])

REFERENCES

Asadi-Pooya AA. Lennox-Gastaut syndrome: a comprehensive review. *Neurol Sci.* 2018;39(3):403-414. [free online resource]

Devinski O, Patel AD, Helen Cross J, et al. Effect of cannabidiol on drop seizures in the Lennox-Gastaut syndrome. *N Engl J Med.* 2018;378:1888-1897.

Ostendorf AP, Ng YT. Treatment-resistant Lennox-Gastaut syndrome: therapeutic trends, challenges and future directions. *Neuropsychiatr Dis Treat.* 2017;13:1131-1140.

Nonepileptic Paroxysmal Neurologic Disorders

TOP 1 0 0

A Very Brief Introduction to Nonepileptic Paroxysmal Neurologic Disorders

Gentlewoman: I have seen her rise from her bed, throw her night-gown upon her, unlock her closet, take forth paper, fold it, write upon't, read it, afterwards seal it, and again return to bed; yet all this while in a most fast sleep. ... (Enter Lady Macbeth, with a taper) Lo you, here she comes! This is her very guise; and, upon my life, fast asleep. Observe her; stand close.

Doctor: You see, her eyes are open.
Gentlewoman: Ay, but their sense is shut. ...

Shakespeare, "Macbeth."

In Macbeth there is a very significant observation on somnambulism. The doctor sees Lady Macbeth get up and begin her somnambulic activity, turns to the other characters on stage, and supposing them better informed than they are, exclaims: "look, her eyes are open." Indeed, in somnambulism, whether the eyes are open or closed is the most important question.

Jean-Martin Charcot[*]

Neurologists are frequently asked to assess patients whose neurologic symptoms have resolved by the time they come for an evaluation. The classic localizationist approach of searching for neurologic signs to localize the lesion has limited applicability since the neurologic examination is normal. Rather, the diagnosis must rely on elucidating the patient's history and comparing it with "illness scripts"—organized mental summaries of the various conditions that cause transient neurologic symptoms.

Foremost, on the list of conditions that cause self-limited focal neurologic deficits is transient ischemic attack or TIA (Chapter 74). TIA is most important to diagnose promptly since it can be a harbinger of stroke, and a timely intervention can forestall lifetime of disability. A number of neurologic diseases of the central and peripheral nervous system can mimic TIAs. Among the most common neurologic mimickers of TIAs are migraine with aura (Chapter 75), benign paroxysmal positional vertigo (Chapter 76), and seizures. No less common are systemic conditions such as syncope, delirium due to infectious or metabolic causes, drug toxicity, hypoglycemia, and panic attack. With the systemic causes, a careful evaluation usually suggests global rather than focal regional brain dysfunction. Rare paroxysmal neurologic disorders may need to be considered based on the specific clinical contexts: episodic ataxia or periodic paralysis point to inherited channelopathies (Chapter 77).

---

[*]Jean-Martin Charcot (1825-1893) was the first professor of diseases of the nervous system at the Salpêtrière Hospital in Paris and a foundational figure in modern neurology. His wide-ranging influence on the field was summed up by his student, Joseph Babinski: "To take away from neurology all the discoveries made by Charcot would be to render it unrecognizable." (Citation in the epigraph is from Goetz CG. Shakespeare in Charcot's neurologic teaching. *Arch Neurol.* 45(8):920.)

The section concludes with a discussion of paroxysmal disorders of sleep—narcolepsy type 1, which manifests with episodic paralysis and hallucinations (Chapter 78), and parasomnias, as illustrated by Lady Macbeth in the epigraphs (Chapter 79).

REFERENCES

Gomez CR, Schneck MJ, Biller J, et al. Recent advances in the management of transient ischemic attacks. *F1000Res.* 2017;6:1893. [free online resource]

Nadarajan V, Perry RJ, Johnson J, Werring DJ. Transient ischaemic attacks: mimics and chameleons. *Pract Neurol.* 2014;14(1):23-31. [free online resource]

74 Transient Ischemic Attack

A self-limited neurovascular syndrome due to temporary focal ischemia of the brain or retina

CORE FEATURES

1. "Strokelike" onset of symptoms.
   Abrupt onset is the most characteristic tempo of illness, but "stuttering" and "crescendo" TIAs are recognized as well.
2. "Negative symptoms" predominate.
   Motor, sensory, and visual deficits rather than "positive" symptoms, such as abnormal movements or visual illusions, are the norm in TIA.
3. Rapid resolution of symptoms.
   Complete resolution of symptoms within 1 hour is expected, and in many patients, symptoms resolve within minutes.
4. "Diffusion restriction" on magnetic resonance imaging (MRI).
   Restricted diffusion—hyperintense/bright signal on diffusion-weighted imaging (DWI) and hypointense/dark signal on apparent diffusion coefficient (ADC) sequences—typically develops within 30 to 120 min following a cerebral infarction. Restricted diffusion is seen in up to 50% of TIA patients whose symptoms self-resolve.
5. Stroke risk factors.
   Stroke risk factors include prior stroke, ischemic heart disease, atrial fibrillation, valvular heart disease, diabetes mellitus, arterial hypertension, hypercholesterolemia, and cigarette smoking. Less commonly, embolism from aortic atherosclerosis and thrombophilic conditions lead to TIAs.

SYNOPSIS

TIA is a fully reversible neurologic syndrome due to temporary focal brain or retinal ischemia. TIA is a challenging diagnosis because presentations are highly variable and include nonspecific sensory or vestibular symptoms. Misdiagnosis has been estimated to occur in as many as 60% of patients. The diagnosis relies on the patient's ability to provide a clear time course of their symptoms and on the clinician's ability to recognize the symptoms as neurovascular in nature.

Despite the self-limited nature of TIAs, brain MRI may demonstrate stigmata of permanent ischemic brain damage in half of the patients. Thus, the distinction between a minor "ischemic stroke" with restricted diffusion but no permanent clinical deficits and transient ischemia without neuroimaging sequelae is not clinically useful. The critical point is that TIAs may be harbingers of cerebral infarctions: approximately 10% of patients with TIAs have a stroke within 90 days and 5% within 2 days of the TIA. Thus, patients with TIAs require urgent evaluation for treatable causes of stroke such as atrial fibrillation and extracranial carotid artery stenosis. Depending on the presumed mechanism, patients with TIA should receive antithrombotic therapy, and the relevant vascular risk factors need to be identified and addressed.

FIGURE

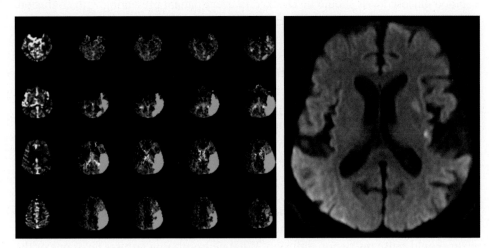

Perfusion-weighted imaging shows prolonged time to peak in the left middle cerebral artery (MCA) territory (left panel). Following mechanical thrombectomy, the patient had only a tiny area of restricted diffusion on MRI (left panel) and a full clinical recovery.

QUESTIONS FOR SELF-STUDY

1. A 65-year-old man presented to the emergency department (ED) with a brief episode of "difficulty speaking." He is uncertain if the problem was in articulating words (dysarthria) or in coming up with the right words (aphasia). During the episode, he was able to type in letters in a text message, but the text was incomprehensible ("dystextia"). Did this patient more likely have aphasia or dysarthria? What is the likely lesion localization?

2. An 80-year-old woman with several vascular risk factors presented to the ED with three episodes of profound right-sided face, arm, and leg weakness without language impairment each lasting for 5 min before fully resolving. What is the likely etiology of this syndrome? What is the name for brief episodes of hemiparesis of vascular origin?

3. One clinical tool that was developed to stratify risk of TIA in patients presenting to ED is the seven-point "ABCD2" score:

No Points	<60 y	Normal	No Speech Deficit/No Unilateral Weakness	<10 min	No Diabetes
1 point	≥60 y	(≥140/90 mm Hg)	Speech disturbance present but no unilateral weakness	10-59 min	Diabetes present
2 points	–	–	Unilateral weakness	≥60 min	–

Patients with a higher score are at a higher risk of stroke. Yet, the American College of Emergency Physicians recommends against using this score to rule out TIA. What are the main limitations of the ABCD2 score that prevent its acceptance by emergency physicians?

4. Hypoglycemia can cause confusion, seizures, and focal neurologic deficits. Thus, blood glucose levels should be checked in every patient presenting with confusion, seizures, or focal neurologic deficits. What are the nonneurologic symptoms and signs of hypoglycemia?

5. A 50-year-old healthy woman presents to the ED after an episode of feeling "out of it," accompanied by palpitations, tingling of both hands, dizziness, sweating, and a sense of impending doom lasting for 15 min. Vitals signs and blood glucose levels are normal. She has had similar episodes in the past and had undergone extensive stroke and cardiac workups, which were unremarkable. What is the likely etiology of her symptoms? What provocative maneuver could be attempted at the bedside to try to replicate her symptoms and confirm your clinical suspicion?

CHALLENGE

A 60-year-old woman presented to the ED following a seizure. MRI of the brain shows an area of diffusion restriction in the left hippocampus. Both stroke and prolonged seizure could cause restriction diffusion. What neuroimaging features favor one or the other diagnosis?

REFERENCES

Coutts SB. Diagnosis and management of transient ischemic attack. *Continuum (Minneap Minn).* 2017;23(1, Cerebrovascular Disease):82-92.

Gomez CR, Schneck MJ, Biller J. Recent advances in the management of transient ischemic attacks. *F1000Res.* 2017;6:1893. [free online resource]

Hextrum S, Biller J. Clinical distinction of cerebral ischemia and triaging of patients in the emergency department. *Neuroimag Clin N Am.* 2018;28:537-549.

75 Migraine Aura

A transient neurologic syndrome that usually precedes or accompanies migraine

CORE FEATURES

1. Visual symptoms.
   Nearly all auras manifest with visual symptoms. Visual symptoms are usually the only symptoms of aura, but they may co-occur with transient sensory symptoms (tingling in limbs, face) and, rarely, language, motor, vestibular, and brainstem transient deficits.
2. Both "positive" and "negative" symptoms are present.
   Examples of "positive" symptoms are "fortification spectra," "flashing lights," or tingling sensation. Examples of "negative symptoms" are visual field defects or numbness. In contrast to aura, positive symptoms are rare in TIA.
3. Symptoms evolve stereotypically over minutes.
   Visual symptoms start in a localized visual field region and spread out to other parts of the visual field during aura. Tingling usually starts over the face and progresses to involve hand and sometimes the trunk and leg on one side of the body. In contrast, symptoms of TIA tend to be more abrupt and do not show such a stereotypic "march" of symptoms.
4. Auras typically resolve within 15 to 30 min.
   Nearly all auras resolve within 60 min. Prolonged auras are very rare and may lead to permanent brain damage ("migrainous infarction").
5. Auras precede or occur during the migraine headache phase.
   Auras are reported by up to 30% of patients with migraines. Auras without migraine ("acephalgic migraine") occur as well, especially among older people with a remote history of migraine ("late-life migraine accompaniments").

SYNOPSIS

Psychologist and behaviorist Karl Spencer Lashley (1890-1958) studied his own migraine auras and proposed that the visual aura was the result of spreading excitation along the occipital cortex at the rate of 3 mm/min. The putative neurophysiologic basis of auras was proposed by the Brazilian scientist Aristides de Azevedo Pacheco Leão (1914-1993), who discovered that electrical or mechanical stimulation of the cerebral cortex causes a wave of extreme depolarization of glial and neuronal cell membranes and a transient increase, followed by a decrease, in cerebral blood flow. Leão's wave of depolarization, which he called "cortical spreading depression" (CSD), proceeds at the same rate as the visual aura, which suggested to him that CSD is the mechanism underlying auras. Moreover, computer simulation of active wave propagation through a model of the visual cortex is able to replicate some of the most characteristic features of auras—fortification spectra and enlarging scotomas (Dahlem MA and Chronicle EP, Prog Neurobiol. 2004;74(6):351-361). The "CSD theory," however, does not readily explain why visual symptoms may be followed by sensory symptoms, nor the rare phenomenon of brainstem auras.

The relationship between CSD and headache is uncertain. CSD can activate trigeminal nociceptive pathways in animal models, which would explain why auras commonly precede the headache phase. However, auras may also coincide or follow the headache. Moreover, most migraines are not accompanied by auras making it unlikely that CSD is required for migraine generation. Interestingly, recent studies implicate CSD as one of the main causative mechanisms of brain injury following trauma and stroke.

FIGURE

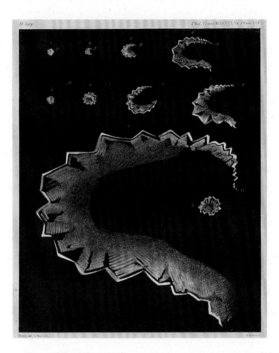

Classic image of expanding of fortification spectra in migraine aura. (Plate XXV 'Stages of Teichopsia' from Hubert Airy, 'On a Distinct Form of Transient Hemiopsia', Philosophical Transactions of the Royal Society of London, 160 (1870).)

QUESTIONS

1. Suggest a reason why visual auras are associated with relatively simple visual phenomena such as fortification spectra and phosphenes but not with the more complex imagery, such as persons or landscapes as in visual hallucinations?
2. Patients may have trouble differentiating monocular vision loss from homonymous hemianopia (vision loss on one side of the visual field). This distinction is important: vision loss in one eye localizes the lesion to the retrochiasmatic portion of the visual pathway, while hemianopsia localizes the lesion to the postchiasmatic portion of the pathway. What questions would you ask the patient to differentiate between these two patterns of visual loss?
3. A 70-year-old man with no prior headache history reports two episodes of slowly losing vision in one eye lasting for a period of half an hour followed by a mild headache. Why is this history not typical of migraine with aura? What diagnoses should be considered for this patient?

4. A 30-year-old woman with a history of migraine reports a peculiar sensation "as if my body has grown larger," which sometimes precedes her migraine headache. What is the name of this phenomenon? Other than migraine aura, what other causes of distorted perceptions of time, space, sound, and body image should be considered?
5. A 20-year-old woman who has migraines with aura and is an active smoker is interested in starting an oral contraceptive pill (OCP). Which class of OCPs are contraindicated in this patient?

CHALLENGE

A 30-year-old man presents following several attacks of unilateral weakness along with scintillating lights and migrainous headache. The weakness lasts several hours and then resolves. Neurologic examination, brain MRI, and a thorough stroke workup are unremarkable. His father suffers from episodic attacks of imbalance that last a few hours but are not accompanied by a headache. Could you suggest a unifying genetic diagnosis for this family?

REFERENCES

Charles A. The migraine aura. *Continuum (Minneap Minn)*. 2018;24(4, Headache):1009-1022.
Fisher CM. Late-life migraine accompaniments as a cause of unexplained transient ischemic attacks. *Can J Neurol Sci*. 1980;7(1):9-17.
Schott GD. Exploring the visual hallucinations of migraine aura: the tacit contribution of illustration. *Brain*. 2007;130(pt 6):1690-1703. [free online resource]

76 Benign Paroxysmal Positional Vertigo

Vertigo due to otolith misplacement in the semicircular canals of inner ear

CORE FEATURES

1. Paroxysms of vertigo that last seconds.
   Vertigo that lasts minutes or more suggests an alternative diagnosis.
2. Vertigo is triggered by a change in position.
   Vertigo usually provoked by rolling in bed or bending the head upwards or sideways.
3. Provocative maneuvers elicit symptoms and signs of benign paroxysmal positional vertigo (BPPV).
   The Epley maneuver replicates symptoms and induces characteristic upbeat-torsional nystagmus in the posterior canal BPPV, which accounts for 90% of BPPV. The supine head roll maneuver replicates symptoms and induces horizontal nystagmus in the horizontal canal BPPV.
4. Normal neurologic examination between attacks.
   Persistent nystagmus or brainstem signs such as ataxia, dysmetria, and cranial nerve deficits are incompatible with the diagnosis of BPPV.
5. Symptoms resolve after canalith repositioning procedure.
   The Epley maneuver is curative after a single treatment in the majority of cases of posterior canal BPPV and in nearly all patients after several sessions. Repositioning maneuvers are also available for horizontal BPPV. Failure to respond to repositioning maneuvers is unusual in BPPV and should lead to a reevaluation of the diagnosis.

SYNOPSIS

Dizziness or vertigo is a common and commonly misdiagnosed symptom. Among patients presenting to EDs with the chief concern of dizziness, nearly half had a reassigned diagnosis on follow-up visits (Royl et al, Eur Neurol. 66(5):256-263). The most important question to answer in patients with vertigo/dizziness is whether the symptoms are likely due to inner ear disease (BPPV, labyrinthitis, Ménière disease), brain pathology (stroke, demyelination, neoplasm), or systemic causes (orthostasis, cardiac arrhythmias, side effects of drugs). The most important clues to the diagnosis are the *time course* of symptoms and *triggers* of symptoms. The terms used by the patient to describe their symptoms—vertigo ("illusory sensation of movement of the self or the surroundings") or "dizziness" ("feeling faint or woozy")—are very helpful in elucidating the cause because patients tend to use these terms interchangeably. The patients with BPPV, a prototypical inner ear cause of vertigo, usually complain of dizziness. To make the diagnosis of BPPV, clinician needs to establish that the patient suffers from an episodic disorder, with brief attacks, triggers by certain movements, and symptom-free periods in between attacks. BPPV symptoms can be replicated with provocative maneuvers, which dislodge the otoliths from the respective canals and cured by repositioning maneuvers that return the otoliths to their place (see the video clip in references). In contrast, vestibular neuronitis, another common cause of vertigo, causes ongoing—not episodic—dizziness/vertigo, that is exacerbated by motion and head turning and makes walking difficult. Vertebrobasilar territory strokes are a relatively uncommon cause of dizziness/vertigo, but one that should not be missed. The presence of brainstem or cerebellar signs alert the clinician to this diagnosis. In suspected cases, brain MRI should be performed urgently. CT of the head has no utility for diagnosing ischemia in the posterior fossa.

FIGURES

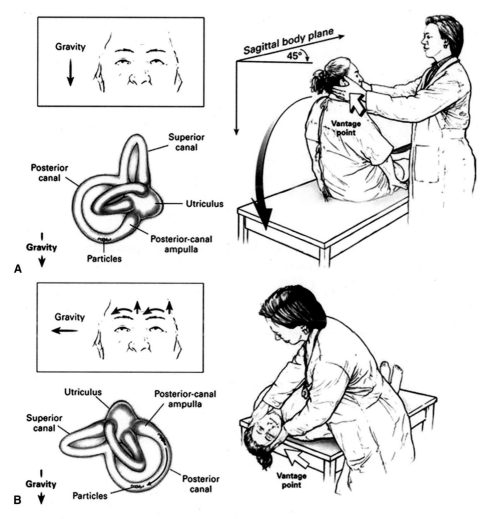

Demonstration of Dix-Hallpike maneuver for diagnosis of posterior of BPPV is shown alongside with presumed location of free-floating debris within the labyrinth. (Reproduced with permission from Bhattacharyya N, Gubbels SP, Schwartz SR, et al. Clinical practice guideline: benign paroxysmal positional vertigo (Update). *Otolaryngol Head and Neck Surg*. 2017;156(3_suppl):S1-S47 © American Academy of Otolaryngology—Head and Neck Surgery Foundation 2017.)

QUESTIONS FOR SELF-STUDY

1. Match each characteristic trigger with the respective disease that causes dizziness:

Hyperventilation	A. Carotid sinus syncope
Rolling over in bed	B. Orthostatic syncope
Getting up from a chair	C. BPPV
Tight collars; shaving	D. Panic attack
Loud sounds; Valsalva maneuver	E. Superior canal dehiscence syndrome

2. A key test to differentiate vertigo due to inner ear disease from vertigo due to brainstem disease is the head impulse test (HIT). This test probes the intactness of the vestibulo-ocular reflex (VOR). Describe how this test is performed and explain how impaired VOR results in a "catch-up saccade" when the head is rotated toward the affected side.

3. Unilateral nystagmus and hearing loss are generally regarded as manifestations of inner ear pathology. Describe a clinical scenario where such "peripheral signs" are due to a brainstem pathology. What neurologic findings would help confirm brainstem localization?

4. The use of vestibular suppressants such as benzodiazepines, antihistamines, or anticholinergics in patients with BPPV is discouraged. Why?

5. A 35-year-old woman presents with sudden-onset vertigo while sitting in a meeting. She also complains of neck and head discomfort on the left side. On arrival to ED, 1 hour after symptom onset, she receives meclizine and hydration, and her symptoms are improved, though not resolved. Screening neurologic examination performed by ED physician is normal except that she is unable to walk unassisted. Provide at least three reasons why this scenario is not compatible with the diagnosis of BPPV. What diagnosis should be suspected in this woman? What imaging studies should be performed to confirm the clinical suspicion?

CHALLENGE

A 50-year-old woman presents with positional paroxysmal vertigo. The clinician suspects BPPV and performs the Dix-Hallpike maneuver, which elicits vertigo and downbeat unilateral nystagmus. Why is this finding not consistent with the diagnosis of BPPV? What is the likely diagnosis? What testing must be done to confirm the diagnosis?

REFERENCES

Bhattacharyya N, Gubbels SP, Schwartz SR, et al. Clinical practice guideline: benign paroxysmal positional vertigo (Update). *Otolaryngol Head Neck Surg*. 2017;156(3_suppl):S1-S47. [free online resource]

Edlow JA, Gurley KL, Newman-Toker DE. A new diagnostic approach to the adult patient with acute dizziness. *J Emerg Med*. 2018;54(4):469-483. [free online resource]

Maneuvers to treat BPPV. https://www.youtube.com/watch?v=KLt2LtISPmQ&feature=youtu.be. [free online resource]

77 Periodic Paralyses

Autosomal-dominant disorders due to mutations in skeletal muscle ion channels

CORE FEATURES

Periodic paralyses (PPs) are characterized by episodes of limb paralysis, which usually start in childhood or adolescence and tend to improve or resolve later in life. The family history of PP may be masked by incomplete penetrance. The table compares PPs associated with low and high serum potassium.

	Hypokalemic PP	Hyperkalemic PP
1. Mean duration of attacks	>2 h; may last days	<2 h; may last minutes
2. Attack triggers	Carbohydrate-rich foods, alcohol, salt; abrupt stopping of strenuous exercise, stress, sleep deprivation	Potassium-rich foods; fasting; cold exposure; abrupt stopping of strenuous exercise, stress, sleep deprivation
3. Serum potassium during the attack	<3.5 mmol/L and may be even <2 mmol/L)	>5 mmol/L
4. Myotonia between attacks	No	Yes, in most patients; evidence of myotonia on electromyography (EMG)[a]
5. Common mutations	Calcium channel (CACNA1S); sodium channel (SCN4A)	Sodium channel (SCN4A)

[a]Spontaneous bursts of motor unit action potentials (MUAPs) of waxing/waning amplitude and frequency.

SYNOPSIS

PPs are "primary channelopathies," a group of genetic disorders that are due to mutations affecting membrane excitability. Neurologic primary channelopathies also include episodic ataxias, familial hemiplegic migraine, paroxysmal dyskinesias, epilepsy syndromes, and episodic pain syndromes. Secondary channelopathies are nongenetic disorders in which the ion channels are affected secondarily by an internal disease process (Lambert-Eaton myasthenic syndrome) or an exogenous cause (magnesium overdose). Some PPs seem to defy this dichotomous characterization into genetic and nongenetic etiologies: patients with thyrotoxic hypokalemic paralysis have predisposing mutations in an ion gene that is influenced by thyroid hormone, and clinical symptoms (paralysis) only become apparent if they experience thyrotoxicosis.

PPs are due to mutations in ion channels responsible for sarcolemmal membrane depolarization in skeletal muscles. Under physiologically stressful conditions, membrane depolarization in PP reaches a threshold beyond which myocytes are unable to contract and paralysis ensues. Attacks can be shortened by gently normalizing serum K^+. In between attacks, patients usually have normal strength, though with age, myopathy and muscle loss may develop. For reasons not entirely clear, the frequency of attacks in both hypoPP and hyperPP attacks can be reduced with carbonic anhydrase inhibitors (acetazolamide and dichlorphenamide).

FIGURE

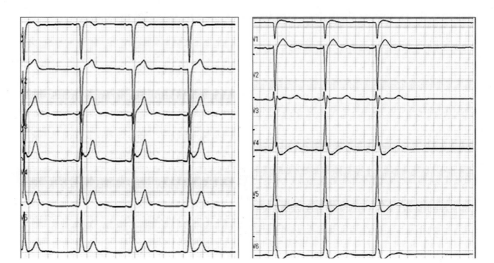

Andersen-Tawil syndrome is a rare autosomal-dominant channelopathy with periodic paralysis and arrhythmias (sustained ventricular arrhythmias, torsade de pointes, and prolonged QT interval). Electrocardiogram (ECG) in a patient with Anderson-Tawil channelopathy before (left) and during (right) the attack shows the disappearance of atrial P-waves during the attack ("atrial standstill") and emergence of prominent U-waves. (Reprinted with permission from Kokunai Y, Nakata T, Furuta M, et al. A Kir3.4 mutation causes Andersen-Tawil syndrome by an inhibitory effect on Kir2.1. *Neurology*. 2014;82(12):1058-1064.)

QUESTIONS FOR SELF-STUDY

1. Two patients are admitted to the ED with generalized weakness and severe hypokalemia. One has a known history or hypoPP and the other has severe diarrhea. What is the difference in total potassium body levels in these two patients? How does this difference impact on the rate of potassium repletion? What could be the consequences of repleting potassium in the patient with hypoPP using a similar protocol as the one used for the patient with gastrointestinal loss?

2. What are key neurologic findings that help differentiate quadriparesis due to myasthenic crisis from quadriparesis due to PP?

3. The American polymath Benjamin Franklin (1706-1790), speaking of Fire Safety, noted that "an ounce of prevention is worth a pound of cure." What advice would you give to a patient with PP to prevent attacks with regard to sleep hygiene; hydration; diet (frequency and composition of meals); exercise (warm-up, warm down, intensity); avoidance of certain medications; anesthesia? What are the similarities and differences in advice to patients with hypoPP and hyperPP?

4. A 40-year-old Vietnamese patient presents to the ED with paralysis of both legs and arms. General examination demonstrates tachycardia, excessive sweating, tremulousness, and mild proptosis. He has no prior history of paralytic attacks. Serum potassium level is 2.1 mM/L (normal >3.6 mM/L). You suspect hypokalemic PP. What laboratory tests are important to obtain, especially given his systemic symptoms and Asian ancestry?

5. A 30-year-old man reports brief episodes of muscle twitching accompanied by imbalance and dysarthria but no weakness. EMG is consistent with neuromyotonia. His father and uncle have similar episodes. Based on the patient's symptoms, where would you guess the defective channels are located? Which channelopathy best fits with this history?

CHALLENGE

When serum potassium level is high, potassium enters into the cells and the skeletal muscle membranes become depolarized. Depolarization of muscle membranes leads to the inactivation of voltage-gated sodium channels, which leads to loss of contractility and paralysis. It is a bit more difficult to understand why low serum potassium levels, which have a hyperpolarizing effect on muscle membranes, can also lead to paralysis. Suggest an explanation for this seemingly paradoxical phenomenon. (Compare your answer with "bistable membrane potential" theory.)

REFERENCES

Ryan DP, Ptácek LJ. Episodic neurological channelopathies. *Neuron.* 2010;68(2):282-292.
Sansone VA. Episodic muscle disorders. *Continuum (Minneap Minn).* 2019;25(6):1696-1711.
Statland JM, Fontaine B, Hanna MG, et al. Review of the diagnosis and treatment of periodic paralysis. *Muscle Nerve.* 2018;57(4):522-530. [free online resource]

78 Narcolepsy Type 1

Hypersomnia associated with loss of hypocretin (orexin) in the hypothalamus

CORE FEATURES

1. Excessive daytime sleepiness.
   Patients wake up rested but feel a need to nap throughout the day.
2. Cataplexy is highly specific to Narcolepsy Type 1 (NT1).
   Cataplexy is defined as involuntary loss of skeletal muscle tone with full preservation of consciousness lasting 1 to 2 min. Cataplexy can be triggered by strong emotions (laughing, crying, surprise).
3. Rapid eye movement (REM) parasomnias.
   REM parasomnias are clinical phenomena that arise as brain transitions between REM sleep and wakefulness. Examples include sleep paralysis (fully aware but unable to move); hallucinations on falling asleep (hypnogogic) or awakening (hypnopompic); and REM behavioral disorder (nonpurposeful behavior while asleep).
4. Positive multiple sleep latency test (MSLT).
   MSLT involves several scheduled short-nap trials during the day. If the patient falls asleep within a mean of 5 minutes of the nap trial start, or enters REM sleep during at least two scheduled nap trials, there is a high likelihood of narcolepsy.
5. Low concentration of cerebrospinal fluid (CSF) hypocretin.
   Hypocretin concentration of <110 pg/mL in CSF is diagnostic of NT1.

SYNOPSIS

NT1 ("narcolepsy with cataplexy") is caused by the loss of cells in the lateral hypothalamus that synthesize hypocretin, a neurotransmitter required for maintaining wakefulness and suppressing REM sleep. Loss of hypocretin leads to excessive daytime sleepiness and REM parasomnias. Cataplexy is thought to be a result of the intrusion of REM sleep paralysis during wakefulness, and some patients may even enter REM sleep following the cataplexy episode. Abnormal activation of the amygdala, which is involved in the processing of emotions and REM sleep regulation, presumably explains why emotions may trigger cataplexy. Narcolepsy is treated with stimulants (modafinil or methylphenidate). Cataplexy may respond to sodium oxybate, selective serotonin reuptake inhibitors (SSRIs), or serotonin-norepinephrine reuptake inhibitors (SNRIs).

NT1 is thought to be an autoimmune disease. It may emerge after infection or vaccination, and nearly all patients with NT1 have the same HLA-DQB1*0602 haplotype. Etiology of narcolepsy without cataplexy, narcolepsy type 2 (NT2), is less clear and may be multifactorial. A subset of patients with NT2 will meet criteria for NT1 if they develop cataplexy or if their CSF hypocretin concentration drops below 110 pg/mL threshold.

FIGURE

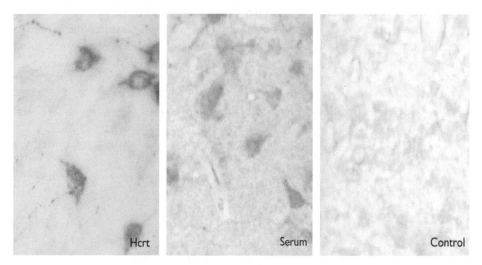

Hypothalamus of a rat stained for hypocretin ("Hcrt," left) shows normal hypocretin-containing neurons. Serum from a patient with NT1 also binds hypocretin-containing neurons ("serum," middle). However, serum from a healthy control does not bind to hypocretin-containing neurons ("control," right). This experiment shows that NT1 patient's serum has antibodies against hypocretin, which are absent in the healthy control. (Reprinted with permission from Knudsen S, Mikkelsen JD, Jennum P. Antibodies in narcolepsy-cataplexy patient serum bind to rat hypocretin neurons. *Neuroreport.* 2007;18(1):77-79.)

QUESTIONS FOR SELF-STUDY

1. How would differentiate cataplexy from an atonic seizure (drop attack)?
2. Cataplexy is a state of muscle atonia. Explain why it does not lead to loss of sphincter tone (bowel and bladder incontinence) as does generalized seizure?
3. Patients with narcolepsy self-report car accidents at a nearly 10-fold rate than the general population. Presence of which symptoms indicate that a patient with narcolepsy should not be driving? (Compare your response to recommendations of the National Highway Traffic Safety Administration referenced below.)
4. An otherwise healthy 40-year-old woman complains of being tired all the time and needing to take frequent naps during the day despite sleeping for more than 10 hours each night. She has no history of sleep paralysis or hallucinations upon falling asleep or upon awakening. MSLT shows markedly decreased latency to sleep but no REM sleep. What is the likely diagnosis?
5. An otherwise healthy 14-year-old has not been able to get out of his bedroom for a week. He does not appear sick, yet spends all day and night sleeping, only waking up for meals. A similar episode occurred 6 months previously, at which time he was admitted to the hospital for evaluation. MRI of the brain and CSF analysis were normal. Polysomnogram showed only prolonged sleep. What is the likely diagnosis?

CHALLENGE

The presence of *DQB1*06:02* allele increases the risk of developing NT1 200-fold—the strongest known association of an HLA haplotype with autoimmune disease. Assuming that the mechanism of NT1 is molecular mimicry, provide a plausible immunologic explanation for why a particular haplotype may be required to generate an autoimmune response to hypocretin-expressing cells in the hypothalamus.

REFERENCES

https://aasm.org/resources/practiceparameters/pp_msltmwt.pdf. [free online resource]

https://www.nhtsa.gov/sites/nhtsa.dot.gov/files/medical20cond2080920690-8-04_medical20cond2080920690-8-04.pdf. [free online resource]

Mahoney CE, Cogswell A, Koralnik IJ, Scammell TE. The neurobiological basis of narcolepsy. *Nat Rev Neurosci.* 2019;20(2):83-93. [free online resource]

79 Sleepwalking and Rapid Eye Movement Behavior Disorder

Parasomnias are abnormal behaviors or experiences arising from sleep

CORE FEATURES

Parasomnias are classified as REM sleep or non-REM sleep parasomnias depending on which stage of sleep they occur. The table compares a non-REM sleep parasomnia—sleepwalking, with a prototypical REM sleep parasomnia—rapid eye movement sleep behavior disorder (RBD).

	Sleepwalking	RBD
1. Age	Up to 30% of children; peak age at onset is 10 years	About 8% of elderly individuals
2. Semiology	Incomplete wakefulness; wandering; more complex behavior, such as driving can be seen	Vocalizations or motor behaviors are often part of "acting out" dreams. Simple movements are most common, but complex and violent behavior can occur
3. Transition to wakefulness	Difficult to awaken, confused, amnestic to event	Easily awakened and quickly oriented
4. Polysomnography	Occurs during slow-wave sleep (non-REM)	Occurs during REM sleep; abnormal muscle activity instead of atonia
5. Associated conditions	Restless legs syndrome (RLS), obstructive sleep apnea, and medications and conditions that cause sleep fragmentation increase risk of sleepwalking	Often a precursor of synucleinopathies (Parkinson disease, dementia with Lewy bodies, multisystem atrophy)

SYNOPSIS

Wakefulness and sleep are mediated via distinct brain circuits. Wakefulness is dependent on specialized nuclei located throughout the brainstem, hypothalamus, and basal forebrain including the locus ceruleus (main neurotransmitter: norepinephrine), pontine tegmental nuclei (acetylcholine), tuberomammillary nucleus (histamine), dorsal raphe nuclei (serotonin), periaqueductal gray (dopamine), and lateral hypothalamus (hypocretin). These nuclei project to the thalami and cerebral cortex to maintain arousal. Non-REM sleep is characterized by little or no eye movements, no dreaming, and normal muscle tone. Non-REM sleep is dependent on a different set of nuclei in the brainstem and hypothalamus, which inhibit the "wakefulness" circuits. REM sleep is characterized by dreaming, rapid eye movements, and paralysis of limb and facial muscles with loss of reflexes. REM sleep is mediated by nuclei in the dorsal pons that inhibit somatic motor neurons to maintain atonia and stimulate cortical areas involved in dreaming. Sleep parasomnias can be conceptualized as "mixed states" in which circuits of wakefulness and sleep operate in parallel rather than sequentially, resulting in a mixture of behaviors and experiences that characterize both wakefulness and sleep. RBD consists of dreaming (as in REM sleep) and normal muscle activity (as in wakefulness). Hence in RBD, patients tend to act out their dreams, while in non-REM parasomnias, the patients engage in rudimentary wakefulness behavior during deep, slow-wave sleep (eg, wondering), and are difficult to transition to wakefulness.

FIGURE

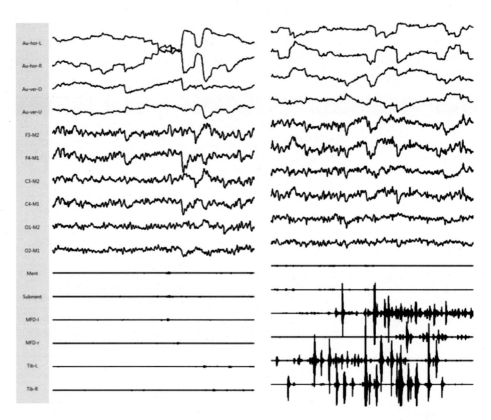

Polysomnogram of normal rapid eye movement (REM) during REM sleep (left panel) is contrasted with REM sleep in a patient with RBD (right panel). In normal REM sleep, there is almost no muscle activity in limb EMG channels (limb atonia), while in RBD, there is phasic EMG activity in both upper and lower extremity muscles during REM sleep. (Reprinted with permission from Högl B, Iranzo A. Rapid eye movement sleep behavior disorder and other rapid eye movement sleep parasomnias. *Continuum (Minneap Minn)*. 2017;23(4, Sleep Neurology):1017-1034.)

QUESTIONS FOR SELF-STUDY

1. Suggest a single question that can serve as a screening tool for diagnosing RBD. (Compare your proposal with the validated REM Sleep Behavior Disorder Single-Question Screen in Postuma RB, et al. *Mov Disord*. 2012;27(7):913-916. [free online resource])

2. A 70-year-old man reports difficulty falling asleep. The primary care provider prescribes zolpidem (Ambien) every night at bedtime (even though a benzodiazepine

receptor agonists are only approved for short-term use). At the next visit, the patient's wife reports that he has gained 10 lb because he wakes up to go to eat in the middle of the night but later denies having eaten. What is the likely diagnosis? What is the likely cause? What medications are associated with the emergence of parasomnias?

3. A 35-year-old man wakes up from sleep, sits in bed, but does not respond to name. He then performs bizarre movements with his legs as if trying to bicycle and then falls back asleep. There is never sleepwalking or vocalizations. In addition to a parasomnia, what other diagnoses should be considered?

4. A 30-year-old healthy man woke up in his home but did not know where he was. His wife reports he was confused and could not tell her who she was but was able to move all limbs. The episode lasted a few minutes. He denies daytime sleepiness and drug or alcohol abuse. What is the most likely diagnosis?

5. Suggest a reason why RBD is a precursor of Parkinson disease but not of Alzheimer disease.

CHALLENGE

Shakespeare describes an unusual parasomnia in a critical scene of *Othello*. Can you find the scene and name the parasomnia?

REFERENCES

Högl B, Iranzo A. Rapid eye movement sleep behavior disorder and other rapid eye movement sleep parasomnias. *Continuum (Minneap Minn)*. 2017;23(4, Sleep Neurology):1017-1034.

Horner RL, Peever JH. Brain circuitry controlling sleep and wakefulness. *Continuum (Minneap Minn)*. 2017;23(4, Sleep Neurology):955-972.

Howell MJ. Parasomnias: an updated review. *Neurotherapeutics*. 2012;9(4):753-775. [free online resource]

Headache
Disorders

TOP 1 0 0

A Very Brief Introduction to Headache Disorders

More than anything in the world the procurator hated the smell of rose oil, and now everything foreboded a bad day, because this smell had been pursuing the procurator since dawn…'Oh, gods, gods, why do you punish me? … Yes, no doubt, this is it, this is it again, the invincible, terrible illness … when half of the head aches, there's no remedy for it, no escape … I'll try not to move my head …

Mikhail Bulgakov*

Headache is a near-universal human symptom. Population surveys document that 99% of women and 93% of men experienced headache at some point in their life. Overwhelmingly, isolated headaches are "primary headaches," migraine or tension-type. But headache can also develop secondary to a variety of neurologic and systemic causes—central nervous system (CNS) infections, cerebrovascular diseases, CNS inflammatory disorders, space-occupying intracranial lesions, head trauma, hypertensive urgency, systemic infections, medication/drug use, intoxication, or withdrawal. The current *International Classification of Headache Disorders* (ICHD third edition) recognizes more than 200 headache diagnoses (https://www.ichd-3.org/).

The critical question when facing a patient with a headache is whether the particular headache can be comfortably assigned to one of the common primary headache categories and treated symptomatically, or warrants additional evaluation for secondary causes. To answer this all-important question, clinicians need to be familiar with the definitions of the main primary headache types—three of the most common ones are discussed in Chapters 80-82—and recognize features that may point to secondary causes ("red flags"). To help remember headache features that should give one pause, one can use the "Neuro-STOP" mnemonic:

- Neurologic symptoms and signs: seizures, depressed consciousness, neck stiffness, papilledema, and persistent focal neurologic deficits.
- Systemic symptoms (fevers, weight loss), systemic diseases (cancer, chronic infection), and systemic conditions (pregnancy and puerperium—at-risk period for eclampsia, pituitary apoplexy, cerebral venous sinus thrombosis). These comorbidities are associated with a number of secondary headaches that should be considered in the differential.
- Thunderclap, maximal at the onset, headache. Must exclude subarachnoid hemorrhage, cervico-cephalic arterial dissection, cerebral venous sinus thrombosis, pituitary apoplexy before assuming it to be a primary thunderclap headache.

---

*Mikhail Afanasievich Bulgakov (1891-1941), a Russian physician-turned-writer, suffered from incapacitating migraines, which find frequent mention in his works. The vivid description of a migraine attack in the character of Pontius Pilate ("*The Master and Margarita*," translation by Richard Pevear and Larissa Volokhonsky) is remarkable for the artistic power and clinical precision. Odor-specific olfactory sensitivity during prodrome, headache worsening with head movements, extreme photophobia, and unilateral "eyelid swelling" due to autonomic dysfunction are all features that may be seen during an attack. The description gives one a feel for the incapacitating nature of this common condition. Highly effective remedies are now available.

- **O**ld age at onset. Primary headaches are very unusual to emerge in persons older than 65 years, and any new-onset headache in this age group raises suspicion for secondary causes, such as giant cell arteritis (GCA), subdural hematoma, or intracranial neoplasm.
- **P**ositional headache. Worsening of headache on getting up or lying down, bending, sneezing, straining, point to increased or decreased intracranial pressure as the cause. Structural causes need to be excluded. Idiopathic intracranial hypertension (IIH) (Chapter 38 in the section on vision disorders) and intracranial hypotension (Chapter 83) should be considered on the differential.

These "red flags" help identify a subset of headache patients who are at higher risk for secondary headaches and may need imaging and other studies. However, the specificity of red flags is not high, and the majority of patients with a "red flag" will have a negative workup.

REFERENCES

Do TP, Remmers A, Schytz HW, et al. Red and orange flags for secondary headaches in clinical practice: SNNOOP10 list. *Neurology.* 2019;92(3):134-144. [free online resource]

https://americanheadachesociety.org/wp-content/uploads/2018/05/NAP_for_Web_-_Headache_Diagnosis___Testing.pdf. [free online resource]

Rasmussen BK, Jensen R, Schroll M, Olesen J. Epidemiology of headache in a general population--a prevalence study. *J Clin Epidemiol.* 1991;44(11):1147-1157.

80 Migraine

Primary, recurrent headache disorder of moderate-to-severe intensity that may be associated with aura

CORE FEATURES

1. Recurrent headaches, usually throbbing rather than pressure-like in quality, last for hours or even days if untreated.
   The *International Classification of Headache Disorders,* 3rd edition (ICHD-3) require a history of at least five prior typical attacks that last 4 to 72 hours (if untreated) for definite migraine diagnosis.
2. Headache usually involves the area of ophthalmic nerve sensory distribution—eye and periorbital region, and frontal and temporal scalp regions.
   The pain usually starts unilaterally and may spread to the other side of the head during the attack. "Sinus pain," due to referred pain from paranasal sinuses, and neck pain, likely due to the convergence of the trigeminal nerve and the upper cervical spinal roots in the trigeminal-cervical complex, are common in migraine.
3. Sensitivity to light, loud sounds, and smells: photophobia, phonophobia, and osmophobia.
   Patients will typically seek a quiet, dark room during attacks.
4. Headache worsened by physical exertion.
   Even walking and head movements exacerbate pain. Patients will try to lie down or avoid moving during the attack.
5. Nausea is reported by about half of patients during the attack; vomiting is much less common.
   Antiemetics are routinely used in the ED as part of a "migraine cocktail" to abort the attack.

SYNOPSIS

There is a tendency to regard migraine as a benign disorder because it is self-limited and patients resume normal activities in between attacks. Yet, estimates of disability-adjusted life years (DALYs) lost due to migraine place it second only to stroke among neurologic disorders. The financial cost of migraine is estimated to be in excess of $20 billion annually in the United States alone. These statistics attest to the disabling nature of migraine as well as high lifetime migraine prevalence (33% of women and 13% of men).

Headache is the most prominent and disabling feature of migraine but is only one phase in a multiphase process. The prodromal phase prior to the onset of headache lasts for hours-to-days and is characterized by a panoply of symptoms including fatigue, impaired concentration, irritability, increase sensitivity to light and touch, and bowel and bladder symptoms. The aura phase, which is present in a minority of patients, usually lasts 15 to 30 min (discussed in Chapter 75). The headache is thought to be due to the activation of trigeminal sensory pathways that innervate the orbits, paranasal sinuses, and frontotemporal dura mater, which explains why migraine manifest with pain in these regions of the cranium. Untreated, headache typically reaches its peak severity within an hour and lasts for several hours or days. Sensitivity to light and sound, so common during migraine headaches, is thought to be the result of the sensitization of third-order neurons in the thalamus in response to trigeminal complex activation. The resolution of headache is followed by the postdrome phase, which is characterized by many symptoms of the prodromal phase—asthenia, somnolence, impaired concentration, photophobia, irritability, and nausea.

The three pillars of migraine management are: (1) Identifying and avoiding migraine triggers and making lifestyle adjustments to minimize headache frequency (regularizing sleep-wake cycles and meals, moderating caffeine intake). (2) Optimizing choice of abortive agents and using them early in the headache phase. These include nonsteroidal anti-inflammatory drugs (NSAIDs), triptans (selective serotonin 5-HT1B/5-HT1D receptor agonists), antiemetics, and calcitonin gene–related peptide (CGRP) blockers. (3) Starting a prophylactic daily medication for patients whose migraines are severe and frequent. Preventative therapies include antihypertensives, antiseizure medications, antidepressants, magnesium citrate, riboflavin, onabotulinumtoxinA (Botox) injections, and nerve blocks. Despite the widespread availability of effective treatments and the disabling nature of migraines, it remains a undertreated condition.

FIGURE

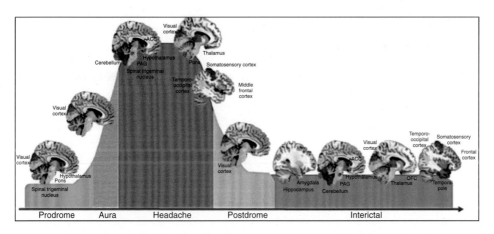

A schematic illustration of the main brain regions implicated in the phases of migraine. ACC, anterior cingulate cortex; OFC, orbito frontal cortex; PAG, periaqueductal gray. (Reprinted with permission from Messina R, Filippi M, Goadsby PJ. Recent advances in headache neuroimaging. *Curr Opin Neurol.* 2018;31(4):379-385.)

QUESTIONS FOR SELF-STUDY

1. Menses trigger migraines in some women. What therapeutic strategy can be employed to minimize the risk of perimenstrual migraine?
2. Why is it not recommended to use abortive agents (NSAIDs and triptans) on a daily or near-daily basis to treat migraine attacks?

3. When choosing a preventative medication for a patient, physicians should consider whether the medication is indicated or contraindicated for the patient's comorbid conditions. Match each preventative migraine medication with the comorbid condition for which it is indicated or relatively contraindicated:

A. Amitriptyline	Indicated: Depression. Contraindicated: Obesity
B. Topiramate	Indicated: Hypertension. Contraindicated: Asthma
C. Propranolol	Indicated: Neuropathic pain, seizures. Contraindicated: Suicidality
D. Gabapentin	Indicated: Seizures. Contraindicated: Kidney stones

4. Migraine is a recurrent episodic disorder, but a small minority of individuals experience "chronification" of migraines leading to daily or near-daily headaches. What are the approved treatments for chronic migraines?

5. CGRP has been consistently shown to be elevated during a migraine attack, and anti-CGRP peptide and anti-CGRP receptor antibodies are effective in preventing migraine. Propose where CGRP may fit in the pathogenesis of migraine.

CHALLENGE

What are the nonheadache migraine variants? How are they treated?

REFERENCES

Dodick DW. Migraine. *Lancet.* 2018;391(10127):1315-1330.

https://americanheadachesociety.org/wp-content/uploads/2018/08/Book_-_Brainstorm_Syllabus.pdf. [free online resource]

Stewart WF, Roy J, Lipton RB. Migraine prevalence, socioeconomic status, and social causation. *Neurology.* 2013;81(11):948-955. [free online resource]

Tension-Type Headache

Recurrent, primary headache of mild-to-moderate intensity

CORE FEATURES

The table contrasts tension-type headache (TTH) with migraine:

	Tension-Type Headache	Migraine Headache
1. Intensity	**Mild-moderate**	Moderate-severe
2. Laterality at onset	**Typically bilateral**	Typically unilateral
3. Headache quality	**Pressure, "vise-like"**	Throbbing, pulsating in most cases
4. Nausea	**No**	In half of patients
5. Worse with motion	**No; patients continue to carry on activities**	Yes; patients prefer to lie down

SYNOPSIS

TTH has the distinction of being the most characterless and least understood of primary headaches. It is also the one most likely to be confused with a secondary headache. For most patients, TTH is just a "regular headache," more of a nuisance than a disruptor of daily living. For this reason, patients with TTH are much less likely to present to the ED or seek neurologic consultation than patients with migraines.

The *Core features* highlight the difference between TTH and migraine, but in reality, features of these two types of headaches overlap. A patient may have severe headaches associated with sensitivity to light that is both bilateral and pressure-like. Differentiation between TTH and migraine is important therapeutically. Migraine shows a favorable response to triptans and CGRP antagonists, while TTH responds best to NSAIDs and caffeine. Preventative medications that work for migraines usually do not prevent TTH (with the exception of certain tricyclic antidepressants that may work for both headache types). Misdiagnosis of migraine as TTH is much more common than the inverse scenario. One likely reason for misdiagnosis is that clinicians are unaware that headaches may be compatible with migraine diagnosis even if not all of the classic migraine-like features are present—ie, not every migraineur will describe their headache as severe, throbbing, unilateral, and associated with nausea and photophobia. Conversely, features that are popularly thought to favor TTH—eg, stress as a headache trigger, neck pain—are just as common among patients with migraine. When in doubt, assume that a severe recurrent headache disorder is migraine rather than TTH.

FIGURE

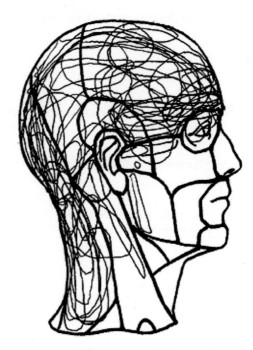

Typical location of tension-type headaches as traced by patients. Pain is concentrated in the neck and pericranial regions. (Reprinted with permission from Svensson P. Muscle pain in the head: overlap between temporomandibular disorders and tension-type headaches. *Curr Opin Neurol.* 2007;20(3):320-325.)

QUESTIONS FOR SELF-STUDY

1. Which three symptoms differentiate migraine from TTH with 98% accuracy? (Compare your answer with Lipton RB, et al. *Neurology.* 2003;61(3):375-382. [free online resource])

2. What nonpharmacologic strategies are effective in decreasing the frequency of TTH?

3. A 70-year-old healthy man with a history of TTH presents to his neurologist with worsening headaches over several weeks. The headache is now more frequent, more severe than before, and lateralizes to the left side, while previously they were bilateral. He reports a blurry vision of a few-second duration in the left eye when he gets up from the bed. What are the most important secondary headaches that must be considered in this context? Which are the most pertinent parts of examination that should be performed and documented? What testing should be pursued?

4. An 80-year-old woman with a distant history of TTH presents to her neurologist with worsening headaches over several weeks. The headache is worse on awakening and with straining (Valsalva). Which secondary headache do these features imply? Which are the pertinent examination findings that need to be documented? What testing should be pursued?

5. TTH-like headaches may result from ingestion or withdrawal from licit or illicit substances. Withdrawal headache may be tricky to diagnose, as patients are not routinely asked about the recently discontinued medications. Name some of the common substances associated with withdrawal headaches. Which diagnostic maneuver may help confirm the diagnosis of substance-withdrawal headaches?

CHALLENGE

A common dilemma for ED physicians is whether a lumbar puncture (LP) is warranted in a patient with an isolated headache. What are the main categories of secondary headaches that are diagnosed with cerebrospinal fluid (CSF) analysis? Which symptoms would you seek to elicit from the patient to decide whether an LP is warranted?

REFERENCES

Bendtsen L, Evers S, Linde M, et al. EFNS guideline on the treatment of tension-type headache – report of an EFNS task force. *Eur J Neurol*. 2010;17(11):1318-1325. [free online resource]
https://americanheadachesociety.org/wp-content/uploads/2018/05/NAP_for_Web_-_Headache_Diagnosis___Testing.pdf. [free online resource]

82 Cluster Headache

Primary recurrent headache, severe in intensity, with prominent autonomic features (rare)

CORE FEATURES

Cluster headache (CH) shares many features in common with migraines, unlike TTH. CH encompasses episodic and chronic phenotypes. CH is unilateral and may be accompanied by nausea, photophobia, and phonophobia. The main features that help distinguish episodic CH from migraine are listed in the table:

	Episodic Cluster Headache	Migraine
1. The rapidity of onset	Usually, takes a few minutes ot build up to maximal pain intensity	Usually, takes more than 20 min to build up to maximal intensity
2. Duration	30-90 min	Several hours to days
3. Autonomic features	Lacrimation (90%), conjunctival injection (75%), nasal stuffiness, rhinorrhea, eyelid ptosis, miosis, eyelid edema	Usually absent
4. Worse with movement	No; patients pace or rock back and forth during an attack	Yes; patients prefer to rest
5. "Clustering of attacks"	Yes; attacks tend to occur during the same time of year and the same time of day	No

SYNOPSIS

Relative to migraine, episodic CH is very rare. It has a prevalence of 1 in 1000, while migraine affects one in three women and one in six men. Yet, relative to other primary headaches that fall under the rubric of trigeminal autonomic cephalalgias (TACs), CH is the most common. All TACs have in common intense unilateral pain in the distribution of the ophthalmic division of trigeminal nerve and ipsilateral autonomic—parasympathetic and sympathetic—features. TACs differ from each other in duration, triggers, and response to treatment. TACs are currently classified into five groups: (1) CH; (2) paroxysmal hemicranias (PH); (3) short-lasting unilateral neuralgiform headache attacks with conjunctival injection and tearing (SUNCT); (4) short-lasting unilateral neuralgiform headache attacks with cranial autonomic symptoms (SUNA); and (5) hemicrania continua (HC). The most striking feature of CH, which is not found in other TACs, is the clustering and periodicity of the attacks. CHs tend to cluster during the same 1 to 3 months each year, often after the summer and winter solstice. Moreover, the headaches often cluster around the same time of the day, often between 1 am and 3 am. Treatments of acute attack include the administration of high-flow 100% oxygen, injectable sumatriptan and CGRP-targeted therapies. Preventative agents, which may be deployed during the cluster period, include calcium channel blockers, lithium, and oral steroids.

FIGURE

A unilateral headache in the location of the ophthalmic division of the trigeminal nerve.

Autonomic features:

- drooping of eyelid (ptosis)
- pupillary constriction (miosis)
- eye redness (conjunctival injection)
- tearing
- unilateral nose stuffiness, rhinorrhea

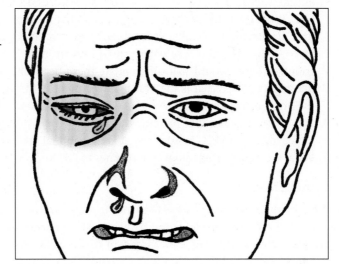

Headache often has circadian rhythmicity, eg, wakes patient from sleep around 2 am.

Patient agitated, getting up to move during the attack.

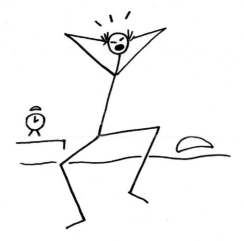

Characteristic features of cluster headache.

QUESTIONS FOR SELF-STUDY

1. Which autonomic features of CH can be attributed to parasympathetic nervous system activation, and which to activation of the sympathetic nervous system?
2. A 40-year-old woman presents with frequent headaches that last about 20 to 30 min and recur more than five times a day. There is no preferred time for the occurrence

of these headaches. There is prominent lacrimation during the attack. She is diagnosed with CH and prescribed galcanezumab (anti-CGRP monoclonal antibody) as an abortive agent and prednisone as a transitional preventative drug. However, the attacks continue unabated. Which clinical features do not fit with the diagnosis of CH? What is the likely correct diagnosis? What medication should be tried to confirm diagnostic suspicion and as a highly effective therapy?

3. SUNCT and SUNA cause paroxysms of severe pain in the trigeminal nerve distribution. How would you differentiate these headache disorders from trigeminal neuralgia (TN)? What is the first-line treatment of SUNCT and SUNA and what is the first-line treatment of TN?

4. It is recommended that patients diagnosed with TACs have brain magnetic resonance imaging (MRI) studies. What is the rationale behind this recommendation?

5. What are nonpharmacologic approaches to CH?

CHALLENGE

A hallmark feature of CH is the tendency to attack around the same time in the 24-hour cycle. A theory that explains the pathogenesis of clustering would thus likely involve brain structures responsible for circadian rhythms. Discuss where the circadian "master clock" is located in the brain and what is the putative link between this structure and CH. Name another primary headache disorder that manifests with clockwork regularity.

REFERENCES

Burish M. Cluster headache and other trigeminal autonomic cephalalgias. *Continuum.* 2018;24(4, Headache): 1137-1156.

https://americanheadachesociety.org/wp-content/uploads/2018/05/NAP_for_Web_-_Cluster___Other_Short-Lasting_Headaches.pdf. [free online resource]

83 Spontaneous Intracranial Hypotension

Secondary headache disorder due to spontaneous leakage of cerebrospinal fluid

CORE FEATURES

1. Headaches that are worse in an upright position and better with the head-down or Trendelenburg position.
   Headaches may have migrainous or TTH-like features and are often accompanied by neck pain and pain between the shoulder blades.
2. Low or low-normal opening CSF pressure.
   Opening pressure of <6 cm H_2O is highly suggestive of spontaneous intracranial hypotension (SIH) (normal opening pressure is 10-18 cm of H_2O). Up to two-thirds of patients with SIH have opening CSF pressures in the low range of normal.
3. Pachymeningeal enhancement on brain MRI.
   Engorgement of cerebral veins and sinuses may lead to smooth pachymeningeal (dural) enhancement. Other characteristic MRI features are "brain sag" (cerebellar tonsillar descent, crowding of the posterior fossa), pituitary gland enlargement, and, less commonly, subdural hygromas or hematomas.
4. Unresponsiveness to headache medications.
   Caffeine may provide temporary relief, but rarely long-lasting benefit.
5. Finding of a spinal CSF leak on computed tomography (CT) myelography or radionuclide cisternography.
   The location of the CSF leak can be determined by injecting contrast in the subarachnoid space and observing where the contrast will emerge. These tests are technically challenging and determine the site of CSF leak in only about half of patients with SIH.

SYNOPSIS

SIH, also known as CSF hypovolemia, clinically resembles post-LP headaches. In low CSF pressure headaches, an upright position typically exacerbates the pain and leads to further "sagging" of the brainstem, while the head-down position relieves the headache. The CSF leak is often "spontaneous" or follows a trivial event, like coughing, sneezing, bending, or a minor fall. The cause of the leak is presumed to be a dural tear from a spondylotic spur in the cervical or thoracic spine, weakness in the dural sac, or meningeal diverticula. The identification of the site of CSF leakage on CT myelography allows one to target epidural autologous blood patch placement. In the absence of an identifiable site, blind epidural blood patches can be tried; the success rate of a blind patch is about 30%.

FIGURE

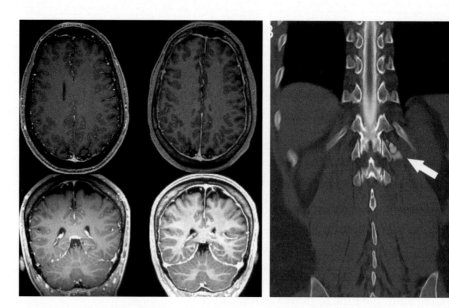

Contrast-enhanced axial and coronal MRI on the left show normal meninges in a 43-year-old man who had brain imaging for multiple sclerosis (MS) surveillance. MR images on the right were taken after he was diagnosed with IIH. Note the new smooth meningeal enhancement in supratentorial and infratentorial compartment. The image of coronal reformatted CT myelogram is from a different patient; it shows a saccular CSF collection (site of CSF leak, arrow) in the left posterior paravertebral soft tissues at the level of T12. (Reprinted with permission from Davagnanam I, Nikoubashman O, Shanahan P. Teaching NeuroImages: nontraumatic spinal CSF leak on CT myelography in a patient with low-pressure headaches. *Neurology.* 2010;75(22):e89.)

QUESTIONS FOR SELF-STUDY

1. Patients with SIH may experience double vision, facial pain, impaired hearing, dizziness, and, in severe cases, depressed consciousness and Parkinsonism. What is the likely neuroanatomic basis for these neurologic symptoms?
2. The table below lists the characteristic features of high and low intracranial pressure. For each characteristic, indicate whether it is seen with SIH or IIH:

	SIH	IIH
Supine position makes headache worse		
Headache worse in the morning		
Transient visual obscurations and pulsatile tinnitus		
Patient is thin or underweight		
Pituitary gland on MRI is distended, but not displaced		

3. Patients with hypermobility disorders, including Ehlers-Danlos and Marfan syndromes, are at increased risk for SIH. Suggest an explanation for this association.

4. A 50-year-old woman complains of positional headaches unresponsive to treatment and clear, colorless discharge from the right nostril. Can you suggest a diagnosis that would explain all of her symptoms? Which test of the nasal discharge could help confirm your clinical suspicion?

5. A 40-year-old man has successful repair of CSF leak for SIH. Soon thereafter, he develops headaches that are worse in the morning hours and when lying down. What could be an explanation for this change in headache pattern?

CHALLENGE

One of the classical brain MRI features of SIH—the presence of low-lying cerebellar tonsils—is also seen with Chiari type 1 malformation. The distinction between these two entities is critical, as patients with SIH who have decompression surgery for presumed Chiari type 1 malformation usually experience considerable worsening of their symptoms. What are the typical symptoms of a Chiari type 1 malformation that are not found in SIH? How would you differentiate Chiari type 1 from SIH by MRI criteria?

REFERENCES

Cullan AM, Grover ML. A 56-year-old woman with positional headache. *Mayo Clin Proc.* 2011;86(6):e35-8. [free online resource]

Friedman DI. Headaches due to low and high intracranial pressure. *Continuum.* 2018;24(4, Headache):1066-1091.

Mokri B. Spontaneous cerebrospinal fluid leaks from intracranial hypotension to ccerebrospinal flid hypovolemia – evolution of a concept. *Mayo Clin Proc.* 1999;74(11):1113-1123. [free online resource]

Infections of
the Central
Nervous System

TOP 1 0 0

A Very Brief Introduction to Infections of the Central Nervous System

> ... those who were under the spell of the coma forgot all those who were familiar to them and seemed to lie sleeping constantly. And if anyone cared for them, they would eat without waking. But those who were seized with delirium suffered from insomnia and were victims of a distorted imagination; for they suspected that men were coming upon them to destroy them, and they would become excited and rush off in flight, crying out at the top of their voices. And those who were attending them were in a state of constant exhaustion.
>
> **Procopius***

Brain infections cause brain malfunction—derangement in cognition, perception, and behavior. The converse, however, is not true: brain malfunction does not mean the patient has a brain infection, as there are many other causes of deranged cerebral function. The question of whether a patient has an infectious or noninfectious encephalopathy is not always easy to answer. When central nervous system (CNS) infection is suspected, a lumbar puncture with thorough cerebrospinal fluid (CSF) investigations is in order. Firm diagnosis of CNS infection requires either isolation of the pathogen from CNS tissue or from CSF, or evidence of an immune response to a specific pathogen in CSF.

A brain infection may be acute (acute viral encephalitis, Chapter 84) or chronic (HIV dementia, Chapter 89). Classic presentations of brain infection are altered mental status, seizures, and focal neurologic deficits, especially if the infection affects a specific brain region (brain abscess, Chapter 86). Bacterial meningitis typically presents acutely with fever, headache, meningismus, and fulminant CSF pleocytosis (Chapter 85), but some organisms induce a more indolent and less dramatic process (Lyme neuroborreliosis, Chapter 87). When patients have signs of infections of both the meningeal and parenchymal compartments, the term "meningoencephalitis" is appropriate.

CNS infections can be of viral, bacterial, mycobacterial, spirochetal, fungal, protozoan, parasitic, or prion (Chapter 91) etiology. Neuroinfections in the advanced market economies are on the decline. They account for less than 3% of inpatient neurology admissions, with about half occurring in immunocompromised hosts. In the emerging economies, "neglected tropical diseases" are highly prevalent, and many of them have prominent neurologic complications. We will discuss one example, neurocysticercosis, which is the most common cause of epilepsy in endemic regions (Chapter 88). Limitations of space prevent us from devoting separate chapters to many of the important neuroinfections of the developing world—tuberculosis, malaria, African

---

*Procopius of Caesarea, a preeminent Byzantine historian of the sixth century, provided an eyewitness account of the first known outbreak of Yersinia pestis in Europe—"the Plague of Justinian." The plague caused multiple pandemics over the centuries, most infamously the Black Death pandemic during the Middle Ages. The citation is from Procopius' *"History of the Wars."*

trypanosomiasis (sleeping sickness), and the many infections that involve neuroana-tomic compartments other than the brain: poliovirus and West Nile virus, which infect the anterior horn cells of the spinal cord; leprosy, a common cause of neuropathy worldwide; trichinosis, a common cause of infectious myositis. Neuroinfections are always important to keep on the differential as many are treatable.

REFERENCES

Tan K, Patel S, Gandhi N, Chow F, Rumbaugh J, Nath A. Burden of neuroinfectious diseases on the neurology service in a tertiary care center. *Neurology*. 2008;71(15):1160-1166.

84 Acute Viral Encephalitis

Viral infection of the brain parenchyma

CORE FEATURES

1. Altered mental status
   Encephalitis causes encephalopathy, behavioral changes, and, in the more severe cases, stupor and coma.
2. Fever (>102°F)
   Fever may precede or follow mental status change.
3. New-onset seizures
   Seizures may be focal or may generalize. A seizure may be clinical or subclinical (epileptiform discharges on electroencephalogram [EEG] in the absence of clinical evidence of seizure activity). Repetitive sharp wave complexes over the temporal lobes and periodic lateralizing epileptiform discharges (PLEDs) are characteristic of herpes simplex virus encephalitis (HSVE).
4. Focal neurologic deficits
   Encephalitis may cause memory loss, ataxia, focal paralysis, or a movement disorder.
5. CSF pleocytosis
   CSF pleocytosis is defined as >5 white blood cells (WBCs)/mm³. In viral encephalitis, pleocytosis is typically lymphocytic predominant and seldom exceeds 1000 WBCs/mm³.

SYNOPSIS

Encephalitis means, brain inflammation' in Greek. Inflammation could be due to an infectious or an autoimmune cause. The most common infectious causes are viral: herpes simplex virus, enterovirus, flavivirus (Japanese encephalitis), and arboviruses (West Nile or dengue). Among the many nonviral etiologies are bacterial (*Listeria, Mycoplasma, Bartonella*), mycobacterial (tuberculosis), spirochetal (*Borrelia burgdorferi*), fungal (*Cryptococcus*), protozoan (*Toxoplasma gondii*), amoebal (*Naegleria fowleri*) infections. Algorithms exist to narrow down the search for infectious agents depending on clinical history (travel history, tick exposures, immunodeficiency) and clinical and paraclinical features (EEG and brain magnetic resonance imagine [MRI] abnormalities). Still, in half of the cases, the infectious etiology remains unknown.

Management of encephalitides consists of supportive measures (ensuring airway patency and hemodynamic stability); control of seizures; measures to decrease intracranial pressure when needed; and parenteral antimicrobials. When HSV encephalitis is suspected, a weight-dose regimen of intravenous acyclovir should be started as early as possible because a delay in treatment correlates with worse outcomes. In a patient with whom no infectious agent is identified, one must consider the possibility of autoimmune encephalitis, which usually responds to corticosteroids and immunomodulation.

FIGURE

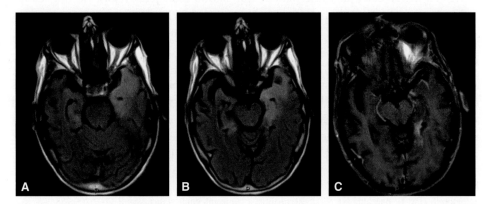

A 77-year-old woman presented with 4 days of cognitive decline and mild fevers. MRI of the brain showed extensive T2-hyperintense lesions in temporal lobes (A and B) with a small area of enhancement (C) suggestive of herpes simplex virus encephalitis (HSVE). HSV was detected in CSF with polymerase chain reaction (PCR) assay, confirming the diagnosis.

QUESTIONS FOR SELF-STUDY

1. Both noninfectious encephalopathy and encephalitis are defined by altered mental status. What are some valuable pointers on the clinical history, neurologic examination, CSF, and brain MRI findings that favor one etiology over the other?
2. A 5-year-old boy presents with fever, irritability, and lethargy. CSF is consistent with encephalitis. His condition deteriorates, and he becomes unresponsive to noxious stimuli. Both pupils become dilated and poorly reactive. What complication of acute encephalitis must be considered in this context? What is your approach to the management of this complication?
3. When evaluating a patient with possible encephalitis, it is important to collect detailed information on travel history, animal exposures, and sick contacts. List the infectious agent(s) that should be considered in the differential diagnosis of encephalitis, if the following risk factors or clinical findings are present:
   a. Hiking through wooded areas in the Northeastern United States during the spring-summer:
   b. History of a cat scratch:
   c. History of wild animal or bat bite:
   d. Recent travel to Africa:
   e. Petechial rash:
4. Explain why measuring pathogen-specific antibody titers during the acute phase and during convalescence (>2 weeks after onset) may enable the retrospective identification of the causative infectious agent of encephalitis.

5. A 10-year-old boy presents with low-grade fever, lethargy, seizures, and abnormal gait. Brain MRI demonstrates several diffuse, poorly demarcated, nonenhancing lesions in the cerebral white matter. CSF shows mild pleocytosis, no oligoclonal bands, and negative meningitis-encephalitis panel. What is the main noninfectious diagnostic consideration? What is the first-line treatment for this condition?

CHALLENGE

A 60-year-old woman successfully treated with intravenous acyclovir for HSVE returns to the ED several weeks following the discharge with worsening mental status and visual hallucinations. Brain MRI shows new T2 lesions in both temporal lobes. What rare complication of herpes encephalitis must be considered in this patient? What test can confirm your suspicion? What is the recommended treatment?

REFERENCES

Solomon T, Hart IJ, Beeching NJ. Viral encephalitis: a clinician's guide. *Pract Neurol.* 2007;7(5):288-305. [free online resource]
Tyler KL. Acute viral encephalitis. *N Engl J Med.* 2018;379(6):557-566.
Venkatesan A, Tunkel AR, Bloch KC, et al. Case definitions, diagnostic algorithms, and priorities in encephalitis: consensus statement of the international encephalitis consortium. *Clin Infect Dis.* 2013;57(8):1114-1128. [free online resource]

85 Acute Bacterial Meningitis

Acute bacterial infection involving the arachnoid meninges and subarachnoid space

CORE FEATURES

1. Fever
   Fever is almost invariably present and is usually >100.4°F. Hypothermia is a rare presentation.
2. Altered mental status
   Most patients are confused or lethargic on presentation and may progress to stupor and coma.
3. Meningismus (signs of meningeal irritation)
   Nuchal rigidity (inability to flex the neck) is the most reliable sign of meningismus. Brudzinski sign is reflex flexion of the patient's hips and knees upon passive flexion of the neck. Kernig sign is a restriction in passive extension at the knee because of the spasm of the hamstring muscles when the hip is flexed 90°. Brudzinski and Kernig signs are highly characteristic of meningismus but are absent in most patients with meningitis.
4. Headache
   Usually severe and generalized and accompanied by photophobia, nausea, and vomiting. "Jolt accentuation" of headache—induced by horizontal rotation of the head at a frequency of 2 to 3 per second—is a specific but not a sensitive sign of meningitis.
5. Neutrophilic CSF pleocytosis
   CSF leukocyte counts of ≥2000 cells/mm³ are predictive of bacterial meningitis, as is neutrophilic predominance. However, lower WBC counts, and even normal CSF, do not exclude this diagnosis. Isolation of bacterial pathogens in the CSF either by cultures (sensitivity of 60%-90% in an untreated patient) or identification of microbial genetic material in CSF by PCR allow for a definitive diagnosis.

SYNOPSIS

The classic triad of bacterial meningitis is fever, nuchal rigidity, and altered mental status. The triad is only present in half of the cases, while fever and encephalopathy can occur in any systemic infection. Tip-off for the diagnosis of bacterial meningitis is the unusual severity of the headache and signs of meningeal irritation. Clinical signs of meningitis may be attenuated or absent in neonates and young children, whose only manifestations may be irritability, poor feeding and decreased muscle tone. All patients with suspected meningitis require an LP unless contraindicated. Bacterial meningitis is associated with robust CSF pleocytosis (>2000 cells/mm³) with neutrophilic predominance, while viral meningitis is lymphocytic-predominant and exhibits a lesser degree of pleocytosis (<1000 cells/mm³). Protein levels in CSF tend to be higher (>2.2 g/L) and glucose levels lower (<1.9 mmol/L) in bacterial compared to viral meningitis, but an absolute distinction is difficult, particularly in early stages. Only a positive culture or PCR identification allows for a definitive diagnosis. Differential diagnosis of meningitis is broad and includes mycobacterial, fungal, protozoal, helminthic, inflammatory, autoimmune, neoplastic causes, and drug-induced aseptic meningitis.

Acute bacterial meningitis is a medical emergency. Long-term sequelae include permanent hearing loss (in children), intellectual disability, paresis, and seizure disorder. It is critical to initiate appropriate antimicrobial therapy within the first hour of presentation. Corticosteroids, administered as adjunctive treatment, significantly reduce the risk of hearing loss and other long-term complications among children.

FIGURE

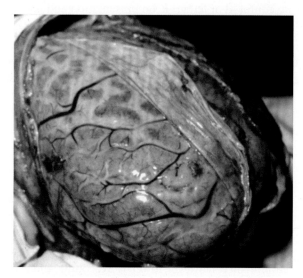

Purulent bacterial meningitis on postmortem. Effective antibiotic therapies have drastically reduced mortality from bacterial meningitis.

QUESTIONS FOR SELF-STUDY

1. There is considerable overlap in the clinical presentations of encephalitis and meningitis. Which findings on examination suggest one diagnosis over the other?
2. What is the likely pathophysiologic explanation for papilledema that may sometimes be observed in bacterial meningitis?
3. An important dilemma in patients with suspected bacterial meningitis is whether it is safe to do a lumbar puncture (LP) without prior brain imaging to rule out an intracranial mass lesion. The conservative approach of always imaging the head first, often results in patients being started on broad-spectrum antimicrobials prior to LP, thereby decreasing the yield of CSF cultures. In most cases of suspected acute meningitis, brain imaging is not required. What are the "red flags" on history or examination that mandate brain imaging prior to performing an LP?
4. CSF glucose concentration of <50% of serum glucose points to the diagnosis of bacterial rather than viral meningitis. Provide an explanation of why the CSF glucose level is lower in cases of bacterial meningitis than in cases of viral meningitis. Name three causes of meningitis associated with very low CSF glucose values.

5. A 30-year-old man presents with fever, headache, and meningismus. CSF is consistent with viral meningitis. CSF PCR for common viral etiologies is negative. Examination discloses white exudates on the tongue and pharynx and generalized lymphadenopathy. What is an important cause of viral encephalitis that should be considered in this patient?

CHALLENGE

PCR is a more sensitive and specific and usually a quicker way to diagnose common infections than traditional bacterial cultures. Yet, CSF culture has a significant advantage over PCR with regard to the choice of antimicrobials. Explain.

REFERENCES

Van de Beek D, Cabellos C, Dzupova O, et al. ESCMID guideline: diagnosis and treatment of acute bacterial meningitis. *Clin Microbiol Infect.* 2016;22(suppl 3):S37-S62. [free online resource]
Logan SA, MacMahon E. Viral meningitis. *BMJ.* 2008;336(7634):36-40. [free online resource]

86 Brain Abscess

Loculated collection of infected brain parenchyma

CORE FEATURES

1. Headache
   Headache is often accompanied by nausea and vomiting. A brain abscess may also cause obstruction of CSF outflow, raised intracranial pressure, and papilledema.
2. Systemic signs of infection are absent in about half of patients
   Patients may not look "sick," though some degree of encephalopathy may be present.
3. Focal neurologic signs are present in approximately half of the patients
   Focal signs correlate with the location and size of the mass lesion.
4. Focal seizures
   Antiseizure therapy is often continued for a year after brain abscess treatment because of the risk of seizure recurrence.
5. Large, space-occupying brain MRI lesion(s) with a predilection for grey-white matter junction and surrounding brain edema may be mistaken for metastases
   The core of a brain abscess often shows diffusion restriction on MRI; bright on diffusion-weighted imaging and dark on apparent diffusion coefficient (ADC). These findings favor brain abscess over a brain tumor.
6. An identifiable infectious source
   Infection usually spreads to the brain either from infected neighboring structures (otitis, mastoiditis, sinusitis, meningitis, dental infection—which can often be detected on brain MRI); hematogenously (pneumonia, infective endocarditis); or as sequelae of trauma or neurosurgical procedure.

SYNOPSIS

Mortality rate from brain abscesses has declined considerably since the introduction of neuroimaging, stereotactic brain biopsies, and broad-spectrum antimicrobials, yet fatal outcomes still occur in 10% to 20% of cases. A brain abscess may be difficult to diagnose in a timely fashion because the classic triad of headache, fever, and focal neurologic deficits is present in only 20% of patients and because brain MRI lesions are easy to mistake for brain tumors. Brain cultures and CSF cultures are positive in only a minority of cases. Definitive diagnosis rests on finding the culprit pathogens on brain biopsy, which should preferably be performed prior to the initiation of antibiotics. The most common organisms found on brain biopsy are streptococci, staphylococci species and Gram-negative enteric bacteria, or multiple species (polymicrobial brain abscess). Treatment of brain abscess involves surgery (excision via craniotomy or stereotactic drainage), prolonged antibiotics and the eradication of primary infection, which may require input from the relevant specialists—otorhinolaryngologist, cardiologist, dentist, and oral surgeon.

FIGURE

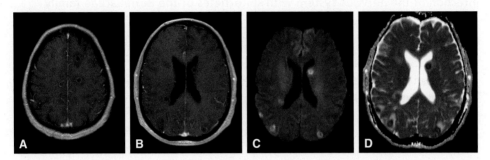

A 55-year-old man with *Staphylococcus intermedius* lung abscess presented to the ED with severe headache and nausea. MRI showed numerous ring-enhancing lesions (A and B) many of which had restricted diffusion (hyperintense on diffusion-weighted imaging [DWI] (C) and hypointense on ADC (D). Diagnosis of bacterial abscess was confirmed with brain biopsy.

QUESTIONS FOR SELF-STUDY

1. Why are fever and systemic symptoms so much less frequent in brain abscess than in bacterial meningitis?
2. An immunosuppressed status is a risk factor for a brain abscess. What are the differences in pathogens causing brain abscess in immunocompetent and immunocompromised patients?
3. Among children, the main risk factor for brain abscess formation is cyanotic congenital heart disease with a right-to-left shunt. Propose an explanation for the propensity for brain abscess in these patients.
4. A brain abscess often appears on MRI as a ring-enhancing lesion. What does the ring of enhancement correspond to on histopathology?
5. A 40-year-old tourist from India present with fevers, chills, and multiple ring gadolinium-enhancing brain lesions on MRI. In addition to neoplasms and bacterial brain abscesses, what other important etiology should be considered in this patient from India?

CHALLENGE

Suggest an explanation for diffusion restriction within a brain abscess core. What disorders, other than stroke, may show diffusion restriction on brain MRI?

REFERENCES

Brouwer MC, Coutinho JM, van de Beek D. Clinical characteristics and outcome of brain abscess: systematic review and meta-analysis. *Neurology.* 2014;82(9):806-813.

Sonneville R, Ruimy R, Benzonana N. An update on bacterial brain abscess in immunocompetent patients. *Clin Microbiol Infect.* 2017;23(9):614-620. [free online resource]

87 Lyme Neuroborreliosis

Infection of the nervous system with spirochetes of the Borreliaceae family

CORE FEATURES

1. *Ixodes* tick bite or a history of exposure to *Ixodes* ticks
   Less than half of patients with Lyme disease recall the history of a tick bite, but all patients with Lyme have a history of being in time and place where *Ixodes* ticks are found.
2. History of erythema migrans ("target rash")
   Erythema migrans occur within days of infection. Other early signs of Lyme infection are fever, headache, fatigue, myalgias, and swollen lymph nodes.
3. Cranial nerve or spinal nerve root involvement
   Neurologic symptoms usually occur within weeks-to-months of exposure, except for peripheral facial palsy which may manifest within 7 to 21 days of exposure. Lyme radiculitis can be easily missed, especially if there is no known history of Lyme infection.
4. Meningitis
   Typically occurs within a few weeks of infection. Mild CSF pleocytosis (50-250 lymphocytes/mm^3) with lymphocytic predominance is characteristic. There is often mild elevation in protein content in CSF, while glucose level is normal.
5. Evidence of an immune response to *Borrelia*
   Within 6 weeks following exposure, infected patients will test positive for Lyme antibodies in serum. Anti–*B. burgdorferi* Abs in CSF are highly specific for neuro-Lyme, but not required for the diagnosis if there is serologic evidence of Lyme infection and clinical syndrome consistent with Lyme neuroborreliosis (LNB).

SYNOPSIS

Lyme disease is caused by spirochetes of the Borreliaceae family, principally *B. burgdorferi* in the United States. These spirochetes are transmitted to humans by the *Ixodes* tick. The transmission requires at least 24 hours of tick attachment, so early discovery and removal of the tick drastically reduce the risk of infection. Systemic symptoms and erythema migrans develop within days of tick bite. Neurologic complications develop later in up to 15% of patients. Facial palsy is the most common complication and accounts for 80% of cranial neuropathies due to LNB, followed by meningitis and radiculitis. Facial palsy in a child or a bilateral peripheral facial palsy in an adult that happens during or soon after "tick season" should raise suspicion of LNB. Inflammation of plexuses (plexitis) and nerves (mononeuropathy, polyneuropathy, mononeuritis multiplex) is rare, and involvement of the brain and spinal cord is rarer yet. MRI may show enhancement of brain and spinal cord meninges, cranial nerves and nerve roots. Enhancing lesion within parenchyma is exceptionally rare.

Treatment of the common neurologic manifestations of Lyme disease (facial palsy, meningitis, radiculitis) can be effected with oral antimicrobials (doxycycline), while the more complicated cases, with brain or spinal cord involvement, may require intravenous antibiotics.

FIGURE

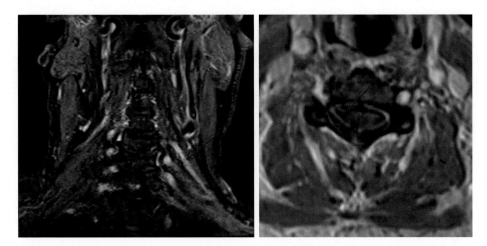

MRI shows enhancement of the roots of brachial plexus (left panel) and dorsal roots (arrowhead) and ventral roots (arrow) within the spinal canal (right panel). (Reprinted with permission from Dabir A, Pawar G. Teaching neuroimages: lyme disease presenting as Bannwarth syndrome. *Neurology.* 2018;91(15):e1459-e1460.)

QUESTIONS FOR SELF-STUDY

1. *Ixodes* ticks transmit not only Lyme disease, the most common vector-borne disease in Europe and North America, but also anaplasmosis (spread by *Ixodes scapularis* or *Ixodes pacificus*) and babesiosis (spread by the *Ixodes scapularis*). What are the recommended measures to reduce the risk of tick-borne infections?

2. The serologic diagnosis of Lyme relies on a two-step procedure. First, total levels of anti-Borrelia antibodies are measured via enzyme-linked immunosorbent assay (ELISA) and then, if the test is positive, the diagnosis is confirmed with Western Blot, which identifies specific IgM and IgG anti-*Borrelia* antibodies. Why should not Western Blot alone be used for testing?

3. Bannwarth syndrome—inflammation of one or more spinal nerve roots in LNB—is often mistaken for a disk herniation. What findings on examination and MRI should prompt a search for an alternative explanation to disk herniation in a patient with radicular pain?

4. Some patients with a history of Lyme disease continue to experience debilitating symptoms such as fatigue, "cognitive fog," and pain, even after an appropriate course of treatment for Lyme (so-called, posttreatment Lyme disease syndrome, PTLDS). Suggest an explanation for these symptoms. Explain why continuous treatment with antibiotics is not indicated for PTLDS.

5. What is the other infamous spirochetal infection that can invade the CNS and cause meningitis, cranial nerve palsies, severe pain, and CSF pleocytosis? Compare and contrast the various neurologic syndromes of this spirochetal infection with that of LNB.

CHALLENGE

Explain why testing for the intrathecal response to a pathogen requires the collection of both serum and CSF samples (the concept of "antibody index").

REFERENCES

Halperin JJ. Neuroborreliosis. *Neurol Clin.* 2018;36(4):821-830.

Lindland ES, Solheim AM, Andreassen S, et al. Imaging in Lyme neuroborreliosis. *Insights Imaging.* 2018;9(5):833-844. [free online resource]

Wormser GP, Dattwyler RJ, Shapiro ED, et al. The clinical assessment, treatment, and prevention of Lyme disease, human granulocytic anaplasmosis, and babesiosis: clinical practice guidelines by the Infectious Diseases Society of America. *Clin Infect Dis.* 2006;43(9):1089-1134. [free online resource]

88 Neurocysticercosis

Brain infection with the cysticerci of *Taenia solium* flatworm

CORE FEATURES

1. Exposure to *Taenia solium* tapeworm
   A person may be exposed to *T. solium* if they live in or travel to the endemic regions (Africa, Asia, South America) or are in a close contact of someone infected with *T. solium*.
2. Seizures in 70% to 90% of patients with neurocysticercosis (NCC)
   NCC accounts for 30% of epilepsy cases in endemic areas. Seizures are usually associated with calcified lesions on brain imaging.
3. Syndrome of increased intracranial pressure (ICP)
   Among patients with active NCC, 25% develop signs of increased ICP because CSF outflow is obstructed by intraventricular cysts or chronic meningeal inflammation. Mass effect from very large cysts in the subarachnoid space ("racemous cysts") can also cause ICP. Isolated headache is common in NCC and by itself does not imply increased ICP.
4. "Hole with a dot" sign on brain MRI
   A cystic lesion on T1 and T2 weighted sequences with a centrally placed bright "dot," which represents the scolex, is pathognomonic for active cysticerci.
5. Soft-tissue calcifications or palpable subcutaneous nodules suggest disseminated cysticercosis
   In patients with seizures and subcutaneous nodules, cysticercosis is a likely unifying diagnosis, but the possibility of seizure disorder being unrelated to cysticercosis should also be considered.

SYNOPSIS

Cysticercosis is one of "neglected tropical diseases," which collectively affect more than 1 billion people in the emerging economy countries (https://www.who.int/neglected_diseases/diseases/en/). Cysticercosis is caused by infection with larva (cysticerci) of the pork tapeworm, *T. solium*. Life cycles of *T. solium* require two hosts (humans and pigs) and a free-living stage. This life cycle can only be maintained in an environment where humans eat pig meat and pigs have access to human feces. When embryonated eggs are ingested by humans, they hatch in the small intestine, penetrate into the bloodstream, spread throughout the body and develop into larva (cysticerci). Many organs can be infected: muscles and skin (hence muscle cysts and calcifications, and subcutaneous nodules), eyes (infection of the retina or vitreous humor), the central nervous system ("hole with a dot" sign on MRI is a picture of a living cysticercus). Only CNS involvement is a significant cause of morbidity, mainly because NCC is such a common cause of epilepsy. NCC may also cause encephalitis, focal neurologic deficits, and dementia, depending on the number and location of cysticerci and the degree of the host response. Enhancement and edema around the cyst indicate that the parasite has been immunologically recognized by the host, while inactive cysticerci are calcified and easily detectable on head computed tomography (CT). The diagnosis of cysticercosis is supported by positive serum enzyme-linked immunoelectrotransfer blot (EITB) assay for the detection of antibodies to *T. solium* antigens. However, the utility of this test is limited since as many as 25% of patients in endemic areas had exposure to *T. solium*, but have no clinical symptoms of NCC. Treatment of NCC with antihelminthic agents (albendazole and praziquantel) should be considered on a case-by-case basis since patients with calcified cysts do not benefit from treatment, while patients with a large number of active cysts may mount a massive immunologic response to dying larva, resulting in rapid neurologic deterioration.

FIGURE

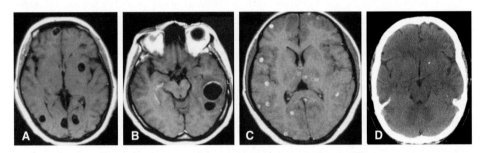

MRI images in (A-C) exemplify cases of vesicular, colloidal, and nodular cysticerci (D) Noncontrast head CT shows two small calcified cysticerci. (A-C, Reprinted with permission from Carpio A, Fleury A, Hauser WA. Neurocysticercosis: five new things. *Neurol Clin Pract*. 2013;3(2):118-125. Copyright © 2013 American Academy of Neurology.)

QUESTIONS FOR SELF-STUDY

1. Where in the patient's body can one see a living, moving cysticercus?
2. A 25-year-old patient born in a small town in rural Guatemala presented with seizures. Head CT showed a large cyst within the brain parenchyma. A repeat CT 2 weeks later shows that the cyst has disappeared. What is the likely explanation?
3. Which EEG findings are not compatible with the diagnosis of NCC-induced epilepsy?
4. Explain why patients with active brain cysticerci who undergo antihelminthic therapy may require adjunct corticosteroid treatment.
5. Match each of the neglected tropical diseases and common parasitic infections with its respective neurologic complications. (Prevalence as of 2019, cited from WHO and CDC.)

   a. Schistosomiasis, aka bilharzia (agent: schistosomes; parasitic blood flukes; transmitted through contaminated freshwater; 218 million people affected).

   b. Leprosy (agent: *Mycobacterium leprae*; mode of transmission unknown; 16 million people affected).

   c. Toxoplasmosis (agent: *T. gondii* parasite; mode of transmission: via cat feces contamination or undercooked meat; 40 million people in the United States may be infected; symptomatic disease is rare).

d. Human African trypanosomiasis, aka "sleeping sickness" (agent: protozoan parasites from genus *Trypanosoma*; transmitted to humans by tsetse fly bites in sub-Saharan Africa; over 10,000 new cases each year).

e. Malaria (agent: *Plasmodium* parasite, transmitted by *Anopheles* mosquitoes in the endemic tropical and subtropical areas of Central and South America, sub-Saharan Africa, and South-East Asia; 216 million cases of malaria worldwide).

   i. Enhancing brain lesions, encephalitis, seizures in the immunocompromised host; vision loss; intellectual disability and blindness in neonates

   ii. Neuropathy, palpable peripheral nerves

   iii. The most common cause of myelitis in the endemic area

   iv. High-grade fevers and teeth-chattering chills, impairment of consciousness, focal neurological signs, and seizures

   v. Rapidly progressive dementia and sleep disorder

CHALLENGE

Based on your understanding of the life cycle of *T. solium*, what practical measures could you propose to limit the spread of this infection in endemic areas? (Compare your response with WHO guidelines cited below.)

REFERENCES

Carabin H, Ndimubanzi PC, Budke CM, et al. Clinical manifestations associated with neurocysticercosis: a systematic review. *Plos Negl Trop Dis*. 2011;5(5):e1152.

Dorny P. Detection and diagnosis. In: Murell D, eds. *WHO/FAO/OIE Guidelines for the Surveillance, Prevention and Control of Taeniosis/Cysticercosis*. 2005. http://www.oie.int/doc/ged/d11245.pdf.

89 HIV-1 Associated Neurocognitive Disorder

Umbrella term for syndromes of cognitive impairment due to infection with human immunodeficiency virus Type 1 (HIV-1)

CORE FEATURES

1. Insidious onset, slowly progressive cognitive decline
   Common early symptoms include attention and memory problems, and impaired executive functions.
2. Affective symptoms, such as apathy, irritability, and depression
3. Motor slowing
   Decreased speed of finger or toe-tapping; Parkinsonian features are common, but not required for the diagnosis of HIV-1–associated neurocognitive disorder (HAND).
4. HIV seropositive
   HAND is due to HIV infection, not due to a secondary infection resulting from the immunocompromised state. CD4 counts are usually not low in HAND patients.
5. Brain MRI shows T2-hyperintense mostly symmetric lesions in the subcortical white matter and basal ganglia
   Similar findings may be seen in vascular aging. Lesions with mass effect and contrast enhancement are not compatible with the diagnosis of HAND.

SYNOPSIS

HIV is a retrovirus estimated to affect more than 40 million people as of 2018. The virus infects and destroys CD4-positive T-cells leading to acquired immunodeficiency syndrome (AIDS), defined as CD4 count of <200 cells/μL or presence of "AIDS-defining" infections or malignancies. HIV enters the CNS via infected lymphocytes early in the infection and may present as mild meningoencephalitis. The introduction of highly effective combined antiretroviral therapy (CART) has drastically reduced the prevalence of HIV-associated opportunistic infections, malignancies, HIV dementia and vacuolar myelopathy that were seen in the advanced stages of immunodeficiency. However, the prevalence of HAND has not decreased in the CART era, and roughly half of HIV-infected patients meet the criteria for HAND. It is unknown whether cognitive impairment in CART-treated patients is a consequence of ongoing, low-grade infection within the CNS or is independent of viral replication. Differential diagnosis of HAND includes AIDS-defining CNS infections and malignancies, psychoactive medications, drug abuse, head trauma, neurodegenerative conditions unrelated to HIV-1, and psychiatric disorders. CSF analysis is not necessary for the diagnosis of HAND but may be necessary to rule out AIDS-defining conditions. In HAND, the CSF routine analyses are essentially normal.

FIGURE

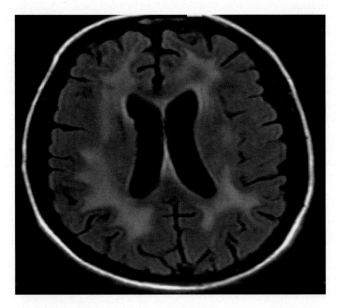

Brain MR fluid-attenuated inversion recovery (FLAIR) sequence shows typical subcortical white matter hyperintensities in a patient with HIV dementia.

QUESTIONS FOR SELF-STUDY

1. Which of the dementias described in the section on disorders of higher cognitive function (Chapters 50-53) does HAND resemble the most?
2. Fill in the correct AIDS-defining infections in the corresponding row of the Table below:
   a. Tuberculous meningitis (organism: *M. tuberculosis*, mycobacterium)
   b. Cryptococcal meningitis (organism: *Cryptococcus neoformans*, a ubiquitous yeast)
   c. Toxoplasma encephalitis (organism: *T. gondii*, an intracellular protozoan parasite)
   d. Cytomegalovirus encephalitis (organism: CMV, herpesvirus)

CNS Infection	Clinical	MRI	Diagnostic Testing
	Subacute onset of focal neurologic deficits; may present as a movement disorder	Multiple ring-enhancing lesions, often in basal ganglia, thalamus, juxtacortical white matter	IgG antibodies against pathogen are sensitive, but non-specific; brain biopsy may be required for diagnosis
	Fever, headache, impaired consciousness, meningismus, lower cranial nerve palsies, focal neurologic signs	Basal leptomeningeal enhancement; parenchymal lesions	CSF pleocytosis, low glucose, high protein; CSF PCR is the gold standard
	Subacute onset of headache, lethargy, fever, malaise	Intracerebral masses, dilated Virchow-Robin spaces, cortical and lacunar infarctions, pseudocysts, hydrocephalus, cerebritis	Antigen in the CSF is highly specific; organism may be found on India ink staining of CSF
	May cause encephalitis, ventriculitis, polyradiculitis, retinitis	Periventricular inflammation or enhancement of meninges and spinal nerve roots	CSF PCR is highly sensitive and specific

3. A 40-year-old man with AIDS is admitted with altered mental status and multiple ring-enhancing lesions on brain MRI. Treatment with sulfadiazine and pyrimethamine is initiated for presumed CNS toxoplasmosis. Over the next 3 weeks, his condition deteriorates. What is the most likely alternative diagnostic consideration? What is the next step in the investigation and management of this patient?

4. Cognitive decline in HIV patients requires evaluation for AIDS-defining conditions that affect the CNS. However, non-AIDS defining infections may coexist with HIV and should be considered on the differential. What treatable infectious causes of cognitive impairment should be sought for in a patient with HIV and dementia?

5. HIV infection may also affect the spinal cord resulting in myelopathies with demyelination of the posterior and lateral funiculi. What other retroviral infection can cause progressive myelopathy? What test is necessary to make the diagnosis?

CHALLENGE

A 50-year-old man with HIV is compliant with CART and has an undetectable serum HIV levels. He develops psychomotor slowing that impairs his daily functioning. CSF analysis reveals very high levels of HIV RNA but is otherwise unremarkable. What is the most plausible explanation for the patient's neurologic decline and CSF findings?

REFERENCES

Eggers C, Arendt J, Hahn K, et al. HIV-1-associated neurocognitive disorder: epidemiology, pathogenesis, diagnosis, and treatment. *J Neurol.* 2017;264(8):1715-1727. [free online resource]

Manji H, Miller R. The neurology of HIV infection. *J Neurol Neurosurg Psychiatry.* 2004;75(suppl 1):i29-35. [free online resource]

90 Progressive Multifocal Leukoencephalopathy

Brain infection with JC virus in immunocompromised individuals

CORE FEATURES

1. Immunocompromised state
   Progressive multifocal leukoencephalopathy (PML) occurs in patients with AIDS; hematologic or solid organ malignancies; organ transplants; autoimmune diseases (systemic lupus erythematosus, rheumatoid arthritis); and with certain immunosuppressive or immunomodulatory medications (natalizumab, mycophenolate mofetil).
2. Progressive focal neurologic deficits
   The common symptoms are cognitive impairment, visual field defect, hemiparesis, dysarthria, and ataxia.
3. Solitary or multifocal lesions in brain MRI
   T2-hyperintense/T1-hypointense lesions, typically without mass effect, are most commonly found in the white matter, but may also be seen in the basal ganglia, thalamus, and brainstem.
4. JC Virus (JCV) in the CSF
   Ultra-sensitive JCV PCR can detect as few as 10 copies of the virus in 1 mL of CSF.
5. Demyelinating lesions with enlarged oligodendroglial nuclei and bizarre astrocytes on brain biopsy
   JC virus can be detected on biopsy by immunostaining of oligodendrocytes with JCV-specific antigen; or more directly by electron microscopy (visualization of particles); or most directly by PCR JCV.

SYNOPSIS

JC virus (JCV, human polyomavirus 2) is present in the kidneys and bone marrow of most adults and has no known pathological effect in either organ ("silent infection"). However, if JCV enters the brain and is able to replicate there, it can cause a potentially fatal disease, PML. In order for a brain infection to occur, JCV must first genetically transform into a neurotrophic strain in the periphery. Then the neurotropic form of the virus crosses the blood-brain barrier (BBB) within infected lymphocytes and infects oligodendrocytes. For the infection to spread in the brain, JCV needs to overcome the normal immune surveillance in the brain. In immunologically competent individuals, the spread of JCV is easily contained, but in patients with defective cellular immunity or impaired immune surveillance, JCV replication will continue unchecked in the brain causing widespread death of oligodendrocytes, demyelination and neuronal death. Rarely, JC virus can infect neurons in the granular cell layer of the cerebellum ("JC virus granule cell neuronopathy") or cortical neurons.

FIGURE

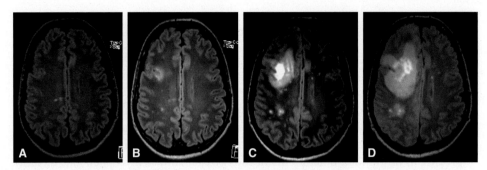

A 44-year-old man with MS developed natalizumab-associated PML. A, MRI prior to PML shows a few demyelinating plaques in the subcortical and juxtacortical white matter. B, The new U-shaped lesion in the right frontal lobe on surveillance MRI is suspicious for PML. The patient was asymptomatic. Natalizumab was discontinued. C, The frontal lesion continues to increase in size. Note "milky way" appearance of several new lesions throughout right and left hemispheres, which likely represent foci of PML. D, The patient was hospitalized with dysarthria and hemiparesis. Note early signs of subfalcine herniation. Intravenous steroids were administered for presumptive immune reconstitution inflammatory syndrome (IRIS) with good effect.

QUESTIONS FOR SELF-STUDY

1. CSF shows pleocytosis in viral encephalitis, but not in PML. Propose an explanation of why the cell count is typically normal or only slightly elevated when a brain infection is caused by the JC virus.

2. A 40-year-old HIV-positive man presents with left hemiparesis. CD4 count is 100 cells/mm³. Brain MRI shows large, nonenhancing T2-hyperintense lesions in the right hemisphere and a smaller T2 hyperintense lesion in the left thalamus. CSF contains 10,000 copies/mL of JCV, confirming the diagnosis of PML. The patient is started on highly active antiretroviral therapy (HAART). Six weeks later, he re-is readmitted with confusion and worsening hemiparesis. Brain MRI shows enhancement and marked increase in the size of both previously seen lesions. What is the likely explanation for this development?

3. A 30-year-old woman diagnosed with multiple sclerosis (MS) is interested in natalizumab therapy. What serum test is required to estimate her risk of developing natalizumab-associated PML?

4. PML and MS are demyelinating disorders. Describe the major differences in how demyelination is effected in these two diseases.

5. Myelin is present in both the central and peripheral nervous systems. Provide an explanation for why the JC virus does not cause demyelination of peripheral nerves.

CHALLENGE

PML can emerge when cellular immunity against JCV is impaired. It follows that restoration of cellular immunity in patients with PML could stop the spread of infection. Propose a mechanism of restoring cellular immunity to JCV in immunocompromised individuals. (Compare your approach with that of Muftuoglu M, et al. cited below.)

REFERENCES

Berger JR, Aksamit AJ, Clifford DB, et al. PML diagnostic criteria: a consensus statement from the AAN Neuroinfectious Disease Section. *Neurology*. 2013;80(15):1430-1438. [free online resource]

Major EO, Yousry TA, Clifford DB. Pathogenesis of progressive multifocal leukoencephalopathy and risks associated with treatments for multiple sclerosis: a decade of lessons learned. *Lancet Neurol*. 2018;17(5):467-480.

Muftuoglu M, Olson A, Marin D, et al. Allogeneic BK virus-specific T cells for progressive multifocal leukoencephalopathy. *N Engl J Med*. 2018;379(15):1443-1451.

91 Creutzfeldt-Jakob Disease

The most common of the human prion brain disorders

CORE FEATURES

1. Rapidly progressive and fatal dementia
   The disease begins with a broad range of behavioral, psychiatric, and autonomic symptoms, followed by global cognitive decline and akinetic mute state within months of onset.
2. Startle myoclonus
   Myoclonic jerk when the patient is startled by a sudden loud clap or some other such stimulus is present in 90% of patients with Creutzfeldt-Jakob Disease (CJD), but not necessarily at the time of onset.
3. High signal on diffusion-weighted imaging (DWI) on MRI in the cortex and deep gray nuclei
   The caudate nucleus and the anterior putamen are the most consistently affected areas.
4. Periodic synchronous biphasic or triphasic sharp wave complexes (PSWC) on EEG
   These findings are seen in most patients with CJD.
5. Elevated levels of protein markers of glial and neuronal damage (14-3-3, Tau, S100b, neuron-specific enolase) in CSF
   These proteins are elevated in CSF in 80% of CJD cases but they are not specific for CJD.

SYNOPSIS

Prions are proteins. They lack genetic material, but can "multiply," spread, and destroy healthy tissue effectively acting as infectious agents. To become a prion, a protein refolds into a form that is capable of inducing refolding in other proteins. Because prions cause neuronal death (apoptosis) without eliciting an immune reaction, they give the brain a highly vacuolated, spongiform appearance. Hence, prion diseases are also known as transmissible spongiform encephalopathies (TSEs).

Prion diseases may spread by contact with contaminated body parts (pituitary hormone extract) or consumption of prion-infected humans (Kuru disease, which is due to consumption of brains of dead people as part of a funeral ritual in New Guinea) or animals (mad cow disease). Prion diseases can be genetically inherited, blurring the boundary between "genetic" and "infectious" disease categories. Currently, five human prion diseases are known: CJD, fatal familial insomnia, Gertsmann-Sträussler-Scheinker syndrome, Kuru, and variable protease-sensitive prionopathy. CJD accounts for about 90% of sporadic cases of prion disease. The mean age of onset of CJD is between 57 and 62 years. It usually presents with rapidly progressive dementia and myoclonus but may start with cortical blindness (Heidenhain variant), cerebellar, extrapyramidal, or thalamic symptoms. Death is expected within 12 months of symptom onset.

FIGURE

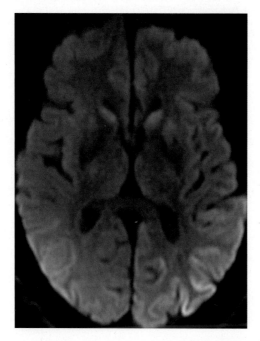

DWI hyperintense signal in bilateral caudate, left putamen and left occipital cortex is suggestive of CJD. CSF markers were reported as "98% probability of CJD."

QUESTIONS FOR SELF-STUDY

1. What is myoclonus? How would you differentiate a patient with myoclonus from a patient with a tremor?
2. Explain the mechanism by which a genetic mutation may cause prion disease.
3. Why does CJD affect the cortex and basal ganglia on MRI? What other conditions may imitate this unusual pattern of injury?
4. In patients with rapidly progressive dementia, it is most important to first rule out potentially reversible autoimmune, metabolic and infectious causes. Name the reversible causes of rapidly progressive dementia.
5. Unique procedures must be followed when operating on a patient with suspected prion disease. The equipment that has been in contact with prion needs to be discarded in a controlled manner (see UK guidelines cited below). Explain why standard decontamination procedures are not adequate when dealing with prions.

CHALLENGE

More than 200 cases of CJD have been attributed to treatment with prion-contaminated human growth hormone. Yet, hardly any cases of CJD have been attributed to blood transfusion, which are many orders of magnitude more common than pituitary hormone treatments. Suggest a reason for the very low risk of prion infection with blood transfusion and high risk with growth hormone treatment.

REFERENCES

Fragoso DC, Gonçalves Filho AL, Pacheco FT, et al. Imaging of Creutzfeldt-Jakob disease: imaging patterns and their differential diagnosis. *Radiographics*. 2017;37(1):234-257.

https://www.gov.uk/government/publications/guidance-from-the-acdp-tse-risk-management-subgroup-formerly-tse-working-group.

Mead S, Rudge P. CJD mimics and chameleons. *Pract Neurol*. 2017;17(2):113-121. [free online resource]

Immune-Mediated Disorders of the Central Nervous System

A Very Brief Introduction to Immune-Mediated Disorders of the Central Nervous System

> We pointed out that the organism possesses certain contrivances by means of which the immunity reaction, so easily produced by all kinds of cells, is prevented from acting against the organism's own elements and so giving rise to … 'horror autotoxicus'.
>
> **Paul Ehrlich***

When contrivances by means of which an immune reaction is prevented from being directed against the organism's own elements fail, autoimmunity—Ehrlich's "horror autotoxicus"—may ensue. Over 100 human autoimmune diseases have been described (https://www.aarda.org/diseaselist/). They collectively affect more than 20 million people in the United States. Some of these autoimmune disorders are directed against specific organs or tissues (alopecia areata is a disease of hair follicles); others are multiorgan diseases (systemic lupus erythematosus). Many autoimmune neurological disorders have already been described elsewhere if they primarily affect a single anatomic compartment: eg, Guillain-Barré syndrome (an autoimmune reaction against peripheral nerves), polymyositis (skeletal muscle), Lambert-Eaton myasthenic syndrome (neuromuscular junction), optic neuritis (optic nerve). This section focuses on multifocal immune-mediated diseases of the central nervous system (CNS). By far the most prevalent disease in this category is multiple sclerosis (MS), a chronic, often disabling disorder that affects almost one million Americans (Chapter 92). MS is characterized by "dissemination in space and time," ie, different parts of the "CNS space" are affected at different time points in the disease. This characteristic is not unique to MS. Other autoimmune and non-autoimmune disorders also exhibit dissemination in space and time. Neuromyelitis optica spectrum disorders (NMOSD; Chapter 93) are relapsing-remitting neuroinflammatory disorders that involve spinal cord, optic nerves, and brain via different immunopathogenic mechanisms than in MS. Systemic autoimmune disorders can cause chronic CNS disease and may be especially challenging to diagnose if the CNS is the first organ to be targeted. A case in point is neurosarcoidosis (Chapter 95), which is notorious for its ability to involve almost any part of the nervous system and mimic many neurologic disorders, including MS. Not all autoimmune diseases are chronic diseases. An example of a monophasic autoimmune CNS disorder, acute disseminated encephalomyelitis (ADEM) is discussed in Chapter 94.

Many of the autoimmune CNS disorders may be brought under sustained remission by appropriately chosen immunosuppressive or immunomodulatory therapies. As is usually the case in medicine, earlier treatment translates into better outcomes. It is essential to correctly diagnose neuroinflammatory disorders at first presentation and offer specific immunotherapy whenever there is a high likelihood of disease recurrence.

---

*Paul Ehrlich (1854-1915)—German-Jewish physician and scientist made seminal contributions to histology, hematology, infectious diseases and was one of the founders of immunology. Ehrlich invented the first successful treatment for syphilis; discovered methylene blue stain and a stain for tuberculous mycobacteria; and anticipated the antibody theory of immunity, among other contributions. Citation is from Collected Papers of Paul Ehrlich (Pergamon, London).

Multiple Sclerosis

Chronic CNS demyelinating disorder

CORE FEATURES

1. Dissemination in time

   There is evidence of episodic focal inflammation (relapses or MRI lesions) and/or ongoing progressive neurodegeneration (deterioration of gait, balance, or cognitive function in the absence of relapses over at least 12 months).

2. Dissemination in the CNS space

   Different parts of the brain, spinal cord, and optic nerves are affected clinically (characteristic neurologic findings referable to different parts of the CNS) and radiologically (MRI lesions in different parts of the brain, optic nerves, and spinal cord).

3. MS-typical MRI lesions in the brain, optic nerves, and spinal cord

   Characteristic lesions are fingerlike projections attached to the ventricular wall (Dawson fingers), lesions along U-fibers (juxtacortical), lesions along cranial nerve roots (brainstem), and lesions in the undersurface of the corpus callosum. Examples of MS-typical lesions are shown in the figure below.

4. Intrathecal inflammation

   Oligoclonal bands (OCBs) in the cerebrospinal fluid (CSF) but not in serum are detected in more than 90% of patients with MS, but also in any infectious and inflammatory CNS disorder. Elevated immunoglobulin (IgG) index, a quantitative marker of intrathecal inflammation, is less sensitive for MS than OCBs.

5. Loss of ganglion cells and axons in the retina

   Optic nerve atrophy is present in most patients with long-standing disease. Loss of ganglion cells and axons can be quantitated by measuring the ganglion cell layer and retinal nerve fiber layer (RNFL) on optical coherence tomography (OCT). Patients with acute optic neuritis show nerve swelling on OCT (increased RNFL thickness) followed by atrophy weeks later.

SYNOPSIS

The mean age of MS presentation is around 30 years of age, but it may also manifest in childhood or in older aged individuals. As in most autoimmune diseases, women are more commonly affected (3-to-1 female-male ratio). Among younger patients, MS almost invariably presents with relapses. Examples of relapses are subacute onset of hemiparesis, brainstem symptoms (internuclear ophthalmoplegia, diplopia), optic neuritis, partial myelitis (ascending numbness and tingling). Symptoms of relapse progress over days-to-weeks, followed by a slow and often incomplete recovery over weeks-to-months and then a period of clinical quiescence of variable duration (remission). The relapses correlate with focal inflammation and demyelination in the characteristic locations of the brain, spinal cord, and optic nerves. During a relapse, there is often contrast-enhancement of lesions on MRI because of a breakdown of the blood-brain barrier. In between relapses, there is often subclinical MRI activity (new lesions without new symptoms), especially in untreated patients. MS is traditionally conceptualized as a two-phase illness with an early relapsing phase and a later progressive phase.

In reality, the pathological processes underlying progression (axonal loss, neurodegeneration) can be detected from the disease onset. With age, the rate of relapses and new lesion formation decreases, while the probability of entering a secondary progressive phase increases. During the progressive phase, there is sustained neurologic deterioration of ambulatory ability, and often of cognitive, cerebellar, and autonomic functions. MRI of the brain and spinal cord do not show many new lesions in the progressive phase, but there is accelerated brain and cord atrophy. The newer approved treatments for MS are extremely effective in suppressing relapses but are only marginally effective in modulating rate of progression.

FIGURES

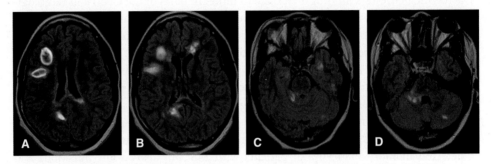

A 25-year-old African-American woman with active MS. FLAIR MRI shows numerous lesions highly characteristic of demyelination. A, Note several oval lesions, one of which has an incomplete ring, as well as U-fiber occipital lesion. B, Juxtacortical, periventricular, and corpus callosum lesions. C, U-fiber and anterior temporal lobe lesions. D, Peripheral pontine, middle cerebellar peduncle, and cerebellar hemisphere lesions.

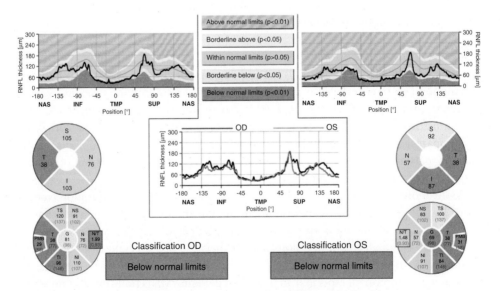

Optical coherence tomography (OCT) in a woman with MS and no visual complaints shows bilateral optic nerve thinning in temporal and inferior quadrants in both eyes.

QUESTIONS FOR SELF-STUDY

1. What are the common brainstem, motor, sensory, and reflex findings in a patient with long-standing MS?

2. Transient worsening of preexisting symptoms—"pseudoexacerbations" are more common in MS than bona fide relapses. Which historical clues favor pseudoexacerbation over a relapse? How does the treatment of a relapse differ from the treatment of a pseudoexacerbation?

3. We do not know what triggers an autoimmune response in MS, but we know that preventing the entry of T- and B-cell lymphocytes into the CNS reduces the number of relapses and new lesions. Match these commonly used disease-modifying therapies (i-iv) in MS with the basic mechanism by which they prevent lymphocyte entry into the CNS (a-d):

   a. Prevents binding of lymphocytes to endothelial cells on brain blood vessels

   b. Prevents egress of lymphocytes from peripheral lymph nodes

   c. Depletes B-cells from the peripheral circulation

   d. Induces apoptosis of T-cells and decreases levels of proinflammatory cytokines

      i. Dimethyl fumarate (Tecfidera)

      ii. Fingolimod (Gilenya)

      iii. Natalizumab (Tysabri)

      iv. Ocrelizumab (Ocrevus)

4. What would you expect to be the ambulatory status of an "average" MS patient after 10, 20, 30, and 40 years of disease? (Compare with Kister I, Chamot E, Salter AR, Cutter GR, Bacon TE, Herbert J. Disability in multiple sclerosis: a reference for patients and clinicians. *Neurology*. 2013;80(11):1018-1024.)

5. Progressive MS typically presents as progressive myelopathy: slow deterioration of ambulatory ability; bowel and bladder dysfunction; and worsening sensory deficits in the legs. Name at least one disorder in immune-mediated, infectious, or vascular categories that can present as progressive myelopathy.

CHALLENGE

Provide a plausible explanation for the high efficacy of disease-modifying therapies in the relapsing phase of MS and their much lesser utility in the progressive phase of MS.

REFERENCES

Kister I. *The Multiple Sclerosis Lesion Checklist*. Fort Washington, PA: Practical neurology; 2018:68-73. Available at https://practicalneurology.com/articles/2018-july-aug/the-multiple-sclerosis-lesion-checklist. [free online resource]

Thompson AJ, Banwell BL, Barkhof F, et al. Diagnosis of multiple sclerosis: 2017 revisions of the McDonald criteria. *Lancet Neurol*. 2018;17(2):162-173.

Thompson AJ, Baranzini SE, Geurts J, Hemmer B, Ciccarelli O. Multiple sclerosis. *Lancet*. 2018;391(10130): 1622-1636.

93 Neuromyelitis Optica Spectrum Disorder

Relapsing CNS inflammatory disorder with a predilection for optic nerves and spinal cord

CORE FEATURES

1. Optic neuritis (ON)
   Compared to ON in MS, ON in patients with NMOSD tends to be more severe, more often bilateral, with longer areas of enhancement of the optic nerves on MRI, and more frequent involvement of the optic chiasm.
2. Severe, longitudinally extensive transverse myelitis (LETM)
   Myelitis that is severe enough to cause inability to walk is typical for NMOSD but atypical for MS. MRI of the spinal cord during the acute phase of NMOSD myelitis shows a large, edematous lesion in the spinal cord that is ≥3 vertebral segments long and may extend into the medulla oblongata.
3. Area postrema syndrome
   Episode of intractable hiccups or vomiting (without other GI symptoms) is suggestive of area postrema syndrome. T2 hyperintense signal in dorsal medulla supports this diagnosis. Area postrema syndrome is seen in 10% to 20% of NMOSD patients, but almost never in MS.
4. Absence of disease progression in between relapses
   Unlike patients with MS who frequently enter progressive phase, patients with NMOSD remain neurologically stable in the absence of relapses.
5. Antibodies to aquaporin-4 (AQP-4) in serum
   Anti-AQP-4 antibody is present in 70% of NMOSD patients and is exquisitely specific for NMOSD. This autoantibody is directed against AQP-4, a water channel located mainly on the astrocytic endfeet, which are part of the blood-brain barrier.

SYNOPSIS

The average age of onset of NMOSD is 40 years, but pediatric and geriatric presentations are described as well. A female predominance is even more striking than in MS (10-to-1 female-male ratio). Optic neuritis and myelitis are the two most common syndromes of NMOSD. Area postrema syndrome is less common but highly suggestive of this diagnosis. The current diagnostic criteria of NMOSD recognize three additional rare clinical syndromes: diencephalic syndrome (hypersomnolence, anorexia, hypothermia), brainstem syndrome (ocular motor dysfunction, long tract signs, ataxia), and cerebral syndrome (encephalopathy, hemispheric symptoms, tumefactive lesions). Clinical and MRI features of NMOSD and MS overlap, but an understanding of the core clinical syndromes and adherence to diagnostic criteria will usually allow for unambiguous differentiation between the two diseases. The correct diagnosis is very important as several MS treatments may precipitate NMOSD relapses. A number of therapeutic strategies—B-cell-depletion, complement inhibition, and IL6 blockade—are highly effective in preventing relapses in NMOSD.

FIGURE

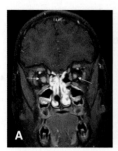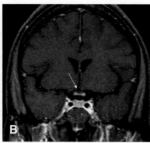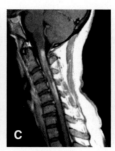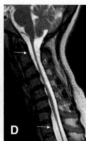

Characteristic MRI appearance of lesions in NMOSD. A, Florid enhancement of optic nerves bilaterally (arrows). B, Enhancement of the optic chiasm (arrow). C, Longitudinally extensive, ring-enhancing spinal cord lesion from C1 to C6. D, Profound segmental cord atrophy in the upper cervical and upper thoracic cord (arrows) in a patient with multiple prior episodes of myelitis and quadriparesis.

QUESTIONS FOR SELF-STUDY

1. What treatments should be used during a severe relapse of NMOSD?
2. The CSF level of glial fibrillary acidic protein, an astrocyte marker, is manyfold higher during a relapse of NMOSD than in a relapse of MS. Why?
3. Eculizumab, a humanized antibody that binds to the terminal complement component C5 and prevents the formation of cytolytic C5b-9 membrane attack complex, is 95% effective in stopping relapses in NMOSD. Propose an explanation for why this drug is highly efficacious in NMOSD but would not be expected to work in MS.
4. A 60-year-old man presents with severe radiating back pain and bilateral leg weakness progressing to complete paraplegia within less than 1 hour. What features of this presentation are atypical for NMOSD myelitis? Which additional diagnoses should be considered in this patient with rapidly progressive paraplegia?
5. A 15-year-old girl presents with painful visual loss. Funduscopy demonstrates bilateral optic nerve swelling. MRI of the brain and orbits shows bilateral enhancement of the optic nerves and no brain lesions. The anti-AQP-4 antibody is negative. The patient is started on intravenous corticosteroids, followed by an oral steroid taper with excellent improvement in her visual acuity. However, at the end of the steroid taper, the ON recurs. What additional antibody test should be obtained in this patient?

CHALLENGE

Since both MS and NMOSD can present with optic neuritis, it would seem like a good idea to measure anti-AQP-4 antibody levels in every patient presenting with optic neuritis independent of other clinical or MRI features "to be on the safe side." Invoking the concepts of pretest probability, likelihood ratio, and baseline rate—NMOSD being about 100-fold less common than MS in Western countries—explain why indiscriminate testing is likely to lead to more misdiagnoses of NMOSD than true diagnoses. (Compare your answer with Kister and Paul cited below.)

REFERENCES

Kister I, Paul F. Pushing the boundaries of neuromyelitis optica: does antibody make the disease? *Neurology.* 2015;85(2):118-119. [free online resource]
Wingerchuk DM, Banwell B, Bennett JL, et al. International consensus diagnostic criteria for neuromyelitis optica spectrum disorders. *Neurology.* 2015;85(2):177-189. [free online resource]

Acute, multifocal, monophasic, inflammatory CNS syndrome; usually pediatric-onset

CORE FEATURES

1. Mean age of onset is 5 to 8 years
   ADEM is distinctly unusual at the extremes of age (children <2 years of age or the elderly).
2. Altered mental status
   Encephalopathy is attributable to immune-mediated brain inflammation, rather than any other cause (infection, seizures, sedating medications).
3. Multifocality of lesions
   Diverse focal neurologic manifestations develop over the course of days. Brain MRI shows multiple large diffuse, poorly demarcated T2-hyperintense lesions dispersed throughout the white and gray matter. Additional lesions may be present in optic nerves and spinal cord.
4. Monophasic course
   The emergence of new symptoms or MRI lesions > 3 months from symptom onset is not compatible with monophasic course.
5. Exclusions of infectious causes
   No infectious organisms are identified in the CSF.

SYNOPSIS

ADEM is a multifocal fulminant inflammatory CNS syndrome that always involves the brain and sometimes the spinal cord and optic nerves as well. In most patients, there is a history of preceding infection, or, much less commonly, a vaccination. ADEM is typically a monophasic disease, but this determination can only be made retrospectively. Many patients with ADEM have autoantibodies against the myelin oligodendrocyte glycoprotein (MOG) or, much less commonly, against AQP-4. In these patients, ADEM may evolve into a chronic relapsing illness—MOG-associated disorder (MOGAD) or NMOSD—and disease-modifying therapy may be necessary to prevent future relapse (especially in NMOSD). ADEM-like presentation may be an inaugural relapse of MS (approximately 10% of patients with seronegative ADEM). When ADEM is the presenting syndrome of a relapsing CNS inflammatory disorder—MS, NMOSD, or MOGAD—the syndromic diagnosis (ADEM) should be replaced by the specific relapsing disorder. The various outcomes of ADEM may be summarized as follows:

Are Autoantibodies Present in Serum?	New MRI Activity > 3 mo of Symptom Onset	Diagnosis
No	No	Likely monophasic ADEM
No	Yes, MS-like lesions	Meets criteria for MS
Yes, AQP4 Ab	Usually not	Meets criteria for NMOSD
Yes, MOG Ab is transiently present	No	Likely monophasic ADEM
Yes, MOG Ab is persistently present	Sometimes	May be relapsing MOGAD

The first-line treatment of ADEM is intravenous corticosteroids, followed by oral corticosteroid taper. Patients unresponsive to intravenous steroids may benefit from intravenous immunoglobulins (IVIG) or plasmapheresis. Severe ADEM may require a course of chemotherapy (cyclophosphamide).

FIGURE

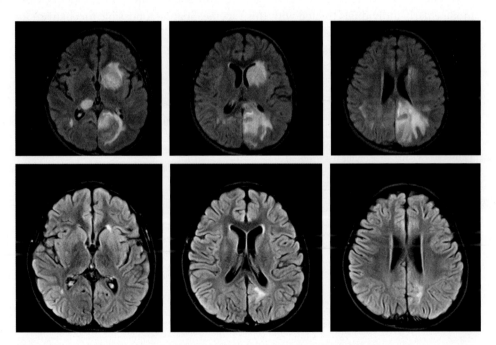

MRI brain of a 5-year-old girl who presented with seizures and unresponsiveness showed large diffuse lesions in gray and white matter of both cerebral hemispheres (upper panel). MRI done 2 years later shows near-complete resolution of the lesions (lower panel). The appearance and disappearance of lesions is typical for ADEM.

QUESTIONS FOR SELF-STUDY

1. Explain why optic neuritis frequently occurs in CNS inflammatory disorders such as ADEM, MS, NMO, or MOGAD, but inflammation of the other cranial nerves is hardly ever observed in CNS inflammatory disorders.
2. Which MRI brain lesions are typical of ADEM and atypical for MS? (Compare your answer with MRI criteria for ADEM. Callen DJ et al. *Neurology*. 72(11):968.)

3. Suggest an explanation for why large T2 lesions in ADEM shrink or disappear on subsequent images.

4. A 25-year-old woman presents with progressive confusion, paranoia, and memory problems for 3 months. Brain MRI shows T2-weighted hyperintense lesions restricted to the medial temporal lobes. CSF is negative for infection. What is the leading diagnosis? Which testing should be done to confirm it?

5. A 35-year-old man with a history of unexplained hearing loss presents with right eye visual blurring and confusion. Brain MRI shows multiple T2-hyperintense lesions throughout the cerebrum. Several large lesions are located in the posterior aspect of the corpus callosum and appear dark on T1-sequences ("T1 holes"). What is the likely diagnosis? What is retinal fluorescein angiography likely to show?

CHALLENGE

The study of an experimental vaccine against Alzheimer disease containing aggregates of synthetic amyloid fragments was stopped following a number of ADEM-like cases among elderly individuals treated with this vaccine. Suggest a possible mechanism for this complication. (Compare your answer with Orgogozo JM, Gilman S, Dartigues JF, et al. *Neurology.* 2003;61(1):46-54.)

REFERENCES

Graus F, Titulaer MJ, Balu R, et al. A clinical approach to diagnosis of autoimmune encephalitis. *Lancet Neurol.* 2016;15(4):391-404. [free online resource]

Pohl D, Alper G, Van Haren K, et al. Acute disseminated encephalomyelitis: updates on an inflammatory CNS syndrome. *Neurology.* 2016;87(9 suppl 2):S38-S45.

Reindl M, Waters P. Myelin oligodendrocyte glycoprotein antibodies in neurological disease. *Nat Rev Neurol.* 2019;15(2):89-102. [free online resource]

95 Neurosarcoidosis

Neurologic complications of sarcoidosis, a multiorgan granulomatous disorder

CORE FEATURES

Nervous system is affected in 5% to 10% of patients with sarcoidosis. The more common neurologic syndromes associated with sarcoidosis are listed in the first three entries:

1. Granulomatous inflammation of the cranial meninges and adjacent structures (cranial nerves and pituitary/hypothalamus)
   Clinical manifestations include facial nerve palsy, optic neuritis, and other cranial nerve neuropathies; subacute-to-chronic meningitis, which may lead to hydrocephalus; endocrinopathies due to infiltration of the hypothalamus-pituitary axis (diabetes insipidus, hyperprolactinemia, hypothyroidism, hypoadrenalism, growth and reproductive hormones deficiencies). On rare occasions, neurosarcoidosis (NS) can cause perivascular granulomatous inflammation within the brain parenchyma.

2. Myelopathy
   Spinal cord involvement manifests as progressive myelopathy and is usually associated with longitudinally extensive lesions with patchy cord enhancement. The involvement of pial meninges, nerve roots, and cauda equina on MRI favors the diagnosis of NS over CNS inflammatory disorders.

3. Peripheral neuropathy and myopathy
   Sarcoid neuropathy is typically asymmetric and multifocal. Painful neuropathic symptoms in the face of normal nerve conduction studies point to small fiber neuropathy. Several patterns of sarcoid myopathy have been described including acute myositis and chronic myopathy.

4. Extraneural manifestations of sarcoidosis outside of nervous tissue
   Sarcoidosis outside of nervous tissue most commonly manifests in the lungs, mediastinal or hilar lymph nodes, and skin (erythema nodosum, lupus pernio, papules, plaques). Biopsy of the affected extraneural tissue is highly advisable to increase diagnostic certainty. However, most patients with NS do not have evident systemic findings on presentation.

5. Histologic evidence of noncaseating epithelioid cell granulomas
   Epithelioid cell granulomas consist of highly differentiated mononuclear phagocytes (epithelioid cells and giant cells) and mostly CD4+ lymphocytes. Biopsy is important to rule out other causes of granulomatous reaction, most importantly mycobacterial or fungal infections. Findings of noncaseating granulomas outside the CNS in conjunction with a clinical syndrome typical of NS are generally sufficient to establish the diagnosis of NS.

SYNOPSIS

Sarcoidosis is the result of multiorgan granulomatous inflammation without an identifiable pathogen. Disease course ranges from mild and self-limited to chronic and disabling. A recent, large-scale study recorded lung involvement in 93% of patients, mediastinal or hilar lymphadenopathy in 77%, skin in 16%, and eye (uveitis) and joints 8% each, but virtually any organ can be involved including the heart, liver, kidneys, spleen (Schupp JC, Freitag-Wolf S, Bargagli E, et al. *Eur Respir J*. 2018;51(1):1700991). NS is estimated to affect 5% to 10% of patients with sarcoidosis. The diagnosis of NS is especially challenging in patients who do not have a history of sarcoidosis. Biopsy of the brain, spinal cord, or meninges is not always practical. It is highly advisable to attempt to identify an accessible affected tissue with the help of whole-body positron emission and computed tomography (PET-CT) and confirm the diagnosis with a biopsy. Corticosteroids are considered first-line treatment, but their long-term use invariably leads to complications. The most promising of the steroid-sparing approaches for NS is infliximab, a TNFα-inhibitor. Because infliximab can exacerbate MS, while approved MS treatments have no utility in NS, it is critical to differentiate NS from MS and target treatment accordingly.

FIGURE

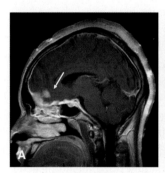 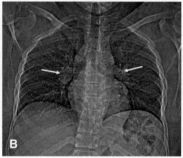 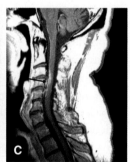

A, Extensive pachymeningeal nodular enhancement predominantly in the anterior cranial fossa (arrow) extending along the floor to the skull base and sella with involvement of the pituitary infundibulum and associated superior displacement of the bilateral prechiasmatic optic nerves. B, The patient had bulky mediastinal lymphadenopathy (arrows). Lymph node biopsy was consistent with sarcoidosis. C, A different patient with pial enhancement along the anterior aspect of the spine (black arrow), enhancement of the anterior nerve roots at C5 and C6, and enhancing lesions in the anterior cervical cord. This patient had no extraneural involvement. Lumbar nerve root biopsy disclosed noncaseating granulomatous inflammation consistent with neurosarcoidosis.

QUESTIONS FOR SELF-STUDY

1. A 40-year-old man with known pulmonary sarcoidosis presents with a protracted history of headaches, impaired smell sensation, bilateral blurry vision, loss of libido, and erectile dysfunction. Funduscopic examination shows bilateral optic nerve edema. Where would you localize the lesion that might account for all of his symptoms? What structures are likely directly affected by NS in this patient?

2. Brain MRI demonstrates extensive pituitary stock involvement in a patient with suspected NS. What endocrine symptoms should the patient be specifically queried about? Which pituitary hormones would you expect to be depressed and which are expected to be elevated in this patient?

3. A 30-year-old woman with biopsy-proven sarcoidosis reports severe fatigue that interferes with her daily functioning. Identify some of the potentially treatable causes

of fatigue related to sarcoid involvement of the lungs, heart, endocrine glands, nervous and muscle tissues.

4. Optic neuritis or progressive myelopathy are two syndromes common to both MS and NS. Name clinical syndromes and neuroimaging findings seen in NS, but not in MS.

5. Name other multiorgan autoimmune diseases that can cause optic neuropathy and myelopathy.

CHALLENGE

A 25-year-old African-American woman, diagnosed with sarcoidosis and hypopituitarism, is compliant with daily hormonal treatment. Following an uncomplicated outpatient surgical procedure, she complains of dizziness, tremulousness, and palpitations. Her blood pressure is very low despite the administration of intravenous fluids. "Stat" chemistries are remarkable for low blood glucose and sodium levels. Explain the likely pathophysiologic mechanism underlying her postoperative decompensation. What is the next best step in management?

REFERENCES

Joubert B, Chapelon-Abric C, Biard L, et al. Association of prognostic factors and immunosuppressive treatment with long-term outcomes in neurosarcoidosis. *JAMA Neurol.* 2017;74(11):1336-1344.

Stern BJ, Royal W III, Gelfand JM, et al. Definition and consensus diagnostic criteria for neurosarcoidosis: from the Neurosarcoidosis Consortium Consensus Group. *JAMA Neurol.* 2018;75(12):1546-1553.

Miscellaneous Section: Neuro-developmental Disorders, Neuro-toxicology, Neuro-oncology

TOP 1 0 0

A Very Brief Introduction to the Miscellaneous Section: Neurodevelopmental Disorders, Neurotoxicology, Neuro-oncology

One cannot embrace the unembraceable.

Koz'ma Prutkov*

The vast subject of clinical neurology cannot be embraced between the covers of a book. Not only important diseases but whole subspecialties must perforce fall outside its purview. The last section of our book provides a sampling of important conditions from the areas of neurology that have not received attention heretofore.

Neurodevelopmental disorders are represented with chapters on Autism Spectrum Disorder (ASD, Chapter 96) and Cerebral Palsy (Chapter 97), the two common syndromes in children with disabilities. ASD is characterized by a deficient ability to communicate and relate to others and by repetitive, stereotypic behaviors. The incidence of ASD has risen dramatically in recent years. Currently, 1 in 60 children in the United States carries this diagnosis. It is unclear to what extent this increase is due to ASD becoming more common rather than loosening of diagnostic criteria, improved recognition through early screening, and parents' desire to obtain special services for a child who is underperforming. Other neurodevelopmental disorders on the differential of ASD—which often coexist with ASD—include intellectual disability, communication disorders, and learning disorders. Cerebral palsy (CP) is a heterogeneous group of disabling, nonprogressive motor disorders. CP is the most common cause of motor disability in children and must be differentiated from progressive motor disorders due to inborn disorders of metabolism and other causes.

Neurotoxicology is a wide area of neurology as hundreds of substances can cause damage to the nervous system. Exposure to certain groups of toxins results in a characteristic constellation of symptoms known as "toxidrome." Neuroleptic malignant syndrome (NMS) and serotonin syndrome (Chapter 98) are examples of toxidromes critical not to miss as they can be effectively managed through discontinuation of the offending medication(s) and supportive measures. Currently, more than 10% of the US population is taking serotonergic antidepressants. NMS and serotonin syndrome are likely to become more prevalent as antidopaminergic and serotonergic drugs come into even wider medical use. The neurology of drugs of abuse is represented by a chapter on opioid intoxication (Chapter 99). Opioid overdose is not a new problem—Aleksey Konstantinovich Tolstoy (1817-1875), Russian poet, dramatist, and one of the creators of the Koz'ma Prutkov character, died from morphine overdose nearly 150 years ago—but in recent decades, it has reached epidemic proportion. At the time of this writing, opioid overdoses cause a greater loss of life in 1 year in the United States than all of US military losses during the two decades of the Vietnam War.

*Koz'ma Prutkov is a pen name for a group of late 19th-century Russian satirists. The quotations are from a collection of aphorisms titled "Fruits of Thought."

This book concludes with a chapter on neuro-oncology. In the interests of brevity, we highlight the five most common presentations of brain tumors rather than describing specific entities (Chapter 100). To cite another Prutkov aphorism: "Better say less, but well."

96 Autism Spectrum Disorder ▬

A neurodevelopmental disorder characterized by deficient sociability and stereotypical behaviors

CORE FEATURES

1. The peak age of diagnosis is 2 to 3 years.
   Subtle deficits—reduced eye contact, lack of response to name, speech delay—are often present before an age of 2 years but may not be recognized. In about one-third of patients, the diagnosis of autism spectrum disorder (ASD) is preceded by language and behavioral regression.
2. Deficient communication skills.
   Language pragmatics is impaired—the child may not understand how to use language as a tool to establish communication and attain one's aims. The child may not initiate interactions or respond appropriately to social overtures by others.
3. Deficient "theory of mind."
   Impaired ability to decipher others' emotions, intentions, thoughts, beliefs, and to see the situation from another's perspective.
4. Inflexibility.
   The child does not like to deviate from established routines. May exhibit an excessive preoccupation with certain objects or topics. May be restricted in the choice of foods.
5. Repetitive, ritualistic, rather than imaginative play.
   For example, instead of pretending to drive a car, a child will obsessively spin the wheels or line up cars. Stereotypic behaviors—hand flapping, twirling, repeating words or phrases—are also highly characteristic of ASD.

SYNOPSIS

ASD is a group of complex neurodevelopment disorders defined by deficient sociability and behavioral peculiarities. ASD is often comorbid with intellectual disability, and about a third of children with ASD are nonverbal. Intellectual abilities may be normal or even overdeveloped in certain areas. Comorbid neurodevelopmental and neurologic diagnoses—sensory integration disorder, Tourette syndrome, epilepsy—are very common. ASD is highly heritable. The risk of ASD in a sibling of a child with ASD is 10-fold higher than in the general population. However, no specific genetic mutations have been found except in "secondary autism" due to tuberous sclerosis complex, fragile X syndrome, Angelman syndrome, and Rett syndrome. Other risk factors for ASD include very premature birth, maternal alcohol abuse, and, to a much lesser extent, older parental age. Screening for ASD is recommended in all children and not just those with risk factors since the condition is common and early intervention with tailored programs such as Applied Behavior Analysis improves long-term outcomes.

QUESTIONS FOR SELF-STUDY

1. An essential early skill for establishing social communication is the ability to initiate and respond to joint attention. How would you test for joint attention in a preverbal child?

2. Concerned parents bring their 2-year-old daughter to be evaluated for ASD. The girl's speech is limited to single, difficult-to-understand words, and she often does not answer when her name is called. Her development is otherwise unremarkable. She is social, likes to play with other children, and exhibits no peculiar behaviors. What evaluation must be performed to exclude a reversible cause of language delay?

3. Both tics and stereotypies can be described as purposeless, repetitive movements, or utterances. How would you differentiate stereotypies from tics? What questions would you ask the patient to determine if the movements are more consistent with tics or stereotypies?

4. Approximately 10% of ASD is secondary to a monogenetic disease. Identifying genetic causes has important implications for genetic counseling. Match these genetic disorders that may manifest with an ASD phenotype with their respective clinical features:

Intellectual disability; large head and large ears; hypotonia; joint hyperextensibility. Only boys affected.	Tuberous sclerosis complex (5%-15% cases have ASD)
Microcephaly; growth failure; seizures; hand wringing; autistic regression in early childhood. Only girls affected.	Fragile X syndrome (30%-50% cases have ASD)
Nonverbal; frequent smiling and laughing; ataxic gait; seizures.	Angelman syndrome
White spots on the skin on Wood lamp examination; facial angiofibromas; MRI brain with focal cortical dysplasia and subependymal nodules.	Rett syndrome

5. A child with ASD is found to have copy number variation (CNV) that have been linked with ASD. What are the implications of this finding with regard to the risk of ASD for the patient's siblings and future children?

CHALLENGE

A 3-year-old child with ASD is brought to the emergency department (ED) with limping and failure to thrive. The mother reports that he has a restricted repertoire of behaviors and lives on a diet of cookies and milk. On examination, he has inflamed gingiva and multiple skin bruises. He refuses to walk but appears to have normal strength in limbs. How can you tie in the patient's clinical presentation with the underlying diagnosis? (Compare your answer with Ma NS, et al. *J Autism Dev Disord.* 2016;46(4): 1464-1470. [free online resource])

REFERENCES

Johnson CP, Myers SM; American Academy of Pediatrics Council on Children With Disabilities. Identification and evaluation of children with autism spectrum disorders. *Pediatrics.* 2007;120(5):1183-1215. [free online resource]

Rapin I, Tuchman RF. Autism: definition, neurobiology, screening, diagnosis. *Pediatr Clin North Am.* 2008;55(5):1129-1146, viii.

97 Cerebral Palsy

Nonprogressive neurodevelopmental group of disorders resulting in motor dysfunction

CORE FEATURES

1. Usually diagnosed before 18 months of age.
   Cerebral palsy (CP) results from brain lesions acquired at the fetal stage or early infancy and becomes manifest during early motor development.
2. Deficits of movement, muscle tone, or motor control of sufficient severity to interfere with daily activities.
   Paretic variants—hemiplegia, diplegia, quadriplegia—are the most common presentations. Dyskinetic (dystonia, athetosis) and ataxic forms are the less common variants of CP.
3. Motor deficits are nonprogressive.
   Deficits become evident when the child fails to reach the expected motor milestones. Early screening for motor deficits, especially in children with risk factors for CP, is recommended as early rehabilitation improves long-term outcomes.
4. Brain MRI demonstrates culprit lesions in approximately 90% of patients.
   Brain MRI is not required but recommended as it helps to clarify the etiology and prognosis. The most common lesion responsible for CP is periventricular leukomalacia, the typical brain injury of prematurity. Other lesions include ischemic stroke or hemorrhage; cerebral malformations; and stigmata of brain infections. Exceptionally, brain MRI may point to a potentially remediable cause (hydrocephalus, brain arteriovenous malformation, subdural hematoma).
5. Comorbid neurodevelopmental diagnoses.
   Half of the patients with CP have intellectual disability, and a significant minority have epilepsy and other neurodevelopmental diagnoses.

SYNOPSIS

CP is the result of brain damage acquired before motor development is complete. The etiologies are traditionally divided into prenatal (prematurity), perinatal (hypoxic injury during delivery), and postnatal (central nervous system [CNS] infection in newborn/infancy period). The lesions are static, and the condition is therefore nonprogressive, though it may appear to be so as infants fall further behind their peers in motor developments. It is therefore not always easy to differentiate abnormal motor development due to a preexisting lesion from abnormal development due to a progressive genetic or neurodegenerative disease. In addition to deficits of motor control, a variety of cognitive, behavioral, communicational, perceptual, hearing, vision, and secondary musculoskeletal (hip displacement) deficits are very common and should be screened for. Known genetic causes of CP account for less than 5% of cases. Thus, genetic screening for Mendelian disorders is presently not recommended unless there are clinical or radiographic findings pointing to a specific genetic etiology (eg, cataracts, chorioretinitis, dysmorphic features, myoclonus, lissencephaly, schizencephaly, and pachygyria).

FIGURE

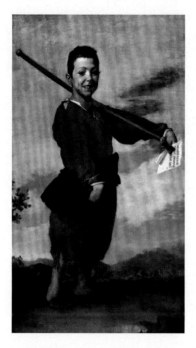

This radiant portrait by Jusepe de Ribera shows a beggar boy with internally rotated arm and flexed right hand and externally rotated right foot—a posture consistent with right hemiparesis. The begging note in the left hands suggests that he may have had difficulty speaking. The diagnosis of cerebral palsy is plausible. (© RMN-Grand Palais / Art Resource, NY.)

QUESTIONS FOR SELF-STUDY

1. Newborns have a limited repertoire of movements and do not obey commands. Which tests on the Dubowitz neurological examination of the full-term newborn could help determine whether a newborn has a focal weakness? What is the most sensitive test for predicting CP in a young infant?
2. Which brain MRI findings predict CP in a newborn? What are the brain MRI predictors of ambulatory versus nonambulatory status in CP?
3. Which historical features related to pregnancy, delivery, and postnatal course indicate that a child is at risk for CP?
4. What screening tests for nonmotor deficits are required in a child with CP? (Compare your answer with Novak et al reference below.)
5. Spasticity, a common problem in CP, is treated with stretching, oral antispasticity medications, Botulinum toxin type A injections, and intrathecal baclofen infusion. One downside of the intrathecal infusion is that pump failure can precipitate acute baclofen withdrawal syndrome. Describe symptoms of baclofen withdrawal.

CHALLENGE

"Constraint-induced movement therapy" is an evidence-based intervention for improving motor function in children with CP. The unaffected side is constrained for weeks with mitts or a sling, while the affected limb is intensively rehabilitated. Describe how the concepts of "learned nonuse" and neuroplasticity may partly explain the effectiveness of constraint-induced movement therapy. (Compare with Zatorre RJ, et al. *Nat Neurosci*. 2012;15(4):528-536. [free online resource])

REFERENCES

Dubowitz L, Ricciw D, Mercuri E. The Dubowitz neurological examination of the full term newborn. *Ment Retard Dev Disabil Res Rev*. 2005;11:52-60.

Novak I, Morgan C, Adde L, et al. Early, accurate diagnosis and early intervention in cerebral palsy: advances in diagnosis and treatment. *JAMA Pediatr*. 2017;171(9):897-907.

Rosenbaum P, Paneth N, Leviton A, et al. A report: the definition and classification of cerebral palsy April 2006. *Dev Med Child Neurol Suppl*. 2007;109:8-14.

98 Neuroleptic Malignant Syndrome and Serotonin Syndrome

Toxidromes associated with iatrogenically induced states of dopaminergic deficiency (NMS) and serotonergic hyperstimulation (serotonin syndrome)

CORE FEATURES

	Neuroleptic Malignant Syndrome	Serotonin Syndrome
1. Exposure to…	Dopamine receptor antagonists (antipsychotics and antiemetics) or withdrawal from dopaminergic agonists ("parkinsonism hyperpyrexia"). Onset within days to weeks of exposure.	Serotonergic agents (antidepressants[a], psychostimulants, opioids, antiemetics, lithium, valproic acid, cocaine, lysergic acid diethylamide [LSD]). Onset usually within hours of initiation, titration, or overdose.
2. Autonomic dysfunction	Temperature often >42°C, sweating, tachycardia, labile blood pressure.	Tachycardia is common; hypertension and fever in the more severe cases.
3. Altered mental status	Delirium is the most common presentation. Other manifestations: psychosis, mutism, stupor, coma.	Delirium, hypomania, agitation usually present. Stupor, coma in the most severe cases.
4. Motor manifestations	"Lead pipe" rigidity (increased tone with passive stretching); catatonia; dystonia; tremors may be seen.	Diffuse hyperreflexia; myoclonus; opsoclonus are highly characteristic. Tremor is common. Rigidity only in severe cases.
5. Elevation in serum creatinine kinase (CK)	Very common; correlates with severity of rigidity; levels often >1000 U/L.	Rare.

[a]MAOIs, monoamine oxidase inhibitors; NDRIs, norepinephrine and dopamine reuptake inhibitors; TCAs, tricyclic antidepressants; SARIs, serotonin antagonist and reuptake inhibitors; SNRIs, serotonin and norepinephrine reuptake inhibitors; SSRIs, selective serotonin reuptake inhibitors.

SYNOPSIS

In neuroleptic malignant syndrome (NMS), there is disruption of dopaminergic pathways involved in central thermoregulation (hyperthermia), nigrostriatal pathways (extrapyramidal symptoms: rigidity and akinesia), and ascending reticular activating system (confusion and impaired level of alertness). Serotonergic pathways also play a role in maintaining alertness, muscle tone, and thermoregulation; hence the clinical manifestations of NMS and serotonin syndrome overlap. Both NMS and serotonin syndrome cause fever, autonomic hyperactivity, altered mental status, and increased muscle tone. However, there are some differences as well: onset in NMS is typically slower than in the serotonin syndrome; there is a greater degree of akinesia and rigidity in NMS and a greater degree of hyperreflexia and myoclonus in the serotonin syndrome; in serotonin syndrome, there are prominent gastrointestinal manifestations (diarrhea), but none in NMS. History of relevant exposure is a critical clue to differentiating the two hyperthermic syndromes. Patients should be asked not only about the medications they are currently taking but also about recently discontinued medications, over-the-counter supplements, and drugs of abuse. Pills found on the scene can be easily identified using the poison control pill identifier site (https://pill-id.webpoisoncontrol.org/#/intro [free online resource]) or contacting poison control center directly (https://www.poison.org/ [free online resource], a free, 24/7 service for toxicologic emergencies).

Early recognition of NMS and serotonin syndrome is essential as these syndromes can be life-threatening if untreated. The first step to correct diagnosis is avoiding the trap of, premature closure' when evaluating a patient with fever, confusion, and leukocytosis. This triad is usually the result of systemic infection but includes many other causes: intoxications (neuroleptic, serotonin, anticholinergic, sympathomimetic syndromes), withdrawal (delirium tremens from alcohol or benzodiazepines), malignant hyperthermia, heatstroke, and malignant catatonia among others. The first steps in managing a toxidrome are supportive care (ensuring respiratory support; cooling; hydration; correcting electrolytes) and discontinuation of the offending medication(s). More specific pharmacologic approaches targeted to the individual toxidrome include reducing hyperadrenergic activation with benzodiazepines; serotonin blockade in serotonin syndrome; and prevention of muscle breakdown with dantrolene in NMS. More invasive techniques such as electroconvulsive therapy, induction of neuromuscular blockade, and intubation are reserved for the most severe cases.

FIGURE

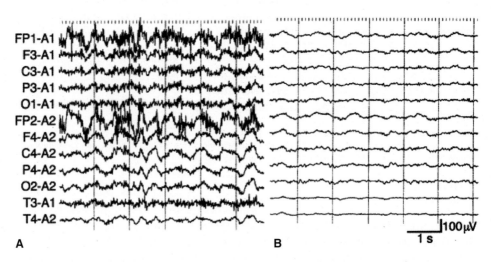

A, Electroencephalography (EEG) in a patient with NMS before injection of diazepam shows continuous, relatively rhythmic delta activities, with artifacts generated by orolingual dyskinesia and blinking. B, Immediately after injection, delta activities diminished and orolingual dyskinesia also improved. (Reprinted with permission from Ihara M, Kohara N, Urano F, et al. Neuroleptic malignant syndrome with prolonged catatonia in a dopa-responsive dystonia patient. *Neurology*. 2002;59(7):1102-1104.)

QUESTIONS FOR SELF-STUDY

1. You are evaluating a patient with confusion and fever. Describe how passive movement of the neck in different directions allows you to differentiate nuchal rigidity (a sign of meningismus) from generalized rigidity due to NMS.

2. A 50-year-old woman presents with confusion, tremulousness, and abnormal jerky eye movements after overdose with an unknown drug. Her medications include sertraline and carbamazepine. How would you differentiate opsoclonus (a sign of serotonin syndrome) from nystagmus (a sign of carbamazepine toxicity)?

3. A 75-year-old woman with mild depression that is well controlled with paroxetine has read in a popular journal that the over-the-counter supplement, L-tryptophan, is a "natural remedy" for depression. Within 4 hours of starting this supplement, she develops fever, tremors, restlessness, and confusion. What is the likely diagnosis? Why is she at risk for this syndrome? What is the pathophysiologic mechanism?

4. Match the agent with the likely mechanism by which it causes serotonergic hyperactivation:

Increased serotonin synthesis	Amphetamines (Adderall, Ritalin)
Increased serotonin release	Triptans (sumatriptan)
Direct serotonin receptor agonist	SSRIs (paroxetine, sertraline)
Inhibition of serotonin reuptake	Cocaine
Decreased serotonin metabolism	Monoamine oxidase B inhibitors (selegiline)

5. Which classic toxidrome causes the patient to become "blind as a bat (dilated pupils), dry as a bone (dry skin), full as a flask (cannot urinate), hot as in Hades (fever), red as a beet (flushed), and mad as a hatter (confusion, hallucinations)"? What is the pathophysiologic explanation for these symptoms? Which toxidrome-specific treatment is indicated to reverse the symptoms?

CHALLENGE

Which toxidromes are characterized by an increase in blood pressure and pulse, and which with a decrease in blood pressure and pulse?

REFERENCES

Francescangeli J, Karamchandani K, Powell M, Bonavia A. The serotonin syndrome: from molecular mechanisms to clinical practice. *Int J Mol Sci.* 2019;20(9):2288. [free online resource]

Rajan S, Kass B, Moukheiber E. Movement disorders emergencies. *Semin Neurol.* 201;39(1):125-136.

Opioid overdose

Opioid toxidrome is usually associated with "recreational" drug use

CORE FEATURES

1. Depressed mental status.
   At lower doses, opioids cause a drowsy and euphoric state, at higher doses—stupor and coma.
2. Depressed respiration.
   Shallow and slow breathing, <12 breath/min, in a "found down" patient is highly suggestive of opioid poisoning.
3. Depressed pupillary size.
   Constricted but reactive pupils—"pinpoint pupils"—are a hallmark of opioid use, but their absence does not preclude the diagnosis of an opioid overdose.
4. Depressed bowel sounds.
   Opioid-induced hypoperistalsis manifests as nausea, vomiting, constipation, and decreased or absent bowel sounds.
5. Rapid symptom reversal with the opioid antagonist (naloxone) is diagnostic of an opioid overdose.
   Escalating doses of naloxone are often needed to achieve adequate respiratory rate. Since naloxone has a shorter half-life than most opioids, patients must be monitored for resedation and respiratory depression after initial improvement.

SYNOPSIS

Opioids are constituents of the poppy plant seeds. They have been widely recognized since antiquity for their analgesic and euphoric properties. But at no time in recorded history has opioid misuse reached such catastrophic proportions as today, with nearly 50,000 fatalities due to opioid overdoses recorded in the United States in 2017. Opioids are popular drugs of abuse because they induce euphoria, which is likely mediated via dopamine release in the mesolimbic system, and anxiolysis, which is likely mediated via stimulation of noradrenergic neurons in the locus ceruleus. Repeated use leads to tolerance and the need to escalate doses to obtain the "high." Opioids are more deadly than other drugs of abuse, such as alcohol or benzodiazepines, because they cause respiratory suppression and pulmonary edema at relatively low doses.

Classic symptoms of "man down" with shallow breathing and pinpoint pupils are not always present with opioid intoxication because patients may abuse multiple substances—sedatives or cocaine along with opioids, which greatly increases risk of fatal outcome, or use substances with opioid and nonopioid properties (eg, opioid agonist tramadol, which also inhibits serotonin reuptake). In addition to the problems directly caused by drug intoxication and withdrawal, patients who abuse drugs are at risk for chronic affective and cognitive disorders as cataloged in the section on substance-related and addictive disorders of the *Diagnostic and Statistical Manual of Mental Disorders Fifth Edition (DSM-5)*. Intravenous and subcutaneous mode of administration allow for the spread of numerous acute and chronic infections—hepatitis B and C; human immunodeficiency virus (HIV); infective endocarditis; abscesses in the brain, epidural space, muscle; osteomyelitis; tetanus; botulism; human T-cell lymphotropic virus type 1 (HTLV-1), etc.

FIGURES

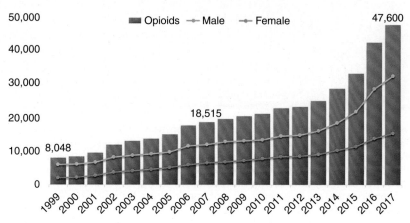

National drug overdose deaths involving any opioid,
Number among all ages, by gender, 1999-2017

Source : Centers for Disease Control and Prevention, National Center for Health Statistics. Multiple cause of death 1999-2017 on CDC WONDER online database, released december, 2018

The opioid epidemic is summarized in the uptrending graph of fatal drug overdoses. (Reproduced with permission from National Overdose Deaths Involving Any Opioid—Number Among All Ages, by Gender, 1999 to 2017.CDC WONDER.)

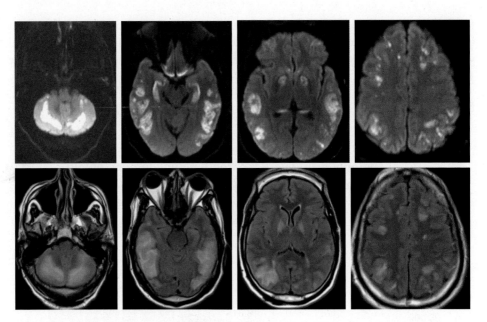

A 56-year-old man presented with agitation and confusion. He had a history of daily heroin inhalation for many years. Diffusion-weighted magnetic resonance imaging (MRI DWI, top raw) and fluid-attenuated inversion recovery (FLAIR, bottom row) show diffuse, mostly symmetrical involvement of the cerebellar white matter, cortical and globus pallidus gray matter, and subcortical white matter consistent with toxic leukoencephalopathy, a rare complication of heroin abuse ("chasing the dragon" leukoencephalopathy).

QUESTIONS FOR SELF-STUDY

1. A 25-year-old man is effectively treated with high doses of naloxone for opioid overdose. He then becomes restless and irritable and develops tachycardia, hypertension, tearing, sweating, abdominal cramping, and diarrhea. What is the probable explanation for these new symptoms?

2. A 35-year-old woman with witnessed drug overdose presents with coma, respiratory depression, and pinpoint pupils. Escalating doses of naloxone fail to improve her mental status. What is a common reason for the lack of response to naloxone in a patient with a typical clinical picture of opioid overdose?

3. A 30-year-old pregnant woman with a history of opioid abuse delivers a healthy-appearing newborn. Two days later, the newborn has a low-grade fever, irritability, poor feeding, and occasional jerky movements of the limbs. Laboratory tests, including complete blood count, electrolytes, liver and thyroid function, and cerebrospinal fluid (CSF) analysis are normal for age. What diagnosis should be considered in this clinical context?

4. Match these common drugs of abuse with respective symptoms and signs of intoxication:

A. Cocaine (benzoylmethylecgonine)	Out-of-body experience, euphoria, dysarthria, ataxia, hyperreflexia, vertical nystagmus
B. Amphetamines	Delusions of grandeur, aggressiveness, tactile hallucinations
C. PCP ("angel dust"; 1-(1-phenylcyclohexyl) piperidine)	Agitation, hallucinations, seizures, sympathetic overdrive (sweating, fever, high blood pressure, tachycardia, mydriasis)
D. Cannabis	Depressed consciousness, slurred speech, ataxia, incoordination, bradycardia, hypotension
E. Barbiturates	Giddiness, a sensation of slowed time, conjunctival injection, increased appetite

5. Drug addiction—"substance abuse disorder" in DSM-5 terminology—is a chronic relapsing disorder characterized by a compulsion to seek and take drugs. But these features are not sufficient to meet the definition of addiction. What are the other two essential elements in the definition of addiction? What questions would you ask to elicit these key features of drug addiction in suspected cases?

CHALLENGE

Urine drug testing for opioids may seem like the obvious test to confirm suspected intoxication, yet many experts recommend against routine urine drug screen in case of a possible drug overdose. Provide an argument for and against drug screening in cases of suspected intoxication. (Compare your responses with the discussion in Pastores SM, et al. *Crit Care Clin.* 2012;28(4):479-498. [free online resource]) When is routine drug screening recommended?

REFERENCES

Boyer EW. Management of opioid analgesic overdose. *N Engl J Med.* 2012;367(2):146-155. [free online resource]
Holstege CP, Borek HA. Toxidromes. *Crit Care Clin.* 2012;28(4):479-498.

Five common presentations of brain tumors are listed below

CORE FEATURES

1. Focal-onset seizures.
   Seizures develop in about one-third of patients with brain tumors. Because seizures may be a presenting symptom of a brain tumor, any new-onset, unprovoked seizure in an adult warrants neuroimaging studies with contrast. The risk of seizures is higher if the brain tumor is a glioma; is slow-growing; and is localized to the cerebral hemispheres.

2. Cognitive changes.
   Psychomotor slowing, forgetfulness, personality changes, lack of initiative, irritability, and emotional lability are the common symptoms that imply global cerebral dysfunction. Focal cortical symptoms—aphasia, apraxia, agnosia, amnesia—are less frequent.

3. Focal neurologic symptoms and signs.
   The more common focal signs are unilateral weakness and numbness, aphasia, homonymous visual field defect, and ataxia. The likelihood of focal symptoms depends on tumor location; size; how destructive it is; whether it is discrete or infiltrative; and how quickly it is growing.

4. Headache.
   Headache occurs in more than half of patients with brain tumors, usually with associated "red flags": focal neurologic or systemic signs; headache upon awakening; change in quality, severity, and location from a preexisting headache; and unremitting nature. Headache as the sole manifestation occurs in a minority of patients. When headaches result from raised intracranial pressure (ICP), they are associated with nausea, vomiting, papilledema, and are usually resistant to analgesics.

5. Brain lesion(s) on MRI.
   A typical appearance of a neoplasm is that of T1-hypointense, T2-hyperintense, enhancing lesion, with surrounding vasogenic edema and mass effect. As the lesion grows, it can cause obstruction of CSF outflow (obstructive hydrocephalus) and herniation syndromes (cingulate gyrus under the falx = subfalcine herniation; uncus of the temporal lobe through the tentorium cerebelli = transtentorial herniation; cerebellar tonsils through the foramen magnum = tonsillar herniation).

SYNOPSIS

In the United States, the lifetime risk of developing a primary brain tumor is 0.5% while the probability of dying from non–brain cancer is about 20%. Up to 30% of patients with disseminated cancer have intracranial involvement on autopsy. Thus, brain metastases are by far the most common cause of brain tumors in the general population. Certain malignancies such as lung and breast cancer and melanoma have a special predilection for the brain. Of the primary CNS tumors, about 75% are either gliomas, which derive from astrocytes and oligodendrocytes, or meningiomas, which derive from meningeal cells. The other tumors derive from the various cells found in the brain—neurons, neuroglial precursor cells, lymphocytes, pinealocytes, choroid plexus, and ependyma. The traditional classification of brain tumors based on histologic appearance of nuclei and cytoplasm, degree of mitotic activity, necrosis, and microvascular proliferation is increasingly supplemented by the more objective genetic classification. Gene defect rather than the cell of origin may be the determining factor in choosing chemotherapy. For example, loss of tumoral O-(6)-methylguanine DNA methyltransferase (MGMT) activity correlates with response to temozolomide and improved survival. As a harbinger of the new era, the FDA approved the first mutation-specific cancer treatment that is agnostic to tissue type in 2017.

FIGURE

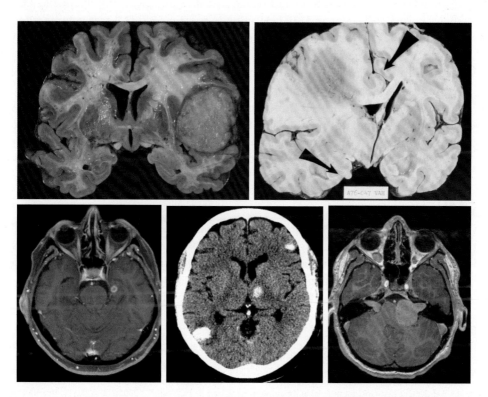

Examples of brain tumors. Left upper panel: Postmortem shows a meningioma. Right upper panel: A large glial tumor in the right frontal lobe with mass effect causing subfalcine and uncal herniation (arrows). Lower left: MRI brain shows a small ring-enhancing lesion at the gray-white junction in the left mesial temporal lobe suspicious for a metastasis in a woman with breast cancer. Lower middle: Multiple hemorrhagic metastasis of melanoma. Lower right: Young woman with neurofibromatosis type 2 and bilateral schwannomas.

QUESTIONS FOR SELF-STUDY

1. Diplopia, tinnitus, hearing impairment, and visual loss may sometimes be "false-localizing" signs. What does this term mean? What is the mechanism(s) by which false-localizing signs are produced?

2. A 60-year-old man with new-onset seizures and two ring-enhancing frontoparietal lobe lesions with brain edema reports weight loss and night sweats for the past few months. What testing should be requested as part of the workup of these brain lesions? What nonneoplastic etiologies should be considered on the differential?

3. A 70-year-old man with metastatic lung adenocarcinoma presents to the ED with subacute-onset headache, double vision, and facial paresis. Noncontrast brain MRI does not disclose any lesions. What is the next step in the workup? Assuming the symptoms are related to the underlying malignancy, what is the likely diagnosis? What laboratory tests should be done to confirm your suspicion?

4. A 60-year-old woman with Hodgkin lymphoma presents with subacute onset of imbalance, nausea, and blurry vision. The examination is remarkable for multidirectional nystagmus, and limb and trunk ataxia. Brain MRI is unremarkable. CSF shows normal cell count and mild elevation in protein content. Large volume cytology and flow cytometry are negative for malignant cells. What is the likely etiology of the acquired cerebellar syndrome in this patient with a known malignancy?

5. MR spectroscopy (MRS) allows for noninvasive detection and quantification of chemicals related to neuronal injury (n-acetyl aspartate), membrane turnover (choline), cellular energy store (creatine), and anaerobic glycolysis (lactate). Explain how MRS may be helpful for grading glial tumors; for assessing response to treatment; and for guiding site for brain biopsy. What other imaging techniques are available to assess for the four "bad H's" of tumors: **H**ypercellularity, **H**igh invasiveness, **H**ypermetabolism, and **H**ypervascularity?

CHALLENGE

One of the challenges in treating brain tumors is that they acquire new oncogenic mutations (genetic evolution) making them more aggressive and less treatment-responsive with time. Think of ways one can keep track of the genetic evolution of brain tumors and adjust treatment accordingly without recourse to a repeat brain biopsy. (Compare with Miller AM, et al. *Nature*. 2019;565(7741):654-658. [free online resource])

REFERENCES

Grant R. Overview: brain tumor diagnosis and management/Royal College of Physicians guidelines. *J Neurol Neurosurg Psychiatry*. 2004;75(suppl 2):ii18–ii23. [free online resource]

Gupta A, Dwivedi T. A simplified overview of World Health Organization classification update of central nervous system tumors 2016. *J Neurosci Rural Pract*. 2017;8(4):629-641. [free online resource]

Jacobs AH, Kracht LW, Gossmann A, et al. Imaging in neurooncology. *NeuroRx*. 2005;2(2):333-347. [free online resource]

Freely Available, High-Quality Internet Resources

1. https://www.ncbi.nlm.nih.gov/pmc/—a repository of full-text articles in biomedical sciences; contains over 2.5 million articles from 2000 to present.
2. https://www.ncbi.nlm.nih.gov/books/NBK1116/— up-to-date reviews of genetic conditions with links to additional resources.
3. https://novel.utah.edu/— neuroophthalmology virtual education library.
4. https://neuromuscular.wustl.edu/—comprehensive, well-organized compendium of neuromuscular conditions.
5. https://www.cdc.gov/—Centers for Disease Control official website is a resource for neuroinfectious disease and other topics related to infectious medicine and public health.
6. https://www.poison.org/—official site of Poison Control center; repository of information on toxicologic emergencies.
7. https://atlas.brain-map.org/—a detailed, annotated human brain atlas.
8. https://stanfordmedicine25.stanford.edu/ and http://mskmedicine.com/clinical-skills/—video resource for improving physical examination skills.
9. https://www.drugbank.ca/—comprehensive drug database.
10. www.medscape.org—excellent disease summaries and up-to-date reviews.
11. https://www.statpearls.com/—thousands of brief, peer-reviewed articles.
12. https://www.merckmanuals.com/professional/neurologic-disorders—virtual medical encyclopedia.
13. Websites of subspecialty societies (https://americanheadachesociety.org/, https://www.epilepsy.com) and disease-specific patient organization (https://www.michaeljfox.org/ for Parkinson Disease, https://www.hda.org.uk/ for Huntington Disease, https://www.alz.org/ for Alzheimer Disease, https://rarediseases.org/ for rare diseases) often contain excellent overviews and provide lists of resources for patients and families.

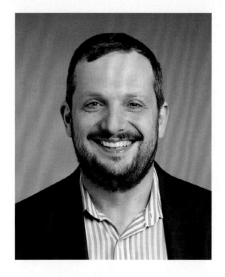

Ilya Kister, MD, FAAN is an Associate Professor of Neurology at NYU Grossman School of Medicine in New York. He specializes in Neuroimmunology and is the Director of NYU Multiple Sclerosis Fellowship and NYU Neuromyelitis Optica Treatment and Research Program. Dr. Kister graduated from Icahn School of Medicine at Mount Sinai, completed Neurology Residency at Albert Einstein College of Medicine and Neuroimmunology Fellowship at NYU Langone (all in New York). Dr. Kister is active in clinical research and has published over 80 peer-reviewed articles and reviews.

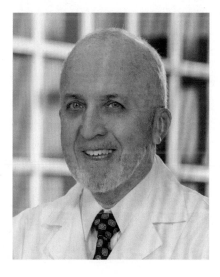

José Biller, MD, FACP, FAAN, FANA, FAHA is Professor of Neurology and Neurological Surgery and Chairperson of the Department of Neurology at Loyola University Chicago Stritch School of Medicine. Dr. Biller is American Board of Psychiatry and Neurology (ABPN) certified (and recertified, including Combined Maintenance of Certification) in Neurology and Vascular Neurology, and certified in Headache Medicine (UCNS).

Dr. Biller served as the Director of the ABPN from 1994 to 2001, and President of the ABPN in 2001, and currently holds the title of Emeritus Director of the ABPN. He is the Editor of the *Journal of Stroke & Cerebrovascular Diseases*, the recent past Chief-Editor of *Frontiers in Neurology*, and an editorial board member and reviewer for an array of other national and international journals and publications. He has published more than 350 peer-reviewed articles, more than 145 book chapters, edited 32 books, and given more than 650 lectures around the world. Dr. Biller earned his medical degree from the School of Medicine at the University of the Republic in Montevideo, Uruguay, where he had postgraduate training in Internal Medicine. He then completed Residency in Neurology at Loyola University Chicago and a Cerebrovascular Research Fellowship at Wake Forest University, Bowman Gray School of Medicine. Dr. Biller was the recipient of A. B. Baker Lifetime Achievement in Neurologic Education Award from the American Academy of Neurology in 2020.

Dr. Biller enjoys history, opera, football (soccer), and is a cinema buff. He treasures spending time with his three grandsons.

Abbreviations

ACC	Anterior cingulate cortex
ADC	Apparent diffusion coefficient
ADEM	Acute disseminated encephalomyelitis
ADHD	Attention-deficit hyperactivity disorder
AIDP	Acute inflammatory demyelinating polyneuropathy
AIDS	Acquired immunodeficiency syndrome
ALS	Amyotrophic lateral sclerosis
AMAN	Acute motor axonal neuropathy
AMSAN	Acute motor sensory axonal neuropathy
AQP-4	Aquaporin-4
ATM	Acute transverse myelitis
BBB	Blood-brain barrier
BG	Basal ganglia
CART	Combined antiretroviral therapy
CCF	Carotid-cavernous fistula
CES	Cauda equina syndrome
CGRP	Calcitonin gene–related peptide
CH	Cluster headache
CIDP	Chronic inflammatory demyelinating polyneuropathy
CIM	Critical illness myopathy
CIP	Critical illness polyneuropathy
CJD	Creutzfeldt-Jakob disease
CMAP	Compound muscle action potential
CMS	Conus medullaris syndrome
CNS	Central nervous system
CSF	Cerebrospinal fluid
CSS	Cavernous sinus syndrome
CT	Computed tomography
DALYs	Disability-adjusted life-years
DAVF	Dural arteriovenous fistula
DM	Diabetes mellitus
DPN	Diabetic sensorimotor polyneuropathy
DWI	Diffusion-weighted imaging
ED	Emergency department
EEG	Electroencephalogram
EITB	Enzyme-linked immunoelectrotransfer blot
ELISA	Enzyme-linked immunosorbent assay
EMG	Electromyography
ET	Essential tremor
FLAIR	Fluid-attenuated inversion recovery
FND	Functional neurologic disorder
GBS	Guillain-Barré syndrome

GCA	Giant cell arteritis
HAART	Highly active antiretroviral therapy
HAND	HIV-1–associated neurocognitive disorder
HC	Hemicrania continua
HD	Huntington disease
HSVE	Herpes simplex virus encephalitis
ICP	Intracranial pressure
ICU	Intensive care unit
IgG	Immunoglobulin
IIH	Idiopathic intracranial hypertension
INO	Internuclear ophthalmoplegia
IRIS	Immune reconstitution inflammatory syndrome
IVIG	Intravenous immunoglobulin
KFR	Kayser-Fleischer ring
LEMS	Lambert-Eaton myasthenic syndrome
LETM	Longitudinally extensive transverse myelitis
LP	Lumbar puncture
LRP4	Lipoprotein receptor–related protein
MOG	Myelin oligodendrocyte glycoprotein
MOGAD	MOG-associated disorder
MRI	Magnetic resonance imaging
MS	Multiple sclerosis
NCC	Neurocysticercosis
NCS	Nerve conduction studies
NM	Nuclear medicine
NMJ	Neuromuscular junction
NMOSD	Neuromyelitis optica spectrum disorder
NPH	Normal-pressure hydrocephalus
NS	Neurosarcoidosis
NSAIDs	Nonsteroidal anti-inflammatory drugs
OCB	Oligoclonal band
OCT	Optical coherence tomography
OFC	Orbito-frontal cortex
ON	Optic neuritis
PAG	Periaqueductal gray
PCR	Polymerase chain reaction
PD	Parkinson disease
PET-CT	Positron emission and computed tomography
PH	Paroxysmal hemicrania
PLEDs	Periodic lateralizing epileptiform discharges
PLMS	Periodic limb movements of sleep
PML	Progressive multifocal leukoencephalopathy
PNS	Peripheral nervous system
PTLDS	Posttreatment Lyme disease syndrome
RAPD	Relative afferent pupillary defect
RLS	Restless legs syndrome

RNFL	Retinal nerve fiber layer
SCA	Superior cerebellar artery
SIH	Spontaneous intracranial hypotension
SIRS	Systemic inflammatory response syndrome
T2DM	Type 2 diabetes mellitus
TAC	Trigeminal autonomic cephalalgia
TN	Trigeminal neuralgia
TSE	Transmissible spongiform encephalopathies
TTH	Tension-type headache
VGCC	Voltage-gated calcium channel
VZV	Varicella-zoster virus
WBC	White blood cells
WE	Wernicke encephalopathy
WES	Whole-exome sequencing

Index

Note: Page numbers followed by "*f*" indicate figures and "*t*" indicate tables.